Cerebral Microbleeds

Pathophysiology to Clinical Practice

Cerebral Microbleeds

Pathophysiology to Clinical Practice

Edited by

David J. Werring

UCL Institute for Neurology, National Hospital for Neurology and Neurosurgery, London, UK

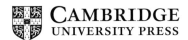

CAMBRIDGE
UNIVERSITY PRESS

CAMBRIDGE UNIVERSITY PRESS
Cambridge, New York, Melbourne, Madrid, Cape Town,
Singapore, São Paulo, Delhi, Tokyo, Mexico City

Cambridge University Press
The Edinburgh Building, Cambridge CB2 8RU, UK

Published in the United States of America by
Cambridge University Press, New York

www.cambridge.org
Information on this title:
www.cambridge.org/9780521198455

First published by Cambridge University Press 2011

Printed in the United Kingdom at the University Press,
Cambridge

*A catalogue record for this publication is available from the
British Library*

Library of Congress Cataloguing in Publication data
Cerebral microbleeds : from pathophysiology to clinical
practice / edited by David J. Werring.
     p. ; cm.
Includes bibliographical references and index.
ISBN 978-0-521-19845-5 (hardback)
1. Brain – Hemorrhage.   I. Werring, David J., 1967–
[DNLM: 1. Cerebral Hemorrhage. WL 355]
RD594.2.C44   2011
616.1′33 – dc22   2010054276

ISBN 978-0-521-19845-5 Hardback

Contents

Section 1 – Historical aspects, detection and interpretation

Section 2 – Mechanisms underlying microbleeds

Section 3 – Microbleeds in relation to specific populations, diseases and neurological symptoms

Contents

Contributors

Rustam Al-Shahi Salman
Division of Clinical Neurosciences, Centre for
Clinical Brain Sciences, University of Edinburgh,
Western General Hospital, Edinburgh, UK

Roland N. Auer
Department of Pathology and Laboratory Medicine,
University of Calgary, Calgary, Alberta, Canada

Samuel Barnes
The Magnetic Resonance Imaging Institute for
Biomedical Research, Detroit, MI, USA

Alexander S. Boikov
The Magnetic Resonance Imaging Institute for
Biomedical Research, Detroit, MI, USA

Sebastian Brandner
Division of Neuropathology, UCL Institute of
Neurology, London UK

Hugues Chabriat
Département of Neurologie, CHU Lariboisière,
Assistance Publique des Hôpitaux de Paris, France

Charlotte Cordonnier
Department of Neurology and Stroke Department,
Lille University Hospital, Lille, France

Martin Dichgans
Institute for Stroke and Dementia Research,
Klinikum der Universität München,
Ludwig-Maximilians-University, Munich, Germany

Steven M. Greenberg
Department of Neurology and Hemorrhagic Stroke
Research Center, Massachusetts General Hospital and
Harvard Medical School, Boston, MA, USA

Simone M. Gregoire
Department of Brain Repair and Rehabilitation, UCL
Institute of Neurology, National Hospital for
Neurology and Neurosurgery, London, UK

E. Mark Haacke
Departments of Radiology and Biomedical
Engineering, Wayne State University and The
Magnetic Resonance Imaging Institute
for Biomedical Research, Detroit, MI, USA

Vladimir Hachinski
Department of Clinical Neurological Sciences,
London, Ontario, Canada

Hans Rolf Jäger
Department of Brain Repair and Rehabilitation, UCL
Institute of Neurology, National Hospital for
Neurology and Neurosurgery, London, UK

M. Ayaz Khan
Department of Neurology and Hemorrhagic Stroke
Research Center, Massachusetts General Hospital and
Harvard Medical School, Boston, MA, USA

Chelsea S. Kidwell
Department of Neurology and Stroke Center,
Georgetown University, Washington, DC, USA

Lenore J. Launer
Intramural Research Program, National Institute on
Aging, Bethesda, MD, USA

Seung-Hoon Lee
Seoul National University Hospital, Seoul, Republic
of Korea

Cheryl R. McCreary
Department of Radiology, University of Calgary,
Calgary, Alberta, Canada

Jaladhar Neelavalli
The Magnetic Resonance Imaging Institute for
Biomedical Research, Detroit, MI, USA

Bo Norrving
Department of Clinical Sciences, Division of
Neurology, Medical Faculty, Lund University, Sweden

Mike O'Sullivan
Cardiff University Brain Research Imaging Centre,
Cardiff University, Cardiff, UK

Gillian Potter
Division of Clinical Neurosciences, Centre for
Clinical Brain Sciences, University of Edinburgh,
Western General Hospital, Edinburgh, UK

Jae-Kyu Roh
Seoul National University Hospital, Seoul,
Republic of Korea

Neshika Samarasekera
Division of Clinical Neurosciences, Centre for
Clinical Brain Sciences, University of Edinburgh,
Western General Hospital, Edinburgh, UK

Rainer Scheid
Max Planck Institute for Human Cognitive and Brain
Sciences, Leipzig, Germany

Varinder Singh Alg
Department of Brain Repair and Rehabilitation, UCL
Institute of Neurology, National Hospital for
Neurology and Neurosurgery, London, UK

Eric E. Smith
Department of Clinical Neurosciences and Hotchkiss
Brain Institute, University of Calgary, Calgary,
Alberta, Canada

Yannie O. Y. Soo
Department of Medicine and Therapeutics, The
Chinese University of Hong Kong, Prince of Wales
Hospital, Hong Kong, SAR

Mark A. van Buchem
C. J. Gorter Center for high field MRI, Department of
Radiology, Leiden University Medical Center, Leiden,
The Netherlands

Wiesje M. van der Flier
Alzheimer Center and Department of Neurology and
Department of Epidemiology & Biostatistics, Vrije
Universiteit Medical Center, Amsterdam, The
Netherlands

Maarten J. Versluis
C. J. Gorter Center for high field MRI, Department of
Radiology, Leiden University Medical Center, Leiden,
The Netherlands

Anand Viswanathan
Department of Neurology and Hemorrhagic Stroke
Research Center, Massachusetts General Hospital and
Harvard Medical School, Boston, MA, USA and
Département of Neurologie, CHU Lariboisière,
Assistance Publique des Hôpitaux de Paris, France

Andrew G. Webb
C. J. Gorter Center for high field MRI, Department of
Radiology, Leiden University Medical Center, Leiden,
The Netherlands

David J. Werring
Department of Brain Repair and Rehabilitation, UCL
Institute of Neurology, National Hospital for
Neurology and Neurosurgery, London, UK

Lawrence K. S. Wong
Department of Medicine and Therapeutics, The
Chinese University of Hong Kong, Prince of Wales
Hospital, Hong Kong, SAR

Foreword

Brain imaging shows us much more than we can understand. This book goes a long way in bridging the gap between seeing and knowing, regarding cerebral microbleeds.

The problem is put in perspective beginning with the classical studies of Charcot and Bouchard and then systematically describing and interpreting subsequent pathological studies. A geography of pathology is reaffirmed, but modified. Although cerebral microbleeds parallel the distribution of the two leading causes of intracerebral hemorrhage, namely hypertensive and cerebral amyloid pathology, their occurrence is not limited to their respective areas of prevalence. Hypertensive hemorrhages typically involve the pons, cerebellum, basal ganglia and thalamus, while vascular amyloid affects the meningeal and cortical vessels. Cerebral microbleeds are found more widely. One can imagine vessels stiffened by hypertension and weakened by amyloid outside the typical subcortical and cortical distribution of hypertensive and amyloid pathology, respectively, where one pathology alone would be asymptomatic but the combination puts the vessels over the threshold for bleeding. It is clear that we have much to learn about what, until recently, we could not see. In the age of falling rates of autopsies, their continuing relevance is heightened by the need to understand the origins and evolution of cerebral microbleeds.

This volume also deals with the occurrence of cerebral microbleeds in the general population, in patients with ischemic stroke and in relation to cognitive impairment. As the resolution and sophistication of brain imaging grows, we will increasingly face the challenge of deciding the clinical relevance of cerebral microbleeds in a given patient. The editors and authors have rendered a great service by collecting, reviewing and evaluating in this volume all that is known. This book will be useful and can be recommended to anyone who relies on brain imaging for diagnosis and decision making.

Vladimir Hachinski, CM, MD, FRCPC, DSc.
Distinguished University Professor

Preface

Cerebrovascular diseases (including symptomatic strokes and vascular cognitive impairment) are arguably the leading cause of death and disability worldwide. About one in three symptomatic strokes are caused by diseases of small perforating arteries, including most cases of spontaneous intracerebral hemorrhage, the most severe and lethal type of stroke. Despite the clear importance of small vessel diseases, many effective interventions (for example endovascular techniques) currently target only disease of large arteries, because small vessels are technically inaccessible and the underlying mechanisms of small vessel diseases remain relatively poorly understood. The importance of small vessel disease is yet further increased because it is the commonest cause of so-called "silent strokes": vascular damage to the brain seen on neuroimaging (or at autopsy) that does not cause an obvious acute stroke syndrome but may have important cumulative effects, particularly on behavior or cognition. Subclinical cerebrovascular disease is revealed by changes on MRI scans, including white matter changes (leukoaraiosis) and small, deep infarcts (lacunes). There is increasing evidence that such silent cerebrovascular disease signifies an increased risk of symptomatic stroke, and plays a key role in cognitive impairment and dementia – perhaps the biggest challenge of all facing aging societies.

Since the first reports, in the late 1990s, of small, black, rounded lesions on gradient-recalled echo MRI scans of patients suffering symptomatic large cerebral hemorrhage, cerebral microbleeds have emerged as an important new imaging manifestation of small vessel diseases. Although new to stroke clinics, the lesions that we now call cerebral microbleeds are probably similar to those described by histopathologists in hypertensive brains affected by macroscopic intracerebral hemorrhage well over a century ago. With the development of MRI techniques that are exquisitely sensitive to the products of bleeding, including gradient echo $T_2{}^*$-weighted and susceptibility-weighted sequences, cerebral microbleeds have been detected in ever-increasing numbers of patients in stroke and cognitive clinics, as well as in population-based samples of healthy older people (up to approximately 40% of healthy community-dwelling individuals over 80 years have microbleeds that are identified with an optimized MRI protocol). As imaging methods improve, with even higher field strength, thinner slices and better tissue contrast, there may come a time when more people have identified microbleeds than do not. There is, therefore, an urgent need to establish their pathophysiological and clinical significance, in all sorts of populations. For example, there is much interest in the concept of prevention and in treatment of high-risk individuals; could cerebral microbleeds have a role in identifying those who would benefit from intensive risk factor management or other new therapeutic approaches to small vessel diseases?

Despite their high prevalence, there remains uncertainty even about the basic question of whether cerebral microbleeds actually have any effect on brain function. So far, it is clear that cerebral microbleeds are common in all stroke populations (more so in intracererbal hemorrhage than ischemic stroke) and are closely linked to the commonest small vessel diseases: hypertensive arteriopathy and cerebral amyloid angiopathy (the latter usually identified in association with intracerebral hemorrhage or Alzheimer's disease). Cerebral microbleeds, therefore, seem likely to play a key role in increasing our understanding of small vessel disease mechanisms, and the link between cerebrovascular disease and neurodegeneration. Another key question is whether microbleeds are a useful tool to assess the risk of intracerebral hemorrhage prior to antithrombotic treatments. This question has particular urgency because intracerebral hemorrhage in older age groups is increasing in incidence compared with other stroke types, probably because of the increasing use of antithrombotic drugs in people with fragile small vessels prone to bleeding.

So, is the time right for a book about cerebral microbleeds? If the interest of a topic can be judged by the number of people writing and publishing articles, then the answer is a resounding "yes." The publication of papers on cerebral microbleeds is increasing at an exponential rate, indicating that cerebral microbleeds have truly captured the attention of cerebrovascular researchers; from the start of 2009 through to mid-2010, over 100 papers relating to cerebral microbleeds have been published. Many studies describe their prevalence and anatomical distribution, or association with clinical or imaging factors; some investigate the physical principles underlying detection, others their pathological basis, and still others describe experimental studies. Because of the diversity of research, studies on cerebral microbleeds have been published in many varied sources. And naturally, as with any emerging technology and its application to clinical medicine, there are areas of uncertainty, debate and sometimes confusion. Methods of detection and quantification are under active development. This book is an attempt to bring all of these sources of information together in a single volume to summarize current knowledge, and controversies, in the field. I have been lucky to be able to assemble a world-class team of authors, all distinguished in their research areas; the contributions of such a diverse team, across many countries and continents, will give different and valuable perspectives.

Each chapter is designed to stand alone, so some repetition between chapters is inevitable and necessary; because the field remains relatively well defined, there will be reference in many chapters to similar early papers and key findings. However, overlap has been minimized as far as possible, so that the book can also be used as a single volume. Although definitive answers to many questions cannot yet be provided, it is hoped that this volume will give a useful synthesis of current understanding and directions for future research. The book is in three sections; the first covers the historical context of cerebral microbleeds, and technical aspects relating to their detection, definition and mapping in the brain. The second considers the mechanisms underlying microbleeds from histopathological studies, epidemiological studies and imaging. The third, and largest, section, discusses microbleeds in the context of different populations and disease groups, and also covers specific clinical settings and questions including cognitive impairment, and the use of antithrombotic medications. The book has been designed to be of interest to all clinical researchers and physicians in the fields of stroke and cognitive impairment, including neurologists, stroke physicians, neuroradiologists, neuropsychologists and vascular scientists. It should provide a useful synthesis of what is currently known about cerebral microbleeds, but more importantly, it will show how many fascinating and clinically important questions remain, and stimulate further research.

David Werring
London, September 2010

Terminology

This book is about radiological lesions corresponding to small areas of bleeding in the brain, commonly referred to as microbleeds. The term microbleed was first coined in 1996 [1], but in subsequent years many different terms have been applied to what seem to be the same thing. These include petechial hemorrhages, silent microbleeds, asymptomatic microbleeds, multi-focal signal loss lesions, dot-like hemosiderin spots, brain microbleeds, cerebral microbleeds, microhemorrhages and microsusceptibility changes. In the interests of consistency, a single term, *cerebral microbleeds* (CMBs), the most frequently used term, has been used throughout this book. The term "microbleed" is not often applied to lesions outside the central nervous system, but it nevertheless seems appropriate to make clear that the lesions being discussed are in the brain. Although a few recent studies have preferred to use the term brain microbleeds (BMBs) [2], these are in the minority.

Cerebral (French *cérébral*, "pertaining to the brain," derived from the Latin *cerebrum*, "the brain") has the advantages of already being widely used and is consistent with much of the other terminology used in hemorrhagic disorders affecting the brain, including intracerebral hemorrhage and cerebral amyloid angiopathy.

References

1. Offenbacher H, Fazekas F, Schmidt R *et al.* MR of cerebral abnormalities concomitant with primary intracerebral hematomas. *AJNR Am J Neuroradiol* 1996;**17**:573–8.

2. Cordonnier C, Al-Shahi SR, Wardlaw J. Spontaneous brain microbleeds: systematic review, subgroup analyses and standards for study design and reporting. *Brain* 2007;**130**:1988–2003.

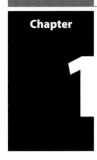

Historical overview

Microaneurysms, cerebral microbleeds and intracerebral hemorrhage

Varinder Singh Alg and David J. Werring

Introduction

Cerebral microbleeds (CMBs) are MRI-defined lesions corresponding to small deposits of blood products (mainly hemosiderin) from previous episodes of bleeding in the brain, usually related to small vessel damage. These CMBs have generated great interest as radiological markers for small vessel diseases prone to bleeding, with the hope that they may contribute to our understanding, diagnosis and clinical management of patients with (or at risk of) larger symptomatic intracerebral hemorrhage (ICH). As CMBs are radiologically identified lesions, they have, by definition, only been widely recognized with the increasing use of advanced magnetic resonance imaging (MRI). Key to our understanding of the pathophysiological and clinical significance of CMBs is determining the histopathological lesions that underlie their characteristic radiological appearance. This has been addressed by only a limited number of MRI–postmortem correlation studies (discussed in Ch. 6). However, much older histopathological studies (which pre-date awareness of MRI-defined CMBs) have described small aneurysmal or hemorrhagic lesions that might shed light on the origin of CMBs, and have shaped current concepts of the pathophysiology of spontaneous ICH. This chapter provides an overview of these pathological studies, which should provide helpful background to some of the chapters in this book, including those discussing CMB histology (Ch. 6), CMBs in relation to hypertensive arteriopathy (Ch. 11) and CMBs in cerebral amyloid angiopathy (CAA; Ch. 12).

Intracerebral hemorrhage may occur from a clear cause, for example trauma, rupture of an arteriovenous malformation or bleeding into a tumor. However, in most cases, no such underlying cause is identified, nor can any large vessel rupture be seen at autopsy.

The underlying arterial pathological processes underlying such "spontaneous" (also termed "primary" or non-traumatic) ICH have been studied since at least the seventeenth century, when Johann Jacob Wepfer (1620–1695) found fragile vessels in relation to a large cerebral hemorrhage, but was unable to identify a point of rupture. Yet, despite a great many studies, using a variety of techniques to study the relationship between small arterial lesions and ICH, even now the question of how ICH occurs remains unsettled and is an important topic for investigation. Understanding the causes of spontaneous ICH is of critical importance in stroke medicine because this type of stroke often leads to death or serious disability, and is becoming more common within aging populations, particularly with the increasing use of antiplatelet and anticoagulant drugs [1]. Only by better understanding the pathophysiological mechanisms underlying ICH can more effective treatments and prevention strategies be developed.

It has long been known that spontaneous ICH is often related to pathological changes of small-caliber cerebral vessels (typically up to approximately 300 mm diameter): the two most important known pathological findings are hypertensive arteriopathy and CAA (these disorders are described in more detail in Chs. 11 and 12). However, rather than being a sufficient "cause" of ICH, it is likely that these arteriopathies interact with other "risk factors," for example acute or chronic hypertension or clotting abnormalities. The proportions of ICH related to these pathological changes in arteries, and exactly how they are modified by chronic or acute environmental risk factors, remain fundamental questions.

Cerebral microbleeds have attracted increasing interest as a new neuroimaging "window" on the small vessel pathologies underlying ICH in vivo, and provide

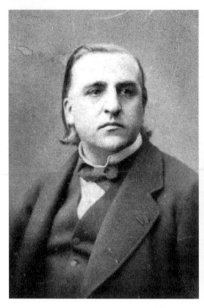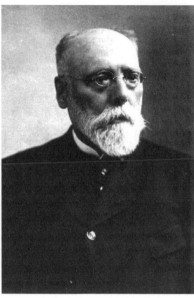

Fig. 1.1 Jean-Martin Charcot (left) and Charles-Joseph Bouchard (right). Charcot (1825–1893) was Professor of Neurology and Anatomical Pathology at the La Salpêtrière Hospital in Paris. He is widely considered to be the "father" of the modern subspecialty of neurology, having made key observations on many diseases including amyotrophic lateral sclerosis and multiple sclerosis. Bouchard (1837–1915) was Charcot's hard-working and ambitious student; he wrote his doctoral thesis on microaneurysms: *Étude sur quelques points de la pathogénie des hémorrhagies cérébrales*. With Charcot's support, Bouchard's career trajectory was meteoric, resulting in his appointment as professor in the school of medicine in Paris. After this, however, their strong ambitious personalities clashed, and this led to a great professional tension between the two men. This conflict resulted in Bouchard famously preventing Josef Babinski, one of Charcot's most gifted young pupils, from passing his examinations. Babinski, despite making fundamental contributions to neurology, including much of the modern neurology examination and his eponymous plantar reflex, never became a professor at the medical school.

a new way to tackle these and other important questions. The methods used to detect, define and map CMBs are discussed in Chs. 2–5. Detailed MRI–postmortem correlation studies of CMBs remain scarce, but the available evidence so far suggests that CMBs are a quite specific radiological marker for small areas of previous bleeding in association with abnormal small vessels affected by hypertensive arteriopathy or CAA [2] (see Ch. 6) To date, histopathological studies have mainly confirmed that CMBs are related to extravasated blood degradation products, sometimes associated with microaneurysms or aneurysm-like lesions. The chapter continues by considering the development of knowledge concerning microaneurysmal and small hemorrhagic lesions in relation to ICH and small vessel diseases, which may be relevant in understanding the origin of radiologically defined CMBs.

Charcot–Bouchard microaneurysms

In their renowned study, published in 1868, Jean-Martin Charcot and his student Charles-Joseph

Bouchard (Fig. 1.1) investigated the cause of spontaneous ICH by careful histopathological analysis of 84 brain autopsies from patients affected by ICH in life. They macerated samples from the fresh ICH cavities in running water to remove unclotted blood and parenchymal brain tissue, then microscopically examined the small arterial vessels associated with the ICH [3]. They described the small parenchymal "miliary" aneurysms that still bear their names; these were much smaller than the saccular aneurysms affecting the circle of Willis, which are involved in subarachnoid hemorrhage, and were suspended upon the vascular filaments made up of the small perforating arteries of the basal ganglia, pons, cerebellum and cerebral white matter (Fig. 1.2) [3,4]. They ascribed the formation of these microaneurysms to "peri-arteritis" and mainly adventitial damage, rather than conventional arteriosclerosis. The hypothesis that has arisen from the work of Charcot and Bouchard is that pathological changes (degenerative or inflammatory, and often associated with arterial hypertension) in small caliber arterioles (up to approximately 300 μm) cause weakening of the wall and microaneurysm formation,

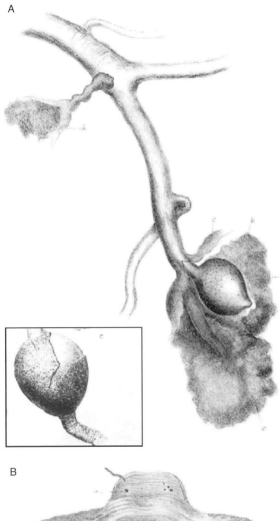

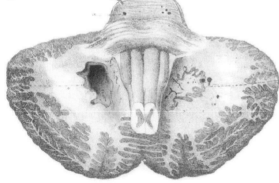

Fig. 1.2 Microaneurysms. (A) Original illustration from Charcot and Bouchard (1868) [3]. A ruptured microaneurysm (miliary aneurysm) is shown (bottom right) with surrounding clot from extravasated blood. Another microaneurysm is also shown (inset, bottom left) without any surrounding clot. A ruptured aneurysm on an arteriole is also shown (top left). (B) Microaneurysms in the pons and the cerebellum from illustrations by Charcot (1881) [4].

which subsequently may rupture to cause ICH. This theory held sway until the early years of the twentieth century, and indeed is still widely accepted. However, subsequent studies have suggested alternative explanations for microaneurysms, including dissection of blood into a diseased segment of arterial wall, false aneurysms (sometimes termed bleeding globes) or even the misinterpretation of complex arteriolar loops or coils as aneurysms. Furthermore, other studies have not been able to consistently find true microaneurysms at the site of macroscopic ICH (e.g. see Fisher [5]). Therefore, although there is no doubt that microaneurysms as described by Charcot and Bouchard occur, many fundamental questions remain regarding their cause, nature, prevalence and role in the pathophysiology of ICH. One problem is that the morphology of aneurysmal abnormalities adjacent to macroscopic ICH may be altered by the anatomical distortion caused by the ICH itself, or by the analysis technique used; even rinsing the hemorrhage in water may lose some of the structure of fragile vessels, while contrast injection injected at necropsy (see below) will only be able to reveal aneurysms with a sufficient size of patent lumen for contrast to reliably enter, or it may cause the development or distortion of some aneurysms. Consequently, even true aneurysms may, by the time of microscopic examination, not conform to the accepted definition of an aneurysm – a vascular dilatation continuous with the wall of the parent artery (and containing all of the arterial wall layers). Furthermore, the value of distinguishing between true and false aneurysms when the arterial wall layers are grossly abnormal (as in many of the studies discussed here) is questionable. These factors, together with variations in terminology, may in part explain the varied and sometimes conflicting conclusions about the nature and significance of microaneurysms in relation to ICH.

Studies of microaneurysms and related lesions are presented in Tables 1.1 and 1.2, in chronological order. In the late nineteenth century, Turner [6] and Eppinger [7] suggested that what Charcot and Bouchard had termed miliary aneurysms were in fact dilatations resulting from the accumulation of blood between the media and adventitia of the affected artery (dissection). Then, with improved histological techniques available at the turn of the twentieth century, Ellis [8] described that the media layer of the vessel wall had completely degenerated at the point of microaneurysmal dilatation and been replaced by connective

Table 1.1 Summary of selected studies on microaneurysms (Charcot–Bouchard aneurysms) in association with hypertension and intracerebral hemorrhage

Study	Year	Reported findings
Charcot and Bouchard [3]	1868	Described tiny swellings along vascular filaments in macerated brain specimens from the cavities of macroscopic ICH; termed these "miliary" aneurysms, and hypothesized they were a result of peri-arteritis and a cause of ICH
Charlewood Turner [6]	1882	Did not find microaneurysms in association with ICH. Suggested dilatations resulted from accumulation of blood between the media and adventitia (dissection)
Eppinger [7]	1887	Like Charlewood Turner, suggested that microaneurysms may, in fact, be dissecting (blood accumulation between the media and adventitia)
Ellis [8]	1909	Described peri-adventitial hematomas with occasional extension into the vessel wall causing dissection
Turnbull [9]	1915	Described "false aneurysms" (bleeding globes?) in association with ICH
Green [10]	1930	Described microaneurysms but speculated that the cause was arteriosclerosis rather than peri-arteritis. Described extravasation of red blood cells into the perivascular (Virchow–Robin) space
Matuoka [11,12]	1939, 1952	Described pseudoaneurysms ("bleeding globes")
Ross Russell [13]	1963	Using microradiographic contrast methods described microaneurysms in brains from elderly hypertensive subjects. The location of aneurysms was not in the vicinity of large ICH, suggesting that microaneurysms cannot be a secondary result of ICH. Described red cells outside the aneurysm with hemosiderin staining
Cole and Yates [14]	1967	Using microradiography demonstrated microaneurysms in association with hypertension. Described collections of hemosiderin pigment adjacent to the aneurysms
Fisher [5]	1972	Described microaneurysms in association with ICH but hypothesized that microaneurysms were not the most important cause of macroscopic ICH because of the small size of the parent artery; described "bleeding globes"
Takabayashi and Kaneko [15]	1983	Electron microscopy of 61 lenticulostriate arteries from patients with ICH. Found only 7 microaneurysms (2 ruptured). Emphasized lipohyalinosis as a cause of rupture, rather than microaneurysms
Wakai and Nagai [16]	1989	Found 5 definite and 2 possible microaneurysms in 14 surgical ICH specimens
Vonsattel et al. [17]	1991	In cerebral amyloid angiopathy reported that patients with ICH had more severe histopathological changes, including thick amyloid deposition and microaneurysms
Challa et al. [18]	1992	Using Bell's modification of the AP techniques, this showed complex arteriolar twists following contrast injection, which could easily be mistaken for microaneurysms and lead to overestimation
Mizutani et al. [19]	2000	Described arterial dissections rather than microaneurysms in lenticulostriate arteries from surgical ICH specimens
Fisher [20]	2003	Serial sections of an acute thalamic hemorrhage showed that it originated from an elongated, thin-walled aneurysmal segment 5 mm in length and 600 mm in diameter; there was a single breech of 1 mm width, allowing continuity between the lumen and the extravasated blood of the ICH
Rosenblum [21]	2003	Serial sections through an acute pontine ICH showed an aneurysm of 1 mm width arising from a parent vessel affected by fibrinoid necrosis. Double lumen with points of rupture in both the inner and outer lumen, suggesting rupture of a dissecting microaneurysm

ICH, intracerebral hemorrhage.

tissue; consequently, the arterial layers expected in a true aneurysm could no longer be seen. In some cases, perivascular hematomas in continuity with the intramural contents gave the appearance of red, grape-like swellings, which Ellis thought could have been mistaken by previous observers for true microaneurysms.

It was, therefore, suggested that progression of an initial intimal lesion allowed blood to dissect into the media and adventitia, with subsequent media degeneration, potentially allowing bleeding into brain parenchyma without invoking the formation of true microaneurysms. Some have even interpreted Ellis's

Table 1.2 Prevalence of microaneurysms (Charcot–Bouchard aneurysms) in hypertension and intracerebral hemorrhage

Study	Year	Number of brains	Controls	Hypertension	Intracerebral hemorrhage
				Prevalence of microaneurysms	
Green [10]	1930	10	–	1/7 (14%)	1/3 (33%)
Ross Russell [13]	1963	54	10/38 (26%)	14/16 (88%)	5/5 (100%)
Cole and Yates [14]	1967	200	7/100 (7%)	46/100 (46%)	18/21 (86%)
Fisher [5]	1972	20	–	13/20 (65%)	NA
Takabayashi and Kaneko [15]	1983	61	–	–	7/61 (11%)
Wakai and Nagai [16]	1989	14	–	–	5/14 (36%)
Challa *et al.* [18]	1992	55	0/20	0/31	0/4
Mizutani *et al.* [19]	2000	12	–	–	0/12
Overall prevalence			**17/158 (11%)**	**74/174 (43%)**	**36/120 (30%)**

work as showing that what had been called microaneurysms might have merely been fragments of blood clot adhering to the adventitia.

In 1930, Green made some similar observations to Ellis, using a different technique to carefully trace the relationship between arterial dilatations and the parent artery [10]. In subjects who had died of ICH, the brain was hardened in formol saline for a few weeks, then thick sections were cut from small tissue blocks to preserve the course of visible arteries; at sites of vascular dilatation, thinner 5 mm slices were cut. Using this method, Green was able to describe in detail a number of microaneurysms including a saccular pontine lesion (Fig. 1.3), with stretching and rupture of necrotic intima and media leading to distension of the adventitia and effusion of red blood cells into the Virchow–Robin (perivascular) space. A fusiform aneurysm showed complete mural thrombosis. While confirming structures compatible with microaneurysms, Green suggested that that the degeneration resulted from intimal arteriosclerosis rather than "peri-arteritis" as had originally been suggested by Charcot and Bouchard.

Later in the twentieth century, new methods of studying the cerebral microvasculature, based on X-ray technology, became available, allowing microaneurysms to be studied without the need for such painstaking work on thin serial sections. In 1963, Ralph Ross Russell set out to study a larger number of subjects with ICH with the aim of further determining the relevance of microaneurysms [13]. In this autopsy study, barium sulfate contrast medium was injected into the basal arteries of the brains from

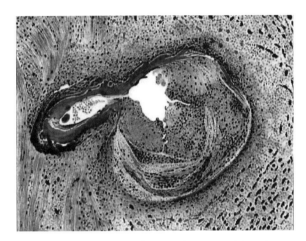

Fig. 1.3 Miliary aneurysm in the pons. There is partial thrombus in the aneurysmal sac, with red blood cells in its proximal portion. There is evidence of recent hemorrhage with deposition of pigment around the aneurysmal sac. These findings are relevant to our understanding of cerebral microbleeds. Hematoxylin and sudan III stain. See the color plate section. (Reproduced with permission from Green, 1930 [10].)

hypertensive and normotensive elderly subjects; after fixing the brain in formalin, microradiography of brain sections was performed to reveal the anatomy of small vessels and microaneurysms, as outlined by the radiopaque tracer. Age and hypertension were found to be strong risk factors for microaneurysms and ICH. In all but 1 of the 16 brains from hypertensive subjects, there were numerous cerebral microaneurysms, ranging in number from 1 to more than 10; by contrast, only 10 of the 38 brains from normotensive subjects had microaneurysms. The microaneurysms, of 300–900 μm diameter, were most often found along

A

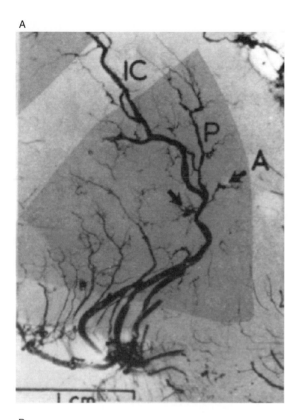

B

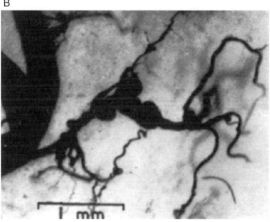

Fig. 1.4 (A) Coronal radiograph of lenticulostriate arteries from an elderly hypertensive subject showing attenuation of small vessels and microaneurysms (arrowed). (B) Enlargement of the same region, showing multiple aneurysms. IC, internal capsule; P, putamen. (Reproduced with permission from Ross Russell, 1963 [13].)

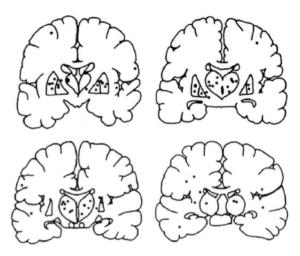

Fig. 1.5 Distribution of microaneurysms in 14 hypertensive brains, in multiple coronal sections, excluding the brainstem and cerebellum. (Reproduced with permission from Ross Russell, 1963 [13].)

tia of the parent vessel. There was abrupt termination of the muscular tissue at the point of origin of the aneurysm, with only disordered remnants of the elastic lamina remaining. Occasionally, there were scattered endothelial cells lining the aneurysmal sac but this was not a prominent feature. Most of the cavities of the aneurysms showed organized layers of fibrin and red blood cells, indicating a degree of thrombosis, as had been observed in some previous studies. Notably, there were often some red cells outside the aneurysm, with many iron-containing macrophages and hemosiderin staining: clearly an observation with relevance for the study of CMBs. The points of rupture were at weakened and diseased points on the parent artery. Interestingly, the distribution of aneurysmal lesions that Ross Russell mapped in the brain (Fig. 1.5) has similarities to the distribution of CMBs seen on some recent MRI studies in hypertensive populations [22] (see Ch. 10).

As discussed, it has been argued that aneurysm-like lesions may result *from* macroscopic ICH, perhaps through small clot fragments adhering to the vessel wall, or from the dissection of blood from outside into the vessel adventitia. However, in Ross Russell's study, the presence of microaneurysm in normotensive brains in the absence of macroscopic ICH argues against this explanation; moreover, the sites of ICH were not the same as those of aneurysms. Therefore, an explanation of Ross Russell's observations is that the lesion begins with rupture of the intimal surface, distending the other arterial wall layers; in a proportion

small lenticulostriate perforating parent arteries of 100–300 mm diameter (Fig. 1.4), and comprised an internal hyaline layer derived from the intima and an outer collagenous layer continuous with the adventi-

of microaneurysms this leads to secondary rupture of the wall with direct leakage of blood from the parent artery lumen into the surrounding parenchyma, causing ICH.

In 1967, Cole and Yates [14] further consolidated the association of microaneurysms with ICH and hypertension: of 100 hypertensive brains examined using an autoradiographic technique, 46 specimens showed the occurrence of microaneurysms, while only 7% of normotensive brains were affected. Aneurysms were mainly along vessels <250 mm in diameter, and once again affected the perforating vessels that irrigate the basal ganglia, pons, cerebellum and white matter. As previously noted, cerebral microaneurysms were more prevalent with increasing age and hypertension. Brains from 13 subjects demonstrated small areas of bleeding outside the vessel wall; all of these brains were from hypertensive individuals. The microaneurysms were surrounded by fresh blood and hemosiderin pigment – once again providing a pathological lesion relevant to the modern MRI finding of CMBs.

Subsequently, Fisher [5] also found microaneurysms and again noted that blood coated the outside of some of them, indicating previous rupture. Hemosiderin-laden macrophages were scattered outside the aneurysm in the surrounding tissue, which suggested chronic, rather than acute, hemorrhage. However, in contrast to previous investigators, Fisher suggested that such microaneurysms were unlikely individually to directly cause macroscopic ICH, but could result in only limited bleeding because of the small size of the parent artery (usually <150 mm). Instead, Fisher suggested that lipohyalinosis-related weak spots along small vessels, rather than microaneurysms, were likely to be an important mechanism for macroscopic ICH (see discussion of "bleeding globes" below).

Subsequent work has also suggested sources of ICH other than microaneurysms. Takebayashi and Kaneko [15] performed electron microscopy studies on a total of 61 ruptured lenticulostriate arteries, 20 from patients undergoing microsurgical hematoma evacuation for large ICH and 41 from autopsy specimens; they found only seven miliary aneurysms, only two of which had ruptured, one in each group. The majority of ruptures were distally located at weak points in severely arteriosclerotic arteries with a diameter of 500–700 mm – considerably larger than the smaller vessels described in association with microaneurysms. It was noted that distal lenticulostriate arteries in

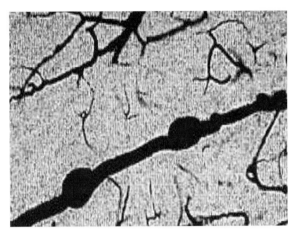

Fig. 1.6 Complex vascular coils and twists, mimicking microaneurysms, revealed using alkaline phosphatase staining. (Reproduced with permission from Challa et al. 1992 [18].)

hypertensive ICH showed marked atrophy, with a "moth-eaten" appearance resulting from the complete obliteration of smooth muscle cells in the media in the middle to distal portions of the artery; rupture occurred at branching sites and the proximal portions showed hardly any medial degeneration. These findings were in agreement with Miller Fisher's emphasis on lipohyalinosis rather than microaneurysms as a common cause of vessel rupture. Mizutani et al. [19] analyzed lenticulostriate arteries from surgical specimens in 12 patients with ICH, and described arterial dissections as the cause of hypertension-related ICH, rather than microaneurysms. By contrast, Wakai and Nagai [16] once again emphasized the role of microaneurysms: they examined surgical specimens of ICH in 14 patients, and in five of these found definite microaneurysms; possible microaneurysms were seen in two cases.

A study using a new histopathological technique developed by Challa and colleagues [18] has been particularly influential in raising doubts about whether microaneurysms are common or relevant as a cause of ICH (Fig. 1.6). In this study, alkaline phosphatase endothelial staining was used to identify miliary aneurysms, using both high-resolution microradiography and light microscopy, in 55 specimens from both hypertensive and normotensive brains. This technique has theoretical advantages over some of the previous methods, including maceration under water, routine paraffin sections and autoradiography following contrast injection. It was suggested by Challa and colleagues that routine paraffin sectioning could underestimate the number of microaneurysms, while injection techniques alone might either fail to reveal very small microaneurysms or lead to misinterpretation of arteriolar twists and overestimate the prevalence of larger microaneurysms. In Challa and colleagues' study [18], no true microaneurysms were seen in any of the cases, including careful sampling of the hematoma cavity in the four brains with hypertension-related ICH. Tracing of vessels in three dimensions revealed that what appeared to be aneurysms were, in fact, complex arteriolar coils and twists, which it was suggested could have mistakenly been interpreted as aneurysms by earlier workers. However, the suggestion of such misinterpretation in Ross Russell's autoradiographic studies does not explain the preferential location of microaneurysms in the basal ganglia [13]; furthermore, in the previous autoradiography studies, systematic analysis of the full thickness of the sections was supplemented by histopathological analysis, making misinterpretation unlikely. It is also possible that alkaline phosphatase is not present in the walls of severely damaged aneurysmal arteriolar walls, leading to underestimation of aneurysm frequency in Challa and colleagues' study. Nevertheless, the logical interpretation of Challa and colleagues' work is that microaneurysms are much less common than had hitherto been thought, and rupture of non-aneurysmal segments of arterial wall, damaged by hypertension, is a more important cause of ICH in hypertensive patients.

Although microaneurysms and ICH have been linked over many years, it is noteworthy that *ruptured microaneurysms as a clear source of bleeding* have very seldom been clearly described in association with acute ICH. Two recent case reports have provided evidence for this and revived interest in microaneurysms as a cause of ICH. In 2003, Fisher reported the histopathological findings in thalamic ICH in a hypertensive patient [20]. An acute 2 cm hemorrhage was sectioned in its entirety to reveal the primary source of bleeding; it originated from an elongated, thin-walled aneurysmal segment 5 mm in length and 600 mm in diameter. The wall had a single breech of 1 mm in width that allowed continuity between the lumen and the extravasated blood of the ICH. In the same year, Rosenblum reported findings from sectioning of a fresh pontine ICH [21]; a blood-filled aneurysm 1 mm in width was found that arose from a parent vessel of approximately 100 μm, affected by fibrinoid necrosis, and with a double lumen. Points of

rupture were seen in both the inner and outer lumen, suggesting that a tiny dissection into the arteriolar wall occurred, with subsequent rupture of this dissecting microaneurysm. The rarity of such reports of bleeding sources may, in part, relate to the destruction of microaneurysms during the acute ICH, or to the requirement for painstaking serial sections through an acute ICH in order to comprehensively assess for microaneurysmal lesions as a cause of the bleeding. These methodological considerations mean that a significant role of microaneurysms in ICH cannot be rejected, based on the available evidence to date.

Pseudoaneurysms or bleeding globes

Soon after the original reports of Charcot and Bouchard, some investigators first suggested that small extravasations of blood adherent to small arteries (not relating to aneurysms) could have been misinterpreted as microaneurysms [9]. These lesions may well have been what Matuoka subsequently termed "bleeding globes": masses of red blood cells enclosing concentric rings of polymerized fibrin from the arterial rupture site [11,12]. The bleeding point was a break in a small (100–200 mm) artery rather than an aneurysmal dilatation. Bleeding globes are generally interpreted as a physiological mechanism to limit the extent of hemorrhage, and the extent to which they are able to do so may have an important effect on the clinical outcome of ICH; indeed they are an important target for modern therapies designed to facilitate fibrin polymerization (e.g. recombinant factor VIIa) [23]. Fisher also clearly demonstrated bleeding globes in 24 ruptured vessels around the perimeter of a small pontine hemorrhage, and he suggested that Charcot and Bouchard's original description of hundreds of aneurysmal structures attached to vascular filaments in the walls of massive ICH might, in fact, have been bleeding globe lesions. Furthermore, the finding of multiple bleeding points around a macroscopic ICH suggested that a weakness of a single vessel or an aneurysm could not be the cause of all of the bleeding. Fisher and others have hypothesized that these findings could result from a hematoma originating from a single small rupture point having an "avalanche" or "domino" mechanical effect on adjacent vessels, causing a spatial spread of bleeding points and continued accumulation of hematoma. The fact that the bleeding points around the hematoma were not affected by severe lipohyalinosis suggested that this sequential mechanical rupture process was more likely than simultaneous separate primary ruptures of small arteries [5]. Bietzke [24] found bleeding globes in 15 cases of ICH at demonstrated break points in the arteries, but conversely suggested that they resulted from small secondary extravasations from arteries that had been torn apart by the force of a stronger macroscopic primary hemorrhage.

Microaneurysms and cerebral amyloid angiopathy

Although the link between microaneurysms and hypertension is not in question, other small vessel pathological processes may also be important in their development and as a cause of ICH. Cerebral amyloid angiopathy is now recognized as a common disorder of elderly populations and is characterized by the deposition of amyloid in cerebral cortical and leptomeningeal small vessels. There is considerable evidence that it is an important cause of ICH and cognitive impairment [25]. Cerebral hemorrhage may occur in CAA with or without the presence of hypertension (since hypertension and CAA are both common as age increases, they must often co-exist).

In autopsy studies of older individuals, CAA may be found without any evidence of ICH, but it is generally recognized clinically by the occurrence of spontaneous lobar ICH. It has been shown that the most severe CAA pathology – with complete arterial wall replacement by amyloid protein, microaneurysm formation and extravasation of blood from the vessel into surrounding brain tissue – is found in association with symptomatic ICH [17]. Less severe angiopathy might be expected to result in no obvious symptoms, or perhaps in cognitive disturbance only. The pathological changes in severe CAA, including perivascular hemosiderin-laden macrophages, are in keeping with the association of multiple lobar ICH and CMBs on MRI with severe CAA on histological studies [26].

How could microaneurysmal lesions relate to cerebral microbleeds?

It is clear that most of the microaneurysmal lesions described since the late nineteenth century, although varying in morphology, have been associated with hypertension, weakened small vessel walls and extravasation of red blood cells. These patterns of perivascular bleeding could be highly relevant in understanding the origin of the MRI appearance of CMBs, which may underpin the well-documented strong association between CMBs and macroscopic ICH (Chs. 10–12). Although large ICH can be easily viewed on non-contrasted CT scans, the small aneurysmal and hemorrhagic lesions discussed above cannot be seen on conventional neuroimaging methods; even the gold standard of catheter angiography is not sensitive to vascular lesions of this size. It has, therefore, been impossible to visualize such lesions in life. Scharf et al. (1994), using T_2 weighted imaging at 1.0 tesla (T) magnetic field strength, found "hemorrhagic lacunes" in a cohort of patients with spontaneous ICH. However, these lesions were probably more substantial hemorrhages (possibly into lacunar infarcts) than those now termed CMBs, because of the relatively low sensitivity of T_2 at low field to blood degradation products. However, since the mid 1990s, gradient-echo T_2^*-weighted MRI sequences have been able to detect very small cerebral hemorrhagic lesions, as small, rounded lesions of low signal intensity, in patients with hemorrhagic and ischemic stroke, hypertension and in healthy elderly subjects [28,29]. In 1996, Greenberg et al. using gradient-echo T_2^*-weighted MRI, reported "petechial hemorrhages" in a cohort of patients diagnosed with CAA [30]. In the same year, Offenbacher et al. reported similar rounded, homogeneous foci of signal loss with diameter of 2–5 mm in 27 of 120 patients with spontaneous ICH, and termed these "microbleeds" [31].

Cerebral microbleeds are particularly common in ICH (and are most prevalent in recurrent cases) [32] suggesting that they may provide clues to the underlying cause and could potentially shed light on the role of microaneurysms. In 1999, the histopathological correlates of CMBs began to be reported [28,33]. In patients with spontaneous ICH, CMBs were histologically characterized by focal accumulations of hemosiderin-containing macrophages [27]. The MRI-negative lesions (seen only on histopathological analysis) were smaller and consisted of only a few macrophages. In hypertensive patients, CMBs were preferentially located in the basal ganglia and thalami, and in these cases the vessels were affected by moderate to severe fibrohyalinosis. Subsequent histopathological studies are limited, but in the majority of cases reported, radiological CMBs were also found to reflect old, small foci of hemorrhage composed of hemosiderin-containing macrophages.

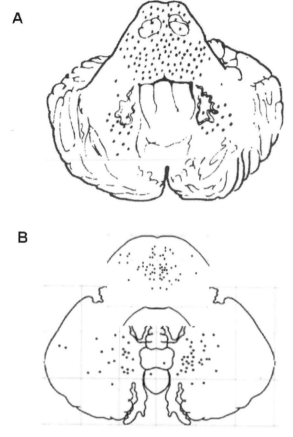

Fig. 1.7 (A) Distribution of microaneurysms in the cerebellum and brainstem of 53 hypertensive patients. (Reproduced with permission from Cole and Yates, 1967[14].) (B) Distribution of cerebral microbleeds in the pons and cerebellum of 164 hypertensive patients. (Adapted from Lee *et al.* 2004 [22].)

could indeed give rise to radiological appearances of CMBs, but the relative contributions of the different lesions to CMBs requires further study. For example, there have been no MRI–pathology correlations in patients with recent ICH to assess whether "bleeding globes" might cause radiological CMBs in relation to macroscopic ICH. The development of increasingly powerful and high-resolution imaging methods (Chs. 2 and 3) could ultimately even allow the different types of microaneurysmal and hemorrhagic lesion to be distinguished in vivo; this could shed important new light on the pathogenesis of ICH, particularly in prospective studies including serial scans.

Many cross-sectional studies have investigated clinical risk factors and associations of CMBs, and these are discussed in detail in subsequent chapters. Typically, in hypertensive patients, CMBs appear in the pons, cerebellum, thalamus and basal ganglia, presumably resulting from lipohyalinosis of small penetrating arterioles. This distribution is strikingly similar to that of microaneurysms in the earlier histological studies of hypertensive individuals, including those by Fisher, Ross Russell, and Cole and Yates, suggesting that the histopathological lesions causing CMBs may overlap with those described so many years earlier. By contrast, in patients diagnosed with CAA on clinical grounds, CMBs are typically found in a lobar distribution, and if exclusively located in such a pattern then the specificity for pathologically proven CAA has been reported to be high [26]. It is hoped that the pattern and burden of CMBs may ultimately be helpful in non-invasively and positively diagnosing and classifying the cause(s) of spontaneous ICH in life. This could spare some patients the need for invasive tests including cerebral angiography or brain biopsy, and allow targeted treatment of the underlying arteriopathy, for example with careful hypertensive control or new amyloid-depleting therapies.

Could CMBs as seen on MRI result from perivascular microbleeding in association with microaneurysms and other small bleeding lesions considered earlier in this chapter? A limited number of studies have correlated MRI-defined CMBs with microaneurysms [34,35] or "pseudoaneurysms" [33]. And, as we have seen, histopathological studies have clearly shown areas of extravasated blood leakage adjacent to microaneurysms [5,10,13,14,36]. Moreover, it is noteworthy that the distribution of microaneurysmal lesions in hypertensive patients in histopathological studies has a striking similarity to that of CMBs in similar hypertensive cohorts (Fig. 1.7), consistent with a shared origin for the histopathological and MRI lesions. Therefore, it seems likely that at least some of the varied aneurysmal and aneurysm-like structures described in this chapter

Conclusions

Uncertainty and controversy continues to surround the pathogenesis of spontaneous ICH and, in particular, the role of microaneurysms. Although the interpretation of the many available studies is challenging because of differences in technical methods and nomenclature, it is clear that spontaneous ICH is often related to two main small vessel arteriopathies: lipohyalinosis of small lenticulostriate perforating vessels and CAA affecting small cortical and leptomeningeal vessels. While microaneurysms have been consistently reported in both of these types of arteriopathy, evidence that they are an important or exclusive cause of spontaneous ICH (with or without hypertension) remains limited, and many studies suggest that arterial rupture is not confined to aneurysm sites but may be related to rupture (sometimes sequentially) at multiple adjacent sites along different vessels of pathologically weak arterial walls. Most studies have shown that abnormal small vessels, with or without microaneurysms, are associated with the extravasation of small collections of blood products, which is highly relevant in the interpretation of CMB lesions on modern MRI studies. These CMBs are now increasingly detected in many populations, leading to an urgent need to know more about their pathogenesis, and whether their presence (or particular patterns) put patients at increased future risk of ICH. Further pathological correlation studies are needed to determine how the distribution and burden of MRI-detected CMBs relate to the histological abnormalities described in this chapter as this will allow a better understanding of their diagnostic and prognostic significance.

Acknowledgement

The authors gratefully acknowledge Professor Sebastian Brandner's critical review of the manuscript.

References

1. Lovelock CE, Molyneux AJ, Rothwell PM. Change in incidence and aetiology of intracerebral haemorrhage in Oxfordshire, UK, between 1981 and 2006: a population-based study. *Lancet Neurol* 2007;**6**:487–93.

2. Greenberg SM, Vernooij MW, Cordonnier C et al. Cerebral microbleeds: a guide to detection and interpretation. *Lancet Neurol* 2009;**8**:165–74.

3. Charcot JM, Bouchard C. Nouvelles recherches sur la pathogenie de l'hemorrhagie cerebrale. *Arch Physiol Norm Pathol* 1868;**642**:110–27.

4. Charcot JM. *Clinical Lectures on Senile and Chronic Diseases.* London: New Sydenham Society. 1881.

5. Fisher CM. Cerebral miliary aneurysms in hypertension. *Am J Pathol* 1972;**66**:313–30.

6. Turner FC. Arteries of the brain from cases of cerebral hemorrhage. *Trans Path Soc London* 1882;**33**:96.

7. Eppinger H. Pathogenesis, histogenesis and etiology of the aneurysms, including the aneurysm equi verminosum: pathological–anatomical studies. *Arch Kiln Chirurg* 1887;**xxxv**(Suppl. 1).

8. Ellis AG. The pathogenesis of spontaneous cerebral hemorrhage. *Proc Path Soc (Phil)* 1909;**12**:197–212.

9. Turnbull HM. Alterations in arterial structure and their relation to syphilis. *Q J Med* 1915;**viii**:201–54.

10. Green FHK. Miliary aneurysms in the brain. *J Pathol Bacteriol* 1930;**33**:71–7.

11. Matuoka S. Studien uber Hirnblutung underweichung. (III Mitteilung). Uber kleine Aneurysmen in den Gehirnen ohne Blutung bezw. Blutungsfreien Hirnpartien. *Trans Soc Pathol Jap* 1939;**29**:449–54.

12. Matuoka S. Histopathological studies on the blood vessels in apoplexia cerebri. *Proceedings of the 1st International Congress of Neuropathology*, Torino, 1952, pp. 222–30.

13. Russell RWR. Observations on intracerebral aneurysms. *Brain* 1963;**86**:425–42.

14. Cole FM, Yates P. Intracerebral microaneurysms and small cerebrovascular lesions. *Brain* 1967;**90**:759–68.

15. Takebayashi S, Kaneko M. Electron microscopic studies of ruptured arteries in hypertensive intracerebral hemorrhage. *Stroke* 1983;**14**:28–36.

16. Wakai S, Nagai M. Histological verification of microaneurysms as a cause of cerebral haemorrhage in surgical specimens. *J Neurol Neurosurg Psychiatry* 1989;**52**:595–9.

17. Vonsattel JP, Myers RH, Hedley-Whyte ET et al. Cerebral amyloid angiopathy without and with cerebral hemorrhages: a comparative histological study. *Ann Neurol* 1991;**30**:637–49.

18. Challa VR, Moody DM, Bell MA. The Charcot–Bouchard aneurysm controversy: impact of a new histologic technique. *J Neuropathol Exp Neurol* 1992;**51**:264–71.

19. Mizutani T, Kojima H, Miki Y. Arterial dissections of penetrating cerebral arteries causing hypertension-induced cerebral haemorrhage. *J Neurosurg* 2000;**93**:859–62.

20. Fisher CM. Hypertensive cerebral hemorrhage. Demonstration of the source of bleeding. *J Neuropathol Exp Neurol* 2003;**62**:104–7.

21. Rosenblum WI. Cerebral hemorrhage produced by ruptured dissecting aneurysm in miliary aneurysm. *Ann Neurol* 2003;**54**:376–8.

22. Lee SH, Kwon SJ, Kim KS, Yoon BW, Roh JK. Cerebral microbleeds in patients with hypertensive stroke. Topographical distribution in the supratentorial area. *J Neurol* 2004;**251**:1183–9.

23. Mayer SA, Brun NC, Begtrup K et al. Efficacy and safety of recombinant activated factor VII for acute intracerebral hemorrhage. *N Engl J Med* 2008;**358**:2127–37.

24. Beitzke H. Die Rolle der kleinen Aneurysmen bei den Massenblutungen des Gehirns. *Verh Dtsch Ges Pathol* 1936;**29**:74–80.

25. Vinters HV. Cerebral amyloid angiopathy. A critical review. *Stroke* 1987;**18**:311–24.

26. Knudsen KA, Rosand J, Karluk D, Greenberg SM. Clinical diagnosis of cerebral amyloid angiopathy: validation of the Boston criteria. *Neurology* 2001; **56**:537–9.

27. Scharf J, Bräuherr E, Forsting M, Sartor K. Significance of haemorrhagic lacunes on MRI in patients with hypertensive cerebrovascular disease and intracerebral haemorrhage. *Neuroradiology* 1994;**36**: 504–8.

28. Fazekas F, Kleinert R, Roob G *et al.* Histopathologic analysis of foci of signal loss on gradient-echo T_2^*-weighted MR images in patients with spontaneous intracerebral hemorrhage: evidence of microangiopathy-related microbleeds. *AJNR Am J Neuroradiol* 1999;**20**:637–42.

29. Roob G, Fazekas F. Magnetic resonance imaging of cerebral microbleeds. *Curr Opin Neurol* 2000;**13**: 69–73.

30. Greenberg SM, Finklestein SP, Schaefer PW. Petechial hemorrhages accompanying lobar hemorrhage: detection by gradient-echo MRI. *Neurology* 1996;**46**:1751–4.

31. Offenbacher H, Fazekas F, Schmidt R *et al.* MR of cerebral abnormalities concomitant with primary intracerebral hematomas. *AJNR Am J Neuroradiol* 1996;**17**:573–8.

32. Cordonnier C, Al-Shahi SR, Wardlaw J. Spontaneous brain microbleeds: systematic review, subgroup analyses and standards for study design and reporting. *Brain* 2007;**130**:1988–2003.

33. Tanaka A, Ueno A, Takayama Y, Takabayashi K. Small haemorrhages and ischemic lesions in association with spontaneous intracerebral hematomas. *Stroke* 1999;**30**:1637–42.

34. Schrag M, McAuley G, Pomakian J *et al.* Correlation of hypointensities in susceptibility-weighted images to tissue histology in dementia patients with cerebral amyloid angiopathy: a postmortem MRI study. *Acta Neuropathol* 2010;**119**:291–302.

35. Tatsumi S, Shinohara M, Yamamoto T. Direct comparison of histology of microbleeds with postmortem MR images: a case report. *Cerebrovasc Dis* 2008;**26**:142–6.

36. Cole FM, Yates PO. The occurrence and significance of intracerebral micro-aneurysms. *J Pathol Bacteriol* 1967;**93**:393–411.

Detection of cerebral microbleeds
Physical principles, technical aspects and new developments

Maarten J. Versluis, Andrew G. Webb and Mark A. van Buchem

Signal loss with cerebral microbleeds

Contrast in MR images reflects differences in tissue magnetic properties such as relaxation times and proton density, and also the type of sequence that is used. Transverse (T_2) and longitudinal (T_1) relaxation times vary for different types of tissue: usually tissue with a long T_1 will appear as low signal on T_1-weighted images and tissue with a long T_2 will appear bright on T_2-weighted images. Relaxation times depend on the distribution of water in tissue and its surroundings. Macromolecular interactions with paramagnetic substances, such as metals in particular, strongly affect relaxation times through the formation of a region of magnetic field inhomogeneity surrounding the paramagnetic center [1]. Of the metals that are commonly present in the human brain, it is considered that only iron in the form of ferritin and hemosiderin is present in sufficient quantities and appropriate oxidation state to be visualized by MRI [2,3]. Histology has shown that cerebral microbleeds (CMBs) contain hemosiderin deposits [4–6], a paramagnetic substance [3]. Therefore, both the T_1 and the T_2 relaxation times are affected by CMBs. In general, a decrease in relaxation times is expected in the presence of hemosiderin. The change in relaxation times depends on, among other factors, the chemical environment and field strength (B_0) and is usually not the same for T_1 and T_2 relaxation [4,7,8]. Shortening of T_1 mainly results from dipole–dipole interactions with individual iron atoms and is proportionally less pronounced at higher field strengths because of the intrinsically longer tissue T_1 values at high field [9]. Shortening of T_2 mainly results from water protons diffusing through the surrounding inhomogeneous field and is enhanced at higher field strengths. Related to changes in T_2, the T_2^* relaxation time is also reduced in the presence of an inhomogeneous magnetic field. The latter includes both static and diffusion-related shortening of relaxation times and will be discussed in more detail below.

The magnetic properties of CMBs cause a local change of the magnetic field in surrounding tissue. The magnetic response of a substance to an external magnetic field (such as generated by an MRI system) is described by the magnetic susceptibility of the tissue, denoted by χ [10,11]. Paramagnetic materials have a value of $\chi > 0$, which results in a local increase in the magnetic field strength, as opposed to diamagnetic materials with a $\chi < 0$. The resulting magnetic field inhomogeneity depends on the exact geometry of the substance and is non-local. An example is shown in Fig. 2.1 for a paramagnetic sphere, approximating the shape of a CMB. A non-local behavior between the CMB and the resulting magnetic field inhomogeneity can be seen, such that the spatial extent of the field changes is much larger than the size of the CMB.

The effect that the generated field inhomogeneity has on T_1 and T_2 relaxation can be modeled using the inner-sphere and outer-sphere mechanisms, respectively. In the inner-sphere mechanism, interactions take place through very close contact between iron and water. Because hemosiderin is a water-insoluble material that is shielded from water by a protein shell [7,12], direct dipole–dipole interactions are limited and, as a result, the corresponding changes in T_1 are small. In the outer-sphere model, in contrast, the distance between the iron and water need not be small to be effective. The iron-containing cores of the CMBs are magnetized by the external magnetic field and a magnetic dipole field is formed around the core (Fig. 2.1A). Surrounding water protons diffuse through the inhomogeneous magnetic

Cerebral Microbleeds, ed. David J. Werring. Published by Cambridge University Press. © Cambridge University Press 2011.

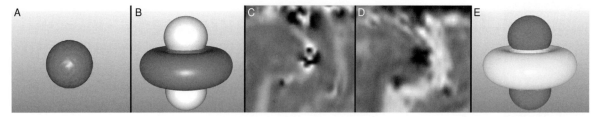

Fig. 2.1 Schematic depiction of a cerebral microbleed (CMB) as a sphere (A) and with the resulting magnetic dipole field changes (B). The white color represents an increase in magnetic field; the gray color corresponds to decreases in magnetic field strength. The net magnetization is decreased for a paramagnetic substance. (C,D) An in vivo example of the phase changes surrounding a CMB (C) and the magnitude signal (D). The shown phase distribution corresponds roughly to the expected phase changes. (E) The dipole field of a diamagnetic sphere is opposite to that of a paramagnetic sphere.

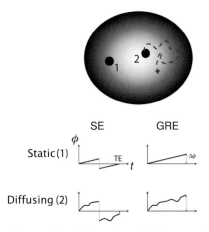

Fig. 2.2 Effect of phase change (ϕ) for static and diffusing spins through an inhomogeneous magnetic field, depicted by 1 and 2, respectively. The change in phase is shown for a spin echo (SE) and a gradient echo (GrE) sequence. The phase reversal in the SE sequence results from the radiofrequency refocusing pulse. The effective phase change ($\Delta\phi$) at time to echo (TE) is different for static and diffusing spins and for SE and GrE sequences. Increased dephasing corresponds to decreased T_2 or T_2^* relaxation times. It can be seen that a GrE sequence leads to the largest phase change and, therefore, the greatest sensitivity for the detection of CMBs.

field and as a result are dephased (Fig. 2.2), which leads to a local reduction in T_2. The amplitude of the magnetic field inhomogeneities increases with field strength and, therefore, the change in T_2 is also dependent on field strength. As a result, the dominating effect of CMBs on the MRI signal will be T_2 shortening, particularly at higher field strengths. The exact amount of dephasing (and T_2 shortening) is related to the tissue properties and geometry and for most in vivo situations it is not possible to calculate it analytically. More comprehensive descriptions of the complex magnetic behavior of hemosiderin and the effect on relaxation times are beyond the scope of this chapter and can be found elsewhere [3,7,10].

In attempts to quantify the actual susceptibility distribution, many different models have been proposed, which relate measurable MRI effects (e.g. signal loss) to the underlying susceptibility distribution. However, for the detection of CMBs it is probably sufficient to use qualitative techniques with a high sensitivity to magnetic field inhomogeneities to provide information on the location and approximate size of the CMB. An important shortcoming of most qualitative techniques, however, is that the source of the change in signal loss is not known. Any magnetic substance will affect transverse and longitudinal relaxation times, including calcifications, iron deposits not related to CMBs, concentration changes of deoxyhemoglobin as well as areas of low water concentration. All these factors can give rise to MRI signal changes that resemble CMBs [13] – so-called microbleed "mimics." A practical approach to interpretation of these mimics is described in Ch. 5. The present chapter will describe some possible technical developments to discriminate between some of the different origins of signal loss.

Sequences sensitive for the detection of cerebral microbleeds

Many different pulse sequences can potentially be used for the detection of CMBs. Most studies use sequences that are sensitive to changes in T_2^* [14,15]; T_2- and T_1-sensitive sequences have also been used to a much lesser extent [16,17]. Because of the very limited use and sensitivity of T_1 sequences for CMBs, these sequences will not be considered in detail here. More recently, there has been increased interest in using not only the magnitude of the MRI signal but also the phase. In most cases, the phase images are combined with the magnitude signal, a technique termed susceptibility-weighted imaging (SWI) [18], to

Table 2.1 Prevalence of cerebral microbleeds in large population-based studies

Study	Field strength (T)	Technique	TR/TE/flip angle resolution	Average age (years) (*n*)	Prevalence (%)	Reference
Austrian Stroke Prevention Study	1.5	2D GRE	620/16/20°, 5 mm slices	60 (280)	6.4	[19]
Japanese study	1.0	2D GRE	1000/30/20°, 0.9 mm × 1.1 mm × 5 mm	54 (450)	3.1	[20]
Japanese Brain Docking Study	1.5	2D GRE	26 ms, 0.9 mm × 1.2 mm × 8 mm	56 (209)	7.7	[21]
Framingham Study	1.0	2D GRE	720/26/30°, 5 mm slices	64 (472)	<75 years: 2.2 >75 years: 12.6	[22]
AGES-Reykjavik study	1.5	2D GRE-EPI	3050/50/90°, 0.85 mm × 0.85 mm × 3 mm	76 (1962)	11.1	[23]
The Rotterdam Scan Study	1.5	3D GRE	45/31/13°, 0.8 × 1.1 mm × 1.6 mm	70 (1062)	60–69 years: 17.8 70–79 years: 31.3 80–97 years: 38.3	[24]

EPI, echo planar imaging; GRE, gradient recall echo; TR, repetition time; TE, echo time; 3D, three dimensional; 2D, two dimensional.

increase the sensitivity to the susceptibility changes caused by CMBs. The development and application of this technique will be described in more detail in Ch. 3. The detection of CMBs is influenced by many parameters, the most important ones being echo time (TE), field strength and sequence type (gradient echo [GRE] or spin echo [SE]). In this section, the different properties of sequences will be described in relation to the sensitivity to detect CMBs. It is important to note that the appearance and size of a CMB on an MR image depends on many sequence parameters, which complicates the definition of general CMB selection criteria.

Table 2.1 gives an overview of sequence parameters that have been used in some large population studies on CMBs.

Sequence type: gradient echo versus spin echo

The dephasing of water protons in tissue surrounding the CMB leads to a decrease in signal magnitude. Part of the dephasing can be *rephased*, resulting in signal recovery when using a SE sequence. The main difference between a SE and a GRE sequence is that the former uses a refocusing radiofrequency pulse while the latter uses only gradients for refocusing. The corresponding transverse relaxation times are called T_2 for SE sequences and T_2^* for GRE sequences. To describe the difference between a SE and GRE sequence, it is convenient to differentiate between static (i.e. non-moving) and diffusing spins. For static spins in an inhomogeneous magnetic field, complete refocusing occurs for a SE sequence and as a result no change in signal magnitude (except for the intrinsic T_2 decay) and phase is observed. The effects of any large-scale background magnetic field gradient are also refocused in a SE sequence. Diffusing spins, however, are not completely refocused, and this results in signal loss, with higher diffusion giving greater signal loss. In contrast to SE sequences, statically dephased spins caused by background magnetic field inhomogeneities are not completely rephased in GRE sequences. Therefore, both static and diffusive dephasing lead to signal loss in GRE sequences and, as a result, the sensitivity for detecting CMBs is increased [17], as shown in Table 2.2.

Figure 2.2 shows the effects of static and diffusive spins on dephasing for a SE and a GRE sequence. Because of these effects, the area of signal loss is larger for a GRE sequence than for a SE sequence, commonly termed "the blooming effect" [13].

Figure 2.3 shows an example of a CMB on T_1-, T_2- and T_2^*-weighted images. The diameter of the CMB is smaller on the T_2-weighted image than on the T_2^*-weighted image and is hardly visible on the T_1-weighted image. This effect can be used to confirm the presence of a microbleed when both SE and GRE images are acquired.

Table 2.2 Comparison of different techniques for detection of cerebral microbleeds

Comparison	Remarks	Outcome	Reference
Field strength: 1.5 vs. 3 T	Identical parameters for 1.5 T and 3 T	Number of CMBs increased by 97%	[25]
	TE = 23 ms for 1.5 T and TE = 16 ms for 3 T	Number of CMBs increased by 28% and contrast increased by 60%	[26]
	Similar parameters for 1.5 T and 3 T	Contrast increased by 48% and diameter increased from 3.09 mm to 3.45 mm	[27]
2D vs. 3D	2D: TE = 25 ms, 5 mm slices 3D: TE = 31 ms, 1.6 mm slices	Number of CMBs increased by 70%	[28]
TE	TE = 10, 17, 23 ms	Size and number of CMBs increases with increasing TE	[29]
Resolution	5 mm vs. 1.5 mm slices	Contrast doubled for thinner slices	[27]
T_2- vs. T_2*-weighted sequence	GRE-EPI: TE = 46 ms SE-EPI: TE = 97 ms	Number of CMBs is doubled for GRE-EPI	[17]
T_2* vs. SWI	SWI involves image processing 2D (T_2*) vs. 3D (SWI) technique	Number CMBs increased by 200% Contrast increased for SWI	[27]
EPI vs. regular T_2*	EPI: TE = 46 ms GRE: TE = 15 ms Scan duration of EPI is 4 s	Contrast remains similar Amount of artefacts is increased	[30]

EPI, echo planar imaging; GRE, gradient recall echo; SE, spin echo; SWI, susceptibility-weighted image; TR, repetition time; TE, echo time; 3D, three dimensional; 2D, two dimensional.

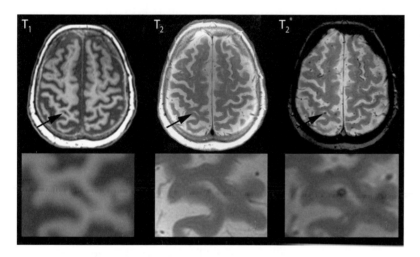

Fig. 2.3 Cerebral microbleed depicted by arrows shown on T_1-, T_2- and T_2*-weighted images. Zoomed in regions are shown on the bottom row. The "blooming" effect is clearly seen by the increased diameter on the T_2*-weighted image compared with the T_2-weighted image.

Large-scale magnetic field inhomogeneities, which occur, for example, at skull–tissue interfaces or close to large veins, are considered to contribute mainly to static dephasing because of their size with respect to the average diffusion distance [31]. The effects of these large inhomogeneities can obscure signal loss caused by CMBs. This detrimental effect is increased when GRE echo planar imaging (GRE-EPI) sequences are used because of the small bandwidth in the phase-encoding direction. The sensitivity of GRE-EPI scans is comparable to that of conventional GRE scans, except for areas close to the skull base, where the number of artefacts hampers CMB detection [17]. The significantly reduced scan duration of GRE-EPI scans could make it a viable alternative in uncooperative patients. Despite these potential problems, GRE sequences are the most widely used for detection of CMBs.

Effect of echo time

In both SE and GRE sequences, the sensitivity to CMBs is, to a large degree, determined by TE. The TE determines on what timescale dephasing occurs; as a result, a long TE leads to more diffusion-related and static dephasing. The area of signal loss increases accordingly, because protons in a larger area surrounding the CMB are dephased, thus leading to a larger decrease in MR signal [29,32]. There are a number of disadvantages when using sequences with a long TE. First, the total signal will decrease through T_2 or T_2^* decay and changes resulting from the CMBs are easily masked by a decrease in the signal-to-noise ratio (SNR) [32]. Second, specifically for GRE sequences, the amount of dephasing caused by large-scale magnetic field inhomogeneities is also increased, specifically obscuring the detection of CMBs near the skull base or near air–tissue interfaces. Typically a TE between 25 and 50 ms is used, but the optimal TE depends strongly on field strength, as shown in Table 2.2. In general a shorter TE can be used at higher field strengths.

Effect of field strength

An intrinsic property of paramagnetic materials is that the internal magnetization of the material increases linearly with the applied field strength, and the amplitude of the resulting field distribution around the material changes accordingly [10]. Therefore, the number and physical extent of dephased spins are related to the field strength; consequently, a higher magnetic field strength results in increased sensitivity for CMB detection. In addition, the intrinsic SNR is increased at higher fields, which increases the sensitivity of CMB detection. However, the sensitivity to large-scale magnetic field inhomogeneities also increases with field strength, which can lead to image artefacts, particularly in the basal forebrain [25]. Overall, the increased sensitivity and SNR at high magnetic field are advantageous in CMB detection, which is illustrated by the increased number of CMBs that are found using higher field strengths (Table 2.2) [25–27,33]. Besides an increase in the number of CMBs, an increase in contrast-to-noise ratio and CMB size is also found [25,27]. These findings indicate that the increased dephasing leads to a more pronounced signal loss, thereby giving rise to greater contrast with respect to surrounding tissue. The use of very high field strengths (i.e. 7 T and above) is discussed below.

Spatial resolution

Smaller voxel sizes minimize not only partial volume effects (i.e. the loss of sensitivity caused by averaging with surrounding tissue) but also the effects of large-scale magnetic field inhomogeneities. More specifically, the use of thinner slices in combination with higher field strengths leads to the detection of more CMBs [13,27,28]. The larger number of CMBs detected in the Rotterdam Scan Study [24] compared with other population-based studies, such as the Framingham Study, the Age Gene/Environment Susceptibility (AGES)-Reykjavik study or the Austrian Stroke Prevention Study [19,22,23] (Table 2.1), can be explained by the use of a high-resolution three-dimensional (3D) technique in the Rotterdam Scan Study compared with two-dimensional (2D) techniques in the other studies. The number of detectable CMBs was increased almost by a factor of two when a conventional 3D sequence was compared with a 2D one [28], and prevalences of 35.5% and 21%, respectively, were found in subjects older than 70 years of age. In addition to providing increased sensitivity, 3D techniques can also be advantageous in terms of SNR efficiency, but usually at the cost of increased scanning times [13].

New sequence and processing developments

The majority of studies that aim to detect CMBs use conventional 2D T_2^*-weighted imaging techniques at 1.5 T with no further processing (Table 2.1). However, the introduction of higher-field scanners and the development of new sequences can provide increased sensitivity for the detection of CMBs. The first reports on CMBs were performed using SE sequences [16] even though the increased sensitivity of GRE sequences for the detection of cerebral hemorrhages was known earlier and had already been compared with SE sequences [34]. However, the use of GRE sequences was limited because of the poor image quality resulting from the large field inhomogeneities. Modern state of the art MRI systems with improved shimming hardware, resulting in a much more homogeneous magnetic field, enables the use of GRE sequences even at high magnetic field strengths. Recently, studies using 3D GRE sequences with higher spatial resolution [28], and more specifically the use of SWI sequences with corresponding post-processing steps [5,17,30,35,36], have been used successfully for CMB detection. In the following section, new sequence and post-processing developments will be discussed.

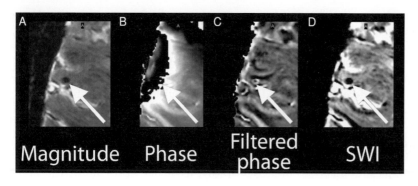

Fig. 2.4 Visualization of a cerebral microbleed (CMB; depicted by arrows) on magnitude, phase, unwrapped (filtered) phase and susceptibility-weighted (SWI) processed data of the same scan. Filtering of the phase images was performed using a 92 × 92 high-pass filter. The CMB is visible on the magnitude as well as on the filtered phase image. The contrast between the CMB and surrounding tissue and the size are increased using SWI processing.

Phase imaging

The MR signal is a complex signal, in that it consists of magnitude and phase components. The magnitude component contains information on the amount of signal and is conventionally the only component used to display MR images. The phase (ϕ) of each voxel in the image contains information directly related to the difference in magnetic field strength (ΔB_0) in that voxel compared with the overall static magnetic field B_0. The phase difference ($\Delta\phi$) in a GRE sequence is given by the following simple formula:

$$\phi = \gamma \Delta B_0 \text{TE} \qquad (2.1)$$

where γ is a physical constant, the proton gyromagnetic ratio. An increase in the local magnetic field strength leads to an increase in the phase. The sum of the different phase shifts of all the spins within a voxel results in a reduction in the magnitude signal compared with the case in which all of the spins have the same phase. Each voxel, therefore, has an effective phase that is governed by the dominant field inhomogeneity within the voxel. As a consequence, smaller voxel sizes give a better definition of the actual phase, because there is less averaging of spins and a more homogeneous field within the voxel. It should also be noted that the signal magnitude contains no information on whether the local magnetic field is higher or lower than B_0: however, this information can be derived from the phase of the signal. Therefore, using the phase images, one can discriminate between paramagnetic and diamagnetic substances, thereby opening up the possibility to differentiate between calcifications (a diamagnetic substance) and CMBs, which are paramagnetic. The former leads to a local magnetic field decrease, whereas the latter results in an increase [37]. The relation is slightly more complicated because of the non-local behavior described above between the exact physical location of a CMB and the resulting phase changes that are present in the image. Figure 2.1 shows the relation between a CMB and the field distribution around a CMB, showing an extended dipole field (compare parts B and C in Fig. 2.1). Therefore, one expects phase differences in the image to extend to voxels surrounding the one in which the CMB is present, and that phase changes in neighboring voxels will be both positive and negative. For a diamagnetic substance, the surrounding dipole field is inverted and is shown in Fig. 2.1D.

One factor that needs to be mentioned is that some basic image processing is needed to display the phase images. If the accumulated phase of a spin represents more than a complete cycle (2π radians or $360°$) a "phase wrap" occurs. From Equation (2.1), the longer the TE, the more likely this is to occur. The TE values used in conventional scans do not result in phase wraps caused by CMBs, but background field inhomogeneities do give large globally varying phase changes, which do produce phase wraps, and these phase wraps can obscure the more subtle effects from CMBs. Therefore, these large-scale magnetic field inhomogeneities need to be removed first from the phase. An efficient way uses high-pass Fourier filtering [38], but more sophisticated approaches that take the origin of the large-scale inhomogeneities into account also exist [39].

Figure 2.4 compares the appearance of a CMB on magnitude data (A) and phase data, before and after removal of large magnetic field inhomogeneities (B and C, respectively), where the local increase in magnetic field strength is visible by the bright appearance on the phase image. In addition, the spatial extent of the resulting phase changes is larger than on the magnitude image.

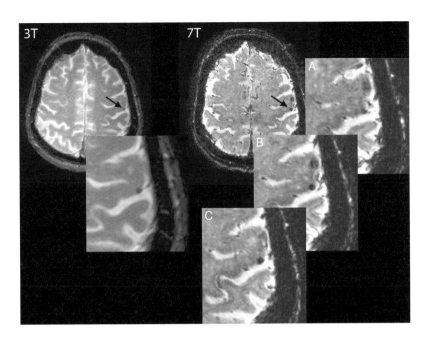

Fig. 2.5 Patient scanned at 3 T and 7 T showing the difference in size. Zoomed in sections from several slcies of 0.6 mm thickness are shown for the 7 T data (A–C), whereas the CMB was visible only on a single slice 4 mm thick on the 3 T image.

Susceptibility-weighted imaging

This SWI technique, which was originally proposed by Haacke [18] for visualization of venous structures, uses a 3D GRE sequence with full-flow compensation on all three axes to avoid phase changes originating from flowing spins. In contrast to conventional GRE sequences, not only the magnitude but also the phase of the complex MR signal is used. To obtain an SWI image, the phase and magnitude data are combined in a post-processing step. A mask is created that suppresses phase changes that are caused by decreases in the magnetic field strength, effectively excluding signal from diamagnetic materials (i.e. calcifications). The resulting phase mask is combined with the magnitude image to enhance signal loss from paramagnetic tissue, including venous structures and CMBs. An example is shown in Fig. 2.4D. An increased contrast for CMB detection from the SWI compared with the magnitude data (Fig. 2.4A) is visible. Several studies have shown an increase in the number of detectable CMBs when using this method [27,30,35]. However, in all these comparative studies, the SWI scan was a high-resolution 3D scan and the regular T_2*-weighted image was a lower resolution 2D technique; consequently, the comparison is not straightforward. The full potential of SWI in the detection of CMBs still needs to be determined [13]. Potential drawbacks of the technique are the longer scanning times required

for the 3D data acquisition and the possibility of introducing image artefacts [30] through remaining background phase errors. This technique will be described in more detail in Ch. 3, which deals exclusively with SWI.

Very-high-field imaging

The recent introduction of human 7 T scanners has led to high quality and high-resolution GRE images of the human brain [40,41], with an increased contrast between gray and white matter. The detection of CMBs could also benefit greatly from the high magnetic field strength, for the reasons described above. Up to now, no studies at 7 T have been published regarding CMB detection. The increased SNR can be used to obtain a smaller voxel size than at lower field strength, and the increased susceptibility effect leads to an increased contrast even at shorter TE values. Figure 2.5 shows an example of a CMB in the same patient scanned at 3 T and 7 T, with approximately the same scan duration for each field strength. Because of the smaller slice thickness of the sequence at 7 T, the CMB is visible on multiple slices. At 3 T, the CMB is only visible on a single slice. In addition, the diameter is increased at 7 T through the increased blooming effect, further increasing the possibilities to detect small CMBs.

References

1. Stankiewicz J, Panter SS, Neema M *et al.* Iron in chronic brain disorders: imaging and neurotherapeutic implications. *Neurotherapeutics* 2007;4:371–86.

2. Schenck JF. Magnetic resonance imaging of brain iron. *J Neurolog Sci* 2003;207:99–102.

3. Schenck JF, Zimmerman EA. High-field magnetic resonance imaging of brain iron: birth of a biomarker? *NMR Biomed* 2004;17:433–45.

4. Thulborn KR, Sorensen AG, Kowall NW *et al.* The role of ferritin and hemosiderin in the MR appearance of cerebral hemorrhage: a histopathologic biochemical study in rats. *AJR Am J Roentgenol* 1990;154:1053–9.

5. Schrag M, McAuley G, Pomakian J *et al.* Correlation of hypointensities in susceptibility-weighted images to tissue histology in dementia patients with cerebral amyloid angiopathy: a postmortem MRI study. *Acta Neuropathol* 2010;119:291–302.

6. Tatsumi S, Shinohara M, Yamamoto T. Direct comparison of histology of microbleeds with postmortem MR images: a case report. *Cerebrovasc Dis* 2008;26:142–6.

7. Brooks RA, Vymazal J, Goldfarb RB *et al.* Relaxometry and magnetometry of ferritin. *Magn Reson Med* 1998;40:227–35.

8. Vymazal J, Brooks RA, Baumgarner C *et al.* The relation between brain iron and NMR relaxation times: an in vitro study. *Magn Reson Med* 1996;35:56–61.

9. Wright P, Mougin O, Totman J *et al.* Water proton T_1 measurements in brain tissue at 7, 3, and 1.5 T using IR-EPI, IR-TSE, and MPRAGE: results and optimization. *Magn Reson Mat Phys Biol Med* 2008;21:121–30.

10. Haacke EM, Cheng NY, House MJ *et al.* Imaging iron stores in the brain using magnetic resonance imaging. *Magn Reson Imaging* 2005;23:1–25.

11. Bos C, Viergever MA, Bakker CJ. On the artifact of a subvoxel susceptibility deviation in spoiled gradient-echo imaging. *Magn Reson Med* 2003;50:400–4.

12. Koorts AM, Viljoen M. Ferritin and ferritin isoforms. I: Structure–function relationships, synthesis, degradation and secretion. *Arch Physiol Biochem* 2007;113:30–54.

13. Greenberg SM, Vernooij MW, Cordonnier C *et al.* Cerebral microbleeds: a guide to detection and interpretation. *Lancet Neurol* 2009;8:165–74.

14. Cordonnier C, Al-Shahi Salman R, Wardlaw J. Spontaneous brain microbleeds: systematic review, subgroup analyses and standards for study design and reporting. *Brain* 2007;130:1988–2003.

15. Fiehler J. Cerebral microbleeds: old leaks and new haemorrhages. *Int J Stroke* 2006;1:122–30.

16. Scharf J, Bräuherr E, Forsting M *et al.* Significance of haemorrhagic lacunes on MRI in patients with hypertensive cerebrovascular disease and intracerebral haemorrhage. *Neuroradiology* 1994;36:504–8.

17. Liang L, Korogi Y, Sugahara T *et al.* Detection of intracranial hemorrhage with susceptibility-weighted MR sequences. *AJNR Am J Neuroradiol* 1999;20:1527–34.

18. Haacke EM, Xu Y, Cheng YN *et al.* Susceptibility-weighted imaging (SWI). *Magn Reson Med* 2004;52:612–18.

19. Roob G, Schmidt R, Kapeller P *et al.* MRI evidence of past cerebral microbleeds in a healthy elderly population. *Neurology* 1999;52:991.

20. Tsushima Y, Tanizaki Y, Aoki J *et al.* MR detection of microhemorrhages in neurologically healthy adults. *Neuroradiology* 2002;44:31–6.

21. Horita Y, Imaizumi T, Niwa J *et al.* [Analysis of dot-like hemosiderin spots using brain dock system.] *No Shinkei Geka* 2003;31:263–7.

22. Jeerakathil T, Wolf PA, Beiser A *et al.* Cerebral microbleeds: prevalence and associations with cardiovascular risk factors in the Framingham Study. *Stroke* 2004;35:1831–5.

23. Sveinbjornsdottir S, Sigurdsson S, Aspelund T *et al.* Cerebral microbleeds in the population based AGES–Reykjavik study: prevalence and location. *J Neurol Neurosurg Psychiatr* 2008;79:1002–6.

24. Vernooij MW, van der Lugt A, Ikram MA *et al.* Prevalence and risk factors of cerebral microbleeds: the Rotterdam Scan Study. *Neurology* 2008;70:1208–14.

25. Scheid R, Ott DV, Roth H *et al.* Comparative magnetic resonance imaging at 1.5 and 3 Tesla for the evaluation of traumatic microbleeds. *J Neurotrauma* 2007;24:1811–16.

26. Stehling C, Wersching H, Kloska SP *et al.* Detection of asymptomatic cerebral microbleeds: a comparative study at 1.5 and 3.0 T. *Acad Radiol* 2008;15:895–900.

27. Nandigam R, Viswanathan A, Delgado P *et al.* MR imaging detection of cerebral microbleeds: effect of susceptibility-weighted imaging, section thickness, and field strength. *AJNR Am J Neuroradiol* 2009;30:338–43.

28. Vernooij M, Ikram MA, Wielopolski PA *et al.* Cerebral microbleeds: accelerated 3D T_2^*-weighted GRE MR imaging versus conventional 2D T_2^*-weighted GRE MR imaging for detection. *Radiology* 2008;248:272–7.

29. Tatsumi S, Ayaki T, Shinohara M *et al.* Type of gradient recalled-echo sequence results in size and

number change of cerebral microbleeds. *AJNR Am J Neuroradiol* 2008;**29**:e13.

30. Akter M, Hirai T, Hiai Y *et al.* Detection of hemorrhagic hypointense foci in the brain on susceptibility-weighted imaging: clinical and phantom studies. *Acad Radiol* 2007;**14**:1011–19.

31. Reichenbach JR, Venkatesan R, Yablonskiy DA *et al.* Theory and application of static field inhomogeneity effects in gradient-echo imaging. *J Magn Reson Imaging* 1997;7:266–79.

32. Gregoire SM, Werring DJ, Chaudhary UJ *et al.* Choice of echo time on GRE T_2*-weighted MRI influences the classification of brain microbleeds. *Clin Radiol* 2010;**65**:391–4.

33. Kikuta K, Takagi Y, Nozaki K *et al.* Asymptomatic microbleeds in moyamoya disease: T_2*-weighted gradient-echo magnetic resonance imaging study. *J Neurosurg* 2005;**102**:470–5.

34. Atlas SW, Mark AS, Grossman RI *et al.* Intracranial hemorrhage: gradient-echo MR imaging at 1.5 T. Comparison with spin-echo imaging and clinical applications. *Radiology* 1988;**168**:803–7.

35. Mori N, Miki Y, Kikuta K *et al.* Microbleeds in moyamoya disease: susceptibility-weighted imaging versus T_2*-weighted imaging at 3 Tesla. *Invest Radiol* 2008;**43**:574–9.

36. Ayaz M, Boikov AS, Haacke EM *et al.* Imaging cerebral microbleeds using susceptibility weighted imaging: one step toward detecting vascular dementia. *J Magn Reson Imaging* 2010;**31**:142–8.

37. Haacke EM, Makki M, Ge Y *et al.* Characterizing iron deposition in multiple sclerosis lesions using susceptibility weighted imaging. *J Magn Reson Imaging* 2009;**29**:537–44.

38. Ogg RJ, Langston JW, Haacke EM *et al.* The correlation between phase shifts in gradient-echo MR images and regional brain iron concentration. *Magn Reson Imaging* 1999;**17**:1141–8.

39. Neelavalli J, Cheng YN, Jiang J *et al.* Removing background phase variations in susceptibility-weighted imaging using a fast, forward-field calculation. *J Magn Reson Imaging* 2009;**29**:937–48.

40. Yao B, Li T, Gelderen PV *et al.* Susceptibility contrast in high field MRI of human brain as a function of tissue iron content. *Neuroimage* 2009;**44**:1259–66.

41. Duyn JH, van Gelderen P, Li T *et al.* High-field MRI of brain cortical substructure based on signal phase. *Proc Natl Acad Sci USA* 2007;**104**:11796–801.

Chapter

3

Susceptibility-weighted imaging

E. Mark Haacke, Alexander S. Boikov, Samuel Barnes,
Jaladhar Neelavalli and M. Ayaz Khan

Introduction

As has been discussed in Ch. 2, imaging cerebral microbleeds (CMB) is possible in MRI thanks to gradient-recalled echo (GRE) imaging methods. These sequences are particularly sensitive to blood products such as hemosiderin (non-heme iron) and to changes in the level of deoxyhemoglobin (heme iron). In the early days of clinical MRI, GRE scanning was usually done in two dimensions (2D) with echo times (TE) limited to a range of 15 to 25 ms at 1.5 T. These limitations were imposed because longer TE values combined with the thick slice 2D scans led to very poor image quality. With the advent of three-dimensional (3D) GRE imaging, it became possible to scan with much smaller voxel sizes and longer TE periods (40, 60 and 80 ms at 1.5 T) while still maintaining good image quality [1], thanks to the decreased dephasing across the now smaller voxels. This early work also recognized the importance of filtered phase images and was the foundation from which the concept of susceptibility-weighted imaging (SWI) was to emerge [2].

Phase data are usually discarded in conventional GRE imaging. This is because phase is sensitive not only to local field inhomogeneities, which are of great interest, but also to all forms of unwanted magnetic field inhomogeneity, including eddy current effects, main magnet effects and air–tissue interface effects. Most of the unwanted phase effects are of low spatial frequency in nature. Therefore, with the appropriate high-pass filtering [2–4], the phase data potentially become quite useful. With both magnitude and phase data at hand, the idea arose [2] to combine them into a single susceptibility-weighted image. These new SWI data showed areas with blood products much better than the magnitude images alone and revealed veins and CMBs as they had never been seen before in vivo [5]. It is, therefore, of interest to compare the

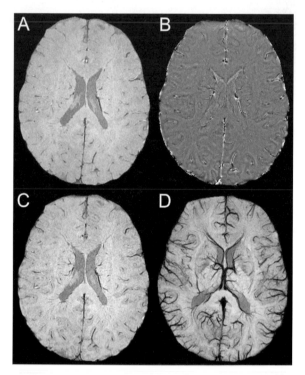

Fig. 3.1 Susceptibilty-weighted image (SWI) data collected at 3 T with an echo time (TE) of 20 ms and a flip angle of 15°, an in-plane resolution of 0.5 mm × 0.5 mm and a slice thickness of 2 mm. (A) Original magnitude image; (B) high-pass filtered phase image; (C) processed SWI single slice; and (D) minimum intensity projection (mIP) over 2 cm. The individual SWI data show an enhancement of the venous information coming from the phase data. This enhancement is best appreciated in the mIP image, which reveals the connectivity of the veins. Often a cerebral microbleed will appear clearly disconnected from the veins, making it easier to appreciate, although this is not always the case.

usual GRE with SWI for CMB detection. Figure 3.1 shows the type of information available with an SWI dataset projected over 10 slices in the central and upper parts of the brain. Figure 3.2 shows a comparison

---

Cerebral Microbleeds, ed. David J. Werring. Published by Cambridge University Press. © Cambridge University Press 2011.

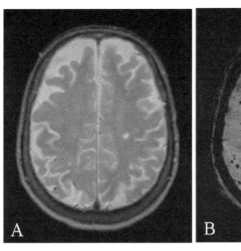 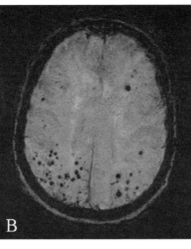

Fig. 3.2 A cerebral microbleed (CMB) is defined more clearly with susceptibilty-weighted imaging (SWI) than with conventional gradient-recalled echo (GRE) T_2*-weighted imaging partly because of the contrast mechanisms and partly because of the higher resolution. (A) The GRE T_2* image contains six detectable CMBs. (B) The corresponding SWI image taken on the same day shows at least a 10-fold increase in detectable CMBs over the GRE image. (Images courtesy of Wolff Kirsch, MD.)

between SWI and a conventional GRE T_2*-weighted scan at 1.5 T for an 88-year-old patient with multiple CMBs.

These CMBs mostly seem to be clinically asymptomatic, although this remains a topic of active investigation, particularly with respect to cognitive impairment (see Chs. 17 and 18). Nevertheless, CMBs appear to be an important new imaging marker for small vessel pathologies and are associated with various imaging and clinical manifestations of cerebrobvascular disease including lacunar infarcts and white matter changes, intracerebral hemorrhage [6–8] and cerebral amyloid angiopathy (CAA) [11]. They are also present in the healthy elderly populations [12]. These aspects are considered in detail in subsequent chapters.

Cerebral microbleeds may also be a source of pathological free iron that could be related to tissue damage [13]. Therefore, the ability to detect even small amounts of iron with a method such as SWI may prove useful in understanding the role iron plays in neurodegenerative diseases, and the role of CMBs in particular.

Cerebral microbleeds are generally considered to be less than 5 to 10 mm in diameter [9]. They consist mostly of hemosiderin [14], which has a large susceptibility effect and hence is easily seen with T_2*-weighted scans such as SWI. In general, CMB contrast and detection is sensitive to many imaging variables, such as field strength, TE [1,15] and resolution [9,16]. The SWI approach is more sensitive in detecting small lesions and bleeds than traditional methods, because it is routinely done at high resolution ($\leq$1 mm³), with long TE values and using the phase image to enhance

contrast. Recent publications have reported a threefold increase in the number of CMBs seen [16] and a sixfold increase in the number of lesions seen [17] using SWI compared with other techniques. Because CMBs can be very small, they are easy to confuse with other structures such as veins (so-called CMB mimics [9]; see Ch. 5), and evaluation of true specificity and sensitivity is challenging in the absence of pathological confirmation of the nature of radiologically defined lesions. The small size of CMBs and the large numbers of CMB mimics have hampered efforts to quantify them automatically. Consequently, methods so far have centered on manually drawing and counting the lesions, or manually defining local thresholds for a small region of interest for their semiautomatic detection [5]. These methods suffer from inter- and intra-observer error [18] and with SWI images, particularly, become extremely time consuming even for evaluating a single patient's data. Recent publications have shown improvements by using standardized rating scales [2,18,19] but further improvement in rapid identification and quantification are desirable.

Application in detection of cerebral microbleeds in mild cognitive impairment and dementia

As an example of the clinical application of SWI, this section describes the use of SWI to monitor CMBs over time in a cohort of elderly patients, 28 of whom were cognitively normal and 75 had mild congnitive impairment (MCI) as defined by the Mayo Clinic Group

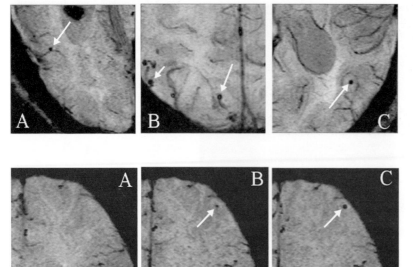

Fig. 3.3 Minimum intensity projection over five slices from three subjects showing the different categories of cerebral microbleed (CMB). (A) A CMB appearing attached to the edge of a vein. (B) A CMB at the end of a vessel (long arrow); not all CMBs are indicated. (C) A "stand-alone" CMB. (Reproduced with permission from [47].)

Fig. 3.4 An example of a cerebral microbleed (CMB) increasing in size. (A) No evidence of a CMB in the first scan. (B) In the second scan, a "stand-alone" CMB appears in the left frontal lobe. (C) In the third scan, the CMB has increased in size. Images are minimum intensity projections over five slices. (Reproduced with permission from Ayaz *et al.* 2010 [5].)

criteria [5]. Participants in the study were evaluated cognitively (bi-yearly) and radiologically (9 months to yearly) over an average follow-up time of 5.5 years (range, 0.5–5.5). Detailed methods for this study have been described elsewhere [3]. In this study, none of the 28 cognitively normal subjects had more than three CMBs. In the 75 subjects with MCI, five had more than three CMBs in both first and last scans, while another subject had more than three bleeds only in the last scan. In five of these six patients, the number of CMBs increased over time and all six went on to develop progressive cognitive impairment. This study raises questions of CMB interpretation; in particular, further discussion about distinguishing a vessel cross-section from a CMB on SWI scans is needed. When attempting to correctly classify a potential CMB, the observer needs to be vigilant about the possibility that it may in fact be a vessel. For example, a vessel parallel to the main field and perpendicular to the image plane would appear as a CMB mimic in a single slice. By cycling back and forth between adjacent slices, a vessel will appear as a shifting, (often elliptical) hypointense cross-section, whereas a CMB will appear as if emerging out of nowhere and will likewise disappear. We have used a guideline that CMBs are taken to be <5 mm in diameter [9,18,20,21]: a CMB (by this definition) may be seen in at most three adjacent 2 mm slices before disappearing (see Ch. 4 for further discussion of CMB size criteria). A long

vessel would appear in more than three slices and/or would be connected to another vessel as seen in the minimum intensity projection (mIP). Using an identical approach, circular regions of signal loss seen at bifurcations of vessels can be discriminated as either CMBs or as vessels. Using these principles, a total of 130 unique CMBs could be counted and were categorized into at least four types: (1) a CMB that appears adjacent to a vessel (Fig. 3.3A); (2) a CMB attached to the end of a vessel (Fig. 3.3B); (3) an isolated CMB with no visible vessel connection (Fig. 3.3C); and (4) a CMB that changes in size over time (Fig. 3.4).

On rare occasions, a very small CMB may be missed in one scan and counted in another scan from another time point. Such a mistake can be avoided when each CMB is tracked scan to scan. Figure 3.5 shows an example of the development of CMBs over the course of approximately 3 years in the parietal lobe.

Another of our observations concerned the range of CMB sizes. Using SWI, we found that most CMB volumes were <33.5 mm^3 (4 mm in diameter) (Fig. 3.6). It is interesting to note that the distribution of these CMBs is well separated from the larger size lesions of ≥4 mm diameter. This is somewhat lower than the cut-off of 5.7 mm diameter recently proposed by Greenberg *et al.* in a cohort of patients with a clinical diagnosis of CAA [21]. The presence of microvascular disease may be hidden even well

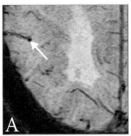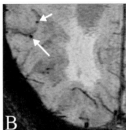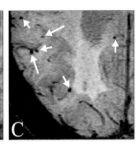

Fig. 3.5 Three time points for the same subject showing the stepwise development of cerebral microbleed (CMB) in the right parietal lobe. (A) A CMB at the end of a vessel (arrow). (B) One year later, the scan reveals a new "stand alone" CMB (short arrow). (C) After a further 9 months, the scan showed four more CMBs (short arrows). Images are minimum intensity projections over five slices. (Reproduced with permission from Ayaz *et al.* 2010 [5].)

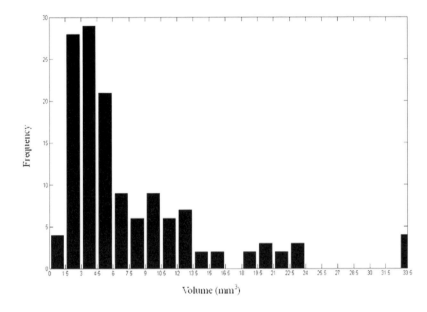

Fig. 3.6 Volume histogram showing a Rayleigh-like distribution for cerebral microbleeds (CMBs) (<33.5 mm^3). Note the sizable gap separating the macrobleeds (≥33.5 mm^3) from CMBs. A majority of the macrobleeds appear to be between 1 and 2 mm in diameter. The use of thinner slices with higher in-plane resolution revealed more macrobleeds than seen with thicker slices. (Reproduced with permission from Ayaz *et al.* 2010 [5].)

below the 1–8 mm^3 peak demonstrated here (Fig. 3.6). Two recent papers studying beta-amyloid plaque in animals and at 7 T both show a large number of very small CMBs that, if plotted here, would have pushed the peak far to the left [22,23]. In the human cadaver brain studies, the images were collected with a 0.3 mm isotropic resolution, opening the door to the discovery of even smaller CMBs than shown in this study. For this reason, we have categorized lesions ≥33.5 mm^3 as macrobleeds. Of the six patients with progressive cognitive impairment that we have studied, four had macrobleeds in frontal, parietal or occipital lobes. These patients were classified as progressive based on their cognitive dementia rating. One subject had major changes in the right frontal lobe of the brain, likely attributable to subarachnoid hemorrhage (Fig. 3.7), an increasingly recognized imaging finding in CAA. Another had two macrobleeds: one in the thalamus on the left side of the brain and the other

in the right side of the brain just above the cerebellum (Fig. 3.8), which appeared to get larger.

Histopathological correlations of cerebral microbleeds detected on susceptibility-weighted imaging

Validation of the radiologically defined CMBs on SWI using either a phantom or a cadaver brain can clarify the nature of underlying lesions (see Chs. 1 and 6). In the case outlined below, we show the histopathological confirmation of a CMB seen with SWI in a cadaver brain (Fig. 3.9). Use of SWI enabled depiction of internal details of another CMB similar to those seen on the cadaver brain photograph (Fig. 3.9B,C). The identity and clinical significance of such internal structure is currently unclear, although it is a testament to the levels of detail possible to achieve with SWI.

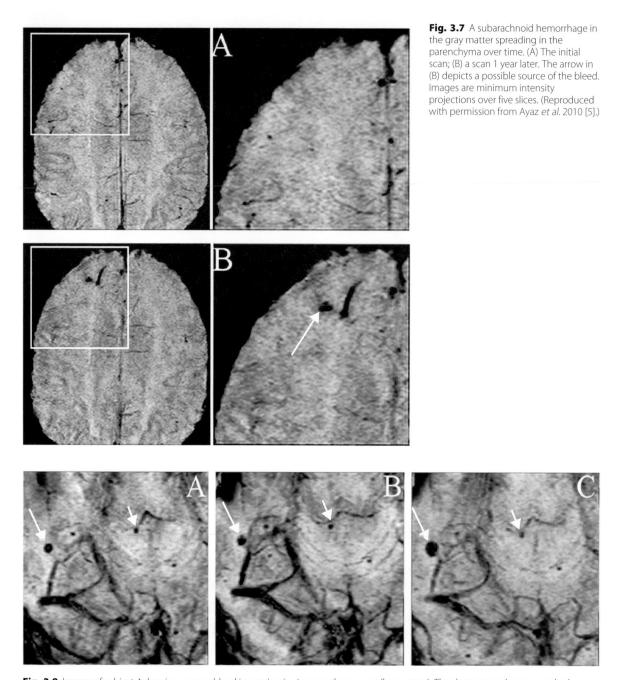

Fig. 3.7 A subarachnoid hemorrhage in the gray matter spreading in the parenchyma over time. (A) The initial scan; (B) a scan 1 year later. The arrow in (B) depicts a possible source of the bleed. Images are minimum intensity projections over five slices. (Reproduced with permission from Ayaz *et al.* 2010 [5].)

Fig. 3.8 Images of subject 4 showing a macrobleed increasing in size over three scans (long arrow). The short arrow shows a cerebral microbleed of constant size, indicating that the macrobleed's larger appearance cannot be blamed on distortion or artefact. Images are minimum intensity projections over five slices. (Reproduced with permission from Ayaz *et al.* 2010 [5].)

"Blooming effects" on susceptibility-weighted imaging

The local fields produced by hemosiderin lead not only to T_2^* signal loss but also to changes in phase.

In our study, we used SWI filtered phase images as a means to detect and map CMBs and to detect changes in iron content [24]. It is possible to have a situation where bleeding occurs so uniformly and diffusely that there are negligible T_2^* effects, but a

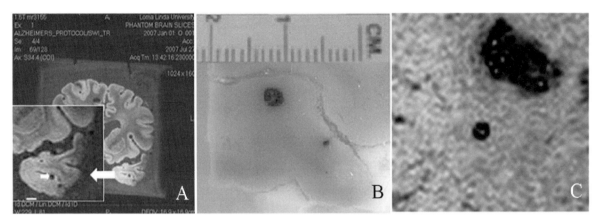

Fig. 3.9 Comparison of a confirmed cerebral microbleed (CMB) in a cadaver brain apparent on susceptibilty-weighted image (SWI) (A) and a histological slide showing an irregular internal composition (B). (C) A different CMB on SWI but one that shows a similar internal irregularity to that shown in (B). (Reproduced with permission from Schrag *et al.* 2010 [26].)

significant phase change makes the bleed visible in SWI when it would not have been in a conventional magnitude GRE image [25]. Generally, as in conventional GRE imaging, there will be a blooming effect or a loss in signal larger than the true size of the object. However, high-resolution imaging and high-pass filtering of the phase images limits the blooming seen in SWI [4,25]. A recent study examining the blooming effect in SWI at 3.0 T in cadaver brains showed it to be quite variable; but the average size on SWI was 1.58 ± 0.75 times the diameter of the actual lesion [26].

Cerebral microbleed "mimics" on susceptibility-weighted imaging

It should be noted that calcifications (sometimes seen in the basal ganglia) can also cause signal loss that can mimic CMBs on GRE T_2^* sequences. Regardless of the fact that CMBs were not found in the basal ganglia in this study (since hypertensive patients were excluded), it is easy to discriminate between calcification and blood products on the SWI high-pass filtered phase images because diamagnetic calcium carbonate appears with the opposite-sign phase with respect to paramagnetic hemosiderin [27]. Even though CMBs are important in identifying CAA, it has also been shown that one can see regions of signal loss in the presence of beta-amyloid plaque in animal models. It may be that it will be possible to see such regions as well with the advent of 7 T and resolution on the order of 200 mm $\times$ 200 mm in-plane [22,23,28]. Technically

these are not CMBs but rather local iron accumulation around the lesions [23].

Sensitivity of susceptibility-weighted imaging for detecting cerebral microbleeds

The high sensitivity of SWI toward detecting CMBs is further exemplified in the following case. A 70-year-old man with a past medical history of diabetes, hypertension and ischemic heart disease was referred for evaluation of recurrent cerebral hemorrhages. The patient had experienced a left temporoparietal cerebral hemorrhage approximately 10 years before presentation. Two months before presentation, the patient underwent coronary artery stent placement and was placed on aspirin and clopidogrel. Within a week, he presented with altered mental status. Computed tomography (CT) without contrast showed a new 3.0 cm $\times$ 2.5 cm intraparenchymal hemorrhage in the left posterior temporoparietal lobe. Before MRI, the patient underwent cerebral angiography, which demonstrated no evidence of arteriovenous malformation or any pathological vascular condition. The MR angiography showed similar negative findings. Although both the T_2^*-weighted GRE (Fig. 3.10A) and SWI image (Fig. 3.10B) showed multiple areas of low signal intensity (consistent with hemosiderin deposition suggesting CMBs) in a cortico-subcortical distribution, SWI showed more numerous lesions with improved apparent contrast. Using the same criteria for counting the small rounded lesions as described

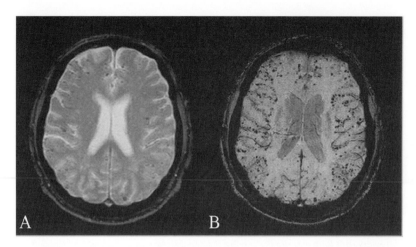

Fig. 3.10 Cerebral amyloid angiopathy (CAA). (A) Axial gradient-recalled echo (GRE) T_2^*-weighted image (repetition time [TR]/echo time [TE], 800/26 ms; section thickness 5 mm; $N_x = 256$, $N_y = 154$) shows some foci of low signal intensity associated with CAA. (B) The corresponding susceptibilty-weighted image (TR/TE 85/35 ms; flip angle 20°; $N_x = 512$, $N_y = 256$; with a resolution of 0.5 mm × 0.5 mm × 2.0 mm, projected over 8 mm) shows many more associated foci of low signal intensity. (Reproduced with permission from [48].)

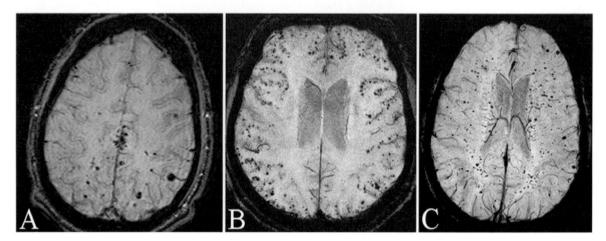

Fig. 3.11 Cerebral damage. (A) Multiple cerebral microbleeds (CMBs) in traumatic brain injury. (B) The CMBs in cerebral amyloid angiopathy are predominantly in gray matter. (C) Radiation damage produces CMBs predominantly in white matter.

above, the SWI projected image had 201 lesions, whereas the GRE-projected image had 74 lesions. Aggregate clinical and imaging findings are highly suggestive of CAA.

Although T_2^*-weighted GRE sequences can detect microhemorrhages, 25% of patients ultimately diagnosed with CAA have no microhemorrhages on conventional T_2^*-weighted GRE images [8,11,29,30]. As SWI becomes more widely used, the diagnosis of CAA may be made even earlier and with higher sensitivity.

Susceptibility-weighted imaging in traumatic brain injury

There are in the order of 1.4 million people a year affected by traumatic brain injury (TBI). For these

patients, CT is the mainstay of imaging in the emergency setting and does a good job detecting major bleeds. However, nearly half of TBI is occult to CT or conventional MRI. We have been imaging patients with both mild and severe TBI and have found that SWI reveals far more CMBs than conventional MRI. One such example is given in Fig. 3.11A. This topic is discussed in detail in Ch. 14.

Susceptibility-weighted imaging and cerebral radiation damage

Radiation damage to blood vessels and radiation necrosis can result from treating tumors and disease with potentially damaging doses of radiation. The effects of radiation on vessel endothelium have been studied using animal models [31]. Smaller vessels such as capillaries appear to be affected first. In some cases, these effects seem to take place over a period of time, perhaps months or years. It may be that this damage can also reverse somewhat; at least some evidence to this effect is presented in an animal model [32]. The effects on the vessels can include fibrinoid build up and narrowing of the lumen, local thrombus blocking the flow, destruction of the elastic fiber, thickening of the overall vessel wall, the presence of dense fibrous connective tissue and a generally abnormal vessel wall. All this might be referred to as a massive fibrous sclerosis effect. Generally, these vascular effects are a form of irradiation-induced occlusive cerebral vasculopathy or angiopathy and can lead to stenoses of even major vessels [33]. Clinical symptoms of these damaged vessels can include stroke, ischemia, headache, dizziness, seizures, cognitive effects, transient ischemic attacks and disordered consciousness.

Most relevant for the SWI studies is the presence of thrombus, telangiectatic vessel change, cavernous angioma and discrete hemorrhages [34,35]. The last were also observed to cause inflammation, sometimes associated with focal ischemia, degeneration of nerve cells and the presence of macrophages [36]. Figure 3.11C shows a comparison of radiation damage along with CMBs seen with TBI (Fig. 3.11A) and CAA (Fig. 3.11B). In this example, the patient had been irradiated for a tumor in the skull base. Interestingly, one paper points out that long-term survivors of brain tumors after whole brain irradiation also suffer cognitive impairment including dementia [37]. The authors claimed that radiation-induced cognitive impairment may be a form of vascular dementia. In this light, it is interesting to compare the results of Fig. 3.11B and 3.11C. The authors also noted that the pathological correlates at autopsy include gliosis, demyelination and, ultimately, white matter necrosis.

Quantification of the magnetic susceptibility of cerebral microbleeds

As discussed, some CMBs change over time, both in size and number. Although phase and $T_2{}^*$ signal loss in magnitude images are very important in identifying CMBs, quantifying changes in these CMBs over time is important to understanding the inter-relationship between their presence, temporal behavior and dis-

ease status. A change in CMB size could indicate either or both of the following scenarios: (1) chronic, but slow deposition of hemosiderin over time from leaky vessels (i.e. an increase in total hemosiderin content in the bleed); (2) dispersion/distribution of already deposited hemosiderin to a larger spatial extent (i.e. an increase in volume of the bleed without any change in total hemosiderin content). In either case, the total amount of iron in the CMB is responsible for the field inhomogeneity and the ensuing signal changes. Hence, direct quantification of the total iron content in the CMB would provide a better quantitative measure for studying changes in CMBs over time. Magnetic susceptibility of the CMB is a direct measure of the amount of iron within, and the process of susceptibility mapping enables this property to be measured using MR magnitude and phase information [38–41].

Phase measured in MR images is a function of size, shape, orientation and the susceptibility of the tissue. Under certain practical assumptions, the shape, size, orientation and susceptibility of the structure can be related to the resultant field perturbation using a simple linear relationship in frequency space [42–44]. Conversely, given the phase information, the magnetic susceptibility distribution information of the tissue can be extracted by regularized inverse processing [40,41]. This is the basis of the susceptibility mapping procedure. Figure 3.12 shows a processed SWI magnitude image (mIP) and the corresponding susceptibility map showing CMBs in a patient with TBI. Although susceptibility mapping provides a unique way of visualizing CMBs and venous vasculature, quantitatively detailed study is yet required to demonstrate accurate susceptibility measurements, with proper understanding of the systematic errors coming from the regularization process, partial voluming, phase aliasing and TE dependence.

Automatic detection of cerebral microbleeds on susceptibility-weighted imaging

We are proposing a semiautomated method of identifying and quantifying CMBs seen on high-resolution SWI scans. This method has four steps: brain "extraction" to remove the skull and background information, statistical thresholding to mark hypointensities, a support vector machine classifier to eliminate noise and

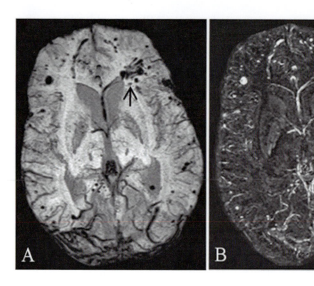

Fig. 3.12 Sheer trauma. (A) Minimum intensity projection processed susceptibilty-weighted image (SWI) projected over 16 mm. (B) Corresponding susceptibility map. The SWI data were collected using a voxel size of 0.5 mm × 0.5 mm × 2 mm with a matrix size of 384 × 512 (phase × readout), flip angle 15°, echo time 20 ms, repetition time 29 ms. The cerebral microbleeds (CMBs) are seen as focal hypointensity spots in (A) and bright spots in the susceptibility map (B) since in the former the magnetic field effects lead to signal loss while in the latter they represent the paramagnetic effect of the blood products. The arrows (black in (A) and white in (B)) point to the sheer injury caused by the head trauma. (Reproduced with permission from [47].)

veins, and, finally, a manual review of results to eliminate the remaining false positives.

Global and local thresholding are performed in an attempt to break the distribution of signal in each region into two separate distributions: one that represents normal brain parenchyma, and one with "low signal" and "probable CMB" information. The global threshold intensity is preset to a value where only structures with low signal are marked as outliers. The local thresholding is performed next in an iterative manner to refine these two distributions. Example images showing potential CMBs are shown in Fig. 3.13A,B. Figure 13A shows the original SWI data and Fig. 13B has the CMBs marked in red.

A number of shape constraints are then supplied and serve as identifying features in a learning algorithm supervised by the support vector machine. The CMBs have a very characteristic shape: they are nearly spherical, making shape features the best positively identifying features. Five different shape features were used: compactness, the three eigenvalues of the covariance matrix and the relative anisotropy calculated from these eigenvalues. In addition to shape features, intensity and size were also used. A total of eight intensity features were calculated for each suspected CMB: minimum, maximum, mean and standard deviation for both the magnitude and phase images. The intensity features helped to further characterize the CMBs and give the classifier algorithm more information to use. Finally, size was also included as a feature. While size alone is not a good criterion for identifying CMBs

[9], other characteristic features (such as shape) might change with the size of the CMB. Having the size information allows the classifier to select the best set of identifying features for each different size of CMB. All true CMBs that were selected by the classifier had a relatively clean and logical boundary, with a minimal amount of extraneous voxels (Fig. 3.13C). The thresholding step had a very high sensitivity of 95%, only missing 6 CMBs out of 126, and the overall sensitivity of the automated method was 81.7%, as an additional 17 bleeds were mistakenly discarded by the classifier. All those points in blue in Fig. 3.13C were the remaining false negatives. These are easily removed during manual review of the results.

Future semiautomated methods hold promise for evaluating large numbers of patients using SWI, and reducing image review times from many hours to less than an hour. These methods can also be made easier by the use of better or additional image information. For example, if high-resolution MR angiographic data were collected postcontrast, the veins and arteries could be excluded based on their bright signal. While co-registration has been used in similar lesion segmentation problems [45], and could be used to remove some CMB mimics [9], it probably would not result in a dramatic improvement in sensitivity, as most of the CMBs are not seen in other MR sequences. It would, therefore, probably be limited to helping to remove false positives and mimics. The CMB mapping methods applicable to GRE T_2^* images and using standardized rating scales are discussed in Ch. 4.

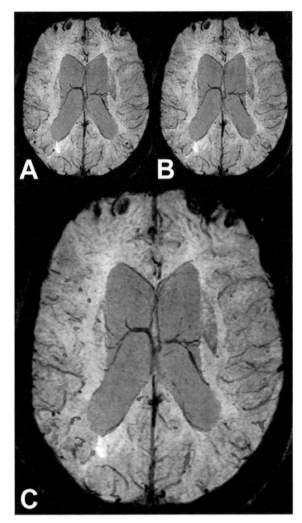

Fig. 3.13 (A) Minimum intensity projection (mIP) over 26 mm of susceptibilty-weighted image (SWI) data. (B) Manually marked true cerebral microbleeds (CMBs) identified using magnitude, phase, SWI and mIP images. (C) Automatically marked suspected CMBs. The yellow CMBs indicate the ones that were missed by the automated methods; the red indicate bleeds that were identified in both methods; and blue are the false positives from the automated methods. The bleeds that were missed by the automated methods (yellow) were erroneously merged with the vein they were adjacent to. See the color plate section.

Conclusions

Susceptibility-weighted imaging has proven to be a very sensitive technique for the identification of CMBs. Increased sensitivity to CMBs may allow assessment of the rate of microhemorrhage development or regression, allowing more precise analysis of the natural history of disease, or better assessment of response to therapy. Early recognition may be advanta-

geous to patients treated with anticoagulant or aspirin therapy in that they are at increased risk for subsequent and possibly fatal hemorrhage [46] (see Ch. 19). Improved detection of microhemorrhage may become particularly important in the diagnosis, management and monitoring of the therapeutic response of patients with CAA, particularly as new therapeutic options, such as low-molecular-weight proteins that reduce amyloid fibril formation, become available. Imaging the brain with SWI requires only 3 to 7 minutes at 3 T and can easily be included in routine neuroimaging protocols.

References

1. Haacke E, Song L, Yablonskiy DA. In vivo validation of the bold mechanism: a review of signal changes in gradient echo functional MRI in the presence of flow. *Int J Imaging Syst Technol* 1995;**6**:153–63.

2. Reichenbach R, Venkatesan R, Schillinger DJ, Kido DK, Haacke EM. Small vessels deoxyhemoglobin in the human MR venography as an intrinsic contrast agent. *Radiology* 1997;**204**:272–7.

3. Wang Y, Yu Y, Li D *et al.* Artery and vein separation using susceptibility-dependent phase in contrast-enhanced MRA. *Radiology* 2000;**670**:661–70.

4. Haacke EM, Xu Y, Cheng YN, Reichenbach R. Susceptibility weighted imaging (SWI). *Magn Reson Med* 2004;**618**:612–18.

5. Ayaz M, Boikov AS, Haacke EM, Kido DK, Kirsch WM. Imaging cerebral microbleeds using susceptibility weighted imaging: one step toward detecting vascular dementia. *J Magn Reson Imaging* 2010;**31**:142–8.

6. Fan YH, Zhang L, Lam WW *et al.* Cerebral microbleeds as a risk factor for subsequent intracerebral hemorrhages among patients with acute ischemic stroke. *Stroke* 2003;**34**:2459–62.

7. Imaizumi T, Horita Y, Hashimoto Y, Niwa J. Dotlike hemosiderin spots on T2*-weighted magnetic resonance imaging as a predictor of stroke recurrence: a prospective study. *J Neurosurg* 2004;**101**:915–20.

8. Greenberg SM, Eng JA, Ning M *et al.* Hemorrhage burden predicts recurrent intracerebral hemorrhage after lobar hemorrhage. *Stroke* 2004;**35**:1415–20.

9. Greenberg SM, Vernooij MW, Cordonnier C *et al.* Cerebral microbleeds: a guide to detection and interpretation. *Lancet Neurol* 2009;**8**:165–74.

10. Vernooij MW, van der Lugt A, Ikram MA *et al.* Prevalence and risk factors of cerebral microbleeds: the Rotterdam Scan Study. *Neurology* 2008;**70**: 1208–14.

11. Walker DA, Broderick DF, Kotsenas AL. Routine use of GRE MRI to screen for cerebral amyloid angiopathy in elderly patients. *AJR Am J Roentgenol* 2004;**182**: 1547–50.

12. Roob G, Schmidt R, Kapeller P *et al.* MRI evidence of past cerebral microbleeds in a healthy elderly population. *Neurology* 1999;**52**:991–4.

13. Gaasch JA, Lockman PR, Geldenhuys WJ, Allen ÆD, Schyf CJ. Brain iron toxicity: differential responses of astrocytes, neurons, and endothelial cells. *Neurochem Res* 2007;**32**:1196–1208.

14. Fazekas F, Kleinert R, Roob G *et al.* Histopathologic analysis of foci of signal loss on GRE T$_2$*-weighted MR images in patients with spontaneous intracerebral hemorrhage: evidence of microangiopathy-related microbleeds. *AJNR Am J Neuroradiol* 1999;**20**:637–42.

15. Gregoire SM, Werring DJ, Chaudhary UJ *et al.* Choice of echo time on GRE T2*-weighted MRI influences the classification of brain microbleeds. *Clin Radiol* 2010; **65**:391–4.

16. Nandigam R, Viswanathan A, Delgado P *et al.* MR imaging detection of cerebral microbleeds: effect of susceptibility-weighted imaging, section thickness, and field strength. *AJNR Am J Neuroradiol* 2009;**30**:338–43.

17. Tong KA, Ashwal S, Holshouser BA *et al.* Radiology hemorrhagic shearing lesions in children and adolescents with posttraumatic diffuse axonal injury: improved detection and initial results. *Radiology* 2003; **227**:332–9.

18. Cordonnier C, Potter GM, Jackson CA *et al.* Development of the brain observer microbleed scale (BOMBS). *Stroke* 2009;**40**:94–9.

19. Gregoire SM, Chaudhary UJ, Brown MM *et al.* The Microbleed Anatomical Rating Scale (MARS): reliability of a tool to map brain microbleeds. *Neurology* 2009;**73**:1759–66.

20. Imaizumi T, Honma T, Horita Y *et al.* Clinical investigation dynamics of dot-like hemosiderin spots on T$_2$*-weighted MRIs associated with stroke recurrence. *J Neuroimaging* 2007;**17**:204–10.

21. Greenberg SM, Nandigam RN, Delgado P *et al.* Microbleeds versus macrobleeds: evidence for distinct entities. *Stroke* 2009;**40**:2382–6.

22. van Rooden SV, Maat-Schieman ML, Nabuurs RJ *et al.* Cerebral amyloidosis: postmortem detection with human 7.0-T MR imaging system. *Radiology* 2009;**253**:788–96.

23. Chamberlain R, Reyes D, Curran GL *et al.* Comparison of amyloid plaque contrast generated by T2-weighted, T* imaging methods in transgenic mouse models of Alzheimer's disease. *Magn Reson Med* 2009;**253**:1158–64.

24. Haacke EM, Ayaz M, Khan A *et al.* Establishing a baseline phase behavior in magnetic resonance imaging to determine normal vs. abnormal iron content in the brain. *J Magn Reson Imaging* 2007; **264**:256–64.

25. Xu Y, Haacke EM. The role of voxel aspect ratio in determining apparent vascular phase behavior in susceptibility weighted imaging. *Magn Reson Imaging* 2006;**24**:155–60.

26. Schrag M, McAuley G, Pomakian J *et al.* Correlation of hypointensities in susceptibility-weighted images to tissue histology in dementia patients with cerebral amyloid angiopathy: a postmortem MRI study. *Acta Neuropathol* 2010;**119**:291–302.

27. Wu Z, Mittal S, Kish K *et al.* Identification of calcification with MRI using susceptibility-weighted imaging: a case study. *J Magn Reson Imaging* 2009; **182**:177–82.

28. Wald LL, Fischl B, Rosen BR. High-resolution and microscopic imaging at high field. In Robitaille P-M, Berliner L (eds.) *Ultra High Field Magnetic Resonance Imaging*. New York: Springer, 2006, pp. 343–71.

29. Greenberg SM. Cerebral amyloid angiopathy: prospects for clinical diagnosis and treatment. *Neurology* 1998;**51**:690–4.

30. Greenberg SM, O'Donnell HC, Schaefer PW, Kraft ME. New hemorrhages: potential marker of progression in cerebral amyloid angiopathy. *Neurology* 1999;**53**:1135.

31. Li Y, Chen P, Haimovitz-Friedman A, Reilly RM, Wong CS. Endothelial apoptosis initiates acute blood–brain barrier disruption after ionizing radiation. *Cancer Res* 2003;**63**:5950–6.

32. Nguyen V, Gaber MW, Sontage MR, Kiania ME. Late effects of ionizing radiation on the microvascular networks in normal tissue. *Radiat Res* 2010;**154**: 531–6.

33. Bitzer M, Topka H. Progressive cerebral occlusive disease after radiation therapy. *Stroke* 1995;**26**: 131–6.

34. Dimitrievich G, Fischer-Dzoga K, Griem M. Radiosensitivity of vascular tissue. I. Differential radiosensitivity of capillaries: a quantitative in vivo study. *Radiat Res* 1984;**99**:511–35.

35. Shobha N, Smith EE, Demchuk AM, Weir NU. Small vessel infarcts and microbleeds associated with radiation exposure. *Can J Neurol Sci* 2009;**36**:376–8.

36. Yoshii Y, Phillips TL. Late vascular effects of whole brain X-irradiation in the mouse. *Acta Neurochirurg* 1982;**84**:87–102.

37. Brown WR, Blair RM, Moody DM *et al.* Capillary loss precedes the cognitive impairment induced by

fractionated whole-brain irradiation: a potential rat model of vascular dementia. *J Neurolog Sci* 2007;**257**: 67–71.

38. McAuley G, Schrag M, Sipos P *et al.* Quantification of punctate iron sources using magnetic resonance phase. *Magn Reson Med* 2010;**63**:106–15.

39. Cheng Y, Neelavalli J, Haacke E. Limitations of calculating field distributions and magnetic susceptibilities in MRI using a Fourier based method. *Physics Med Biol* 2009;**54**:1169–98.

40. de Rochefort L, Brown R, Prince M, Wang Y. Quantitative MR susceptibility mapping using piece-wise constant regularized inversion of the magnetic field. *Magn Reson Med* 2008;**60**:1003–9.

41. Haacke EM, Cheng NY, House MJ *et al.* Imaging iron stores in the brain using magnetic resonance imaging. *Magn Reson Imaging* 2005;**23**:1–25.

42. Salomir R, Senneville B, Moonen C. A fast calculation method for magnetic field inhomogeneity due to an arbitrary distribution of bulk susceptibility. *Concepts Magn Reson* 2003;**198**:26–34.

43. Deville G, Bernier M, Delrieux J. NMR multiple echoes observed in solid 3He. *Phys Rev* 1979;**19**: 5666–88.

44. Marques JP, Bowtell R. Application of a Fourier-based method for rapid calculation of field inhomogeneity due to spatial variation of magnetic susceptibility. *Concepts Magn Reson* 2005;**25**:65–78.

45. Lao Z, Shen D, Liu D *et al.* Computer-assisted segmentation of white matter lesions in 3D MR images using support vector machine 1. *Acad Radiol* 2008;**15**: 300–13.

46. Passero S, Burgalassi L, D'Andrea P. Recurrence of bleeding in patients with primary intracerebral hemorrhage. *Radiology* 2009;**253**:788–96.

47. Haacke EM, Reichenbach JR (eds.) *Susceptibility Weighted Imaging: Basic Concepts and Clinical Applications.* Wiley-Blackwell, 2011.

48. Haacke EM, DelProposto ZS, Chaturvedi S *et al.* Imaging Cerebral Amyloid Angiopathy with Susceptibility-Weighted Imaging. *AJNR* 2007; **28**:316–317.

Defining and mapping cerebral microbleeds

Simone M. Gregoire and David J. Werring

Introduction

Cerebral microbleeds (CMBs) are an increasingly common radiological finding in stroke, neurological and general medical practice. Finding CMBs in the brain can raise a number of clinical questions regarding the safety of antithrombotic drugs, the risk of recurrent symptomatic intracerebral hemorrhage (ICH), cognitive decline and clinical deterioration. As well as the presence or number of CMBs, their anatomical distribution (e.g. lobar versus deep) is likely to be important in interpreting the cause and clinical relevance of CMBs, particularly as a means to diagnose small vessel arteriopathies (including cerebral amyloid angiopathy [CAA]) non-invasively in life. In order to tackle these questions, it is important to be able to reliably define and map CMBs in the brain. This may be challenging because of the many other lesions seen on MRI with similar morphological or signal characteristics (CMB mimics, discussed in more detail in Ch. 5).

Although there has been general agreement on the radiological properties of CMBs, there has until recently been a lack of standardized specific criteria with which to define them. Many research units have used in-house CMB rating methods, and although reliability (intra- and inter-observer agreement) has been reported, the exact methods used (detailed CMB definition criteria, anatomical boundaries, etc.) have not usually been fully described. A standardized approach with clearly described criteria for CMBs and their anatomical location may be helpful in improving reliability and allowing results from different centers to be compared. There are, at the time of writing, two published CMB rating scales that have been validated in hospital cohorts of stroke patients. This chapter considers the radiological criteria for defining CMBs and then discusses these standardized rating scales.

The potential for automatically detecting and mapping CMBs in future is discussed briefly at the end of the chapter.

How should cerebral microbleeds be defined?

Since the emergence of MRI techniques allowing the detection of CMBs, definitions of the MRI criteria for identifying CMBs have varied. However, all studies have used features relating to shape (described variously as rounded, dot-like, ovoid, spherical), size (small) and signal characteristics on MRI sensitive to susceptibility effects (dark or black, and of homogeneous signal). Using these criteria, most radiological lesions defined as CMBs do correspond to hemosiderin deposition in relation to pathologically abnormal small vessels [1,2], sometimes related to microaneurysms (see Ch. 1 for a discussion of microaneurysms and Ch. 6 for a discussion of histopathology in relation to CMBs). Although many papers have described the various radiological features used to distinguish CMBs, the first consensus criteria for their identification were not published until 2009 [3]. On appropriate MRI sequences (typically gradient-recalled echo [GRE] $T_2{}^*$ or susceptibility-weighted imaging [SWI]), CMBs are defined as round or ovoid (rather than linear or curvilinear) foci of homogeneous signal intensity loss. This definition has the purpose of excluding larger ICHs ("macrobleeds"), subarachnoid blood or siderosis, specific secondary causes of bleeding (e.g. arteriovenous malformations or tumors) and non-hemorrhagic causes of low signal (e.g. mineralization, regions of air–bone susceptibility-related signal loss). These and other common mimics of CMBs are considered further in Ch. 5. There has so far been general agreement on a CMB cut-off size

---

Table 4.1 Recommended criteria for the identification of cerebral microbleeds

Criterion	Rationale
1. Black on T_2*-weighted MRI	To ensure the lesion is paramagnetic and likely to contain blood degradation products
2. Round or ovoid lesions (rather than linear)	To exclude blood vessels and distinguish microbleeds from subarachnoid blood (the latter may have separate relevance for diagnosing small vessel arteriopathies)
3. Blooming effect on T_2*-weighted MRI	Ensures that the lesion has susceptibility effect
4. Devoid of signal hyperintensity on T_1-weighted or T_2-weighted sequences	To avoid misclassifying some mimics, including cavernous malformations (bright on T_2), metastatic melanoma (bright on T_1)
5. At least half of lesion surrounded by brain parenchyma	To include very superficial cortical lesions, which may be seen in cerebral amyloid angiopathy
6. Distinct from other mimics such as iron or calcium deposits, bone or vessel flow voids	A reminder to consider these mimics
7. Clinical history excluding traumatic diffuse axonal injury	To avoid mixing secondary traumatic microbleeds with spontaneous CMBs caused by cerebrovascular disease

Source: from Greenberg *et al.,* 2009 [5].

of 5–10 mm in diameter on standard GRE T_2* MRI sequences, although in some studies, the minimum diameter used was 2 mm [4]. However, it should be appreciated that the measurement used for a radiological lesion is not a true reflection of the actual size of the CMB; because of the "blooming" effect of the MRI signal at the lesion border [3], the actual tissue lesion size is usually considerably smaller, and generally significantly less than approximately 5 mm [2]. Some recent lines of evidence suggest that a rigid size definition for CMBs should not be emphasized. First, CMB size may be affected by imaging parameters including magnetic field strength and MR sequence characteristics, including the echo time (TE). Post-processing techniques including SWI (Ch. 3) can further increase the size, conspicuity and number of CMBs detected [1]. Indeed, the smallest CMBs (<1 mm) can be magnified to up to threefold on SWI or high-resolution three-dimensional GRE T_2* sequences because of the blooming effect [2]. Therefore, if an absolute size criterion is applied, the definition of CMBs even in the same subject could markedly change depending on which MRI sequence has been used. Second, a recent study of lesion volumes in 46 patients with probable CAA showed that brain hemorrhage volumes in this population did not form a single continuum between CMBs and macrobleeds. Rather, they showed a clearly bimodal distribution with a cut-off point of 5.7 mm, which interestingly falls within the lower end of the most commonly used CMB upper cut-off size of 5–10 mm [5]. Whether this finding holds true in other populations of patients with CMBs (e.g. with ischemic stroke) requires further investigation. For the

moment, it remains reasonable to assume that radiological lesions much larger than approximately 5–10 mm should not be considered to be CMBs. Based on the principles discussed above, consensus MRI diagnostic criteria for CMBs have been proposed [1] and are shown in Table 4.1. Note that these criteria do not include any indication of size for CMB identification.

Cerebral microbleed quantification and mapping

Rationale for cerebral microbleed mapping

Mapping CMBs gives information on the burden of CMBs in different anatomical regions in the brain. Quantifying the number of CMBs may be relevant in exploring their relationship with other quantitative imaging or clinical data and for prognostic purposes (e.g. it might be hypothesized that a higher CMB burden might be associated with worse prognosis). Moreover, their categorization into relevant anatomical regions may be important for the diagnosis of small vessel arteriopathies in life (including hypertensive arteriopathy, CAA and CADASIL [cerebral autosomal dominant arteriopathy with subcortical infarcts and leukoencephalopathy]) [1,5–7]. Cerebral microbleeds may have a preferential location for the deep or lobar (superficial) regions, which it is hypothesized indicates the likely underlying vascular pathology [7]. Cerebral amyloid angiopathy typically affects the superficial leptomeningeal arterioles and is expected to be characterized by the occurrence of CMBs and ICH mainly in lobar locations [1,7,8], whereas hypertensive microangiopathy is hypothesized to be associated with ICH and CMBs primarily in the deep areas (deep hemispheric and infratentorial locations) [1]. If a positive diagnosis and classification of the arteriopathy underlying spontaneous ICH is made (rather than simply diagnosis by exclusion of underlying causes, including arteriovenous malformations) this could potentially obviate the need for diagnostic angiography in some cases, though this approach may be challenging to test in clinical practice. Some recent evidence suggests that CAA is a particular risk for warfarin-related [9,10] or antiplatelet-related [11–13] ICH, so reliable diagnosis of CAA in life could have a direct impact on antithrombotic treatment decisions.

However, it should be appreciated that CAA and hypertensive arteriopathy often co-exist, particularly in older populations, and the interpretation of a "mixed" lobar and deep distribution of CMBs presents a challenge for interpretation. Ultimately, the only way to definitively establish the pathological cause of certain patterns of CMBs is by further study of MRI–pathology correlations [1,2]. There is a clear need for further work to address this question. Chapters 11 and 12 discuss CMBs in relation to CAA and hypertensive arteriopathy, respectively, in more detail.

If CMBs do have a direct effect on brain function, through the surrounding tissue damage that may be associated with them, disordered blood vessel function, or disturbance of function of surrounding nervous tissue, then their location may be important. Therefore, mapping their distribution may help in the investigation of how CMBs impact on clinical measures (e.g. cognitive tests). Evidence that CMB location is important in determining their clinical effects remains limited; nevertheless, case–control studies have reported associations with CMB location and cognition; for example, CMBs in the frontal lobes and basal ganglia have been associated with frontal executive impairment in patients at a stroke clinic [14], while CMBs in the thalamus have been associated with post-stroke emotional lability [15]. In a two-center CADASIL cohort, CMBs in the frontal lobes showed a borderline effect on global cognitive scores [16]. However, the strong associations of CMBs with other MRI manifestations of small vessel disease (e.g. lacunes, white matter changes) mandates careful studies considering all of the relevant MRI markers in larger populations. Quantitative mapping of CMBs may also help to assess the prognosis or progression of vascular cognitive impairment [17] or the responses to

new treatment strategies designed to prevent vascular dementia.

Despite the undoubted challenges, systematically mapping CMBs should help to provide reliable information on CMB distribution and allow the investigation of regional correlations between CMBs, other MRI indicators of cerebrovascular pathology and clinical factors.

Rationale for the use of standardized visual rating scales for cerebral microbleeds

Like white matter changes (leukoaraiosis) [18], CMBs are recognized as an MRI correlate of small vessel pathology. Over many years, white matter changes on MRI have been extensively investigated, and a number of rating scales have been developed to assess their severity and location [19]. These have been shown to have good inter-rater reliability and continue to be widely used. While volumetric quantification of white matter changes is considered superior to rating scales in assessing the burden of disease, rating instruments continue to be used because of their practicality and applicability to standard clinical datasets. Since awareness of CMBs is much more recent, few standardized instruments have yet been developed, and there has been great inconsistency in the methods and reporting of reliability in CMB studies to date. Investigators have used a wide variety of MRI sequences and rating methods for CMBs, the characteristics of which varied greatly or were inconsistently reported. The level of observer agreement varies considerably across recent studies. A summary of the differences in MRI specifications, brain CMB size definitions and reports of inter- and intra-observer reliability in recent cohort studies (published in 2009) is shown in Table 4.2. In 13 out of 21 studies (62%), there was no report of the reliability of their CMB measures. Variations in methods included differences in MRI sequences, in CMB defining criteria and in observers' training background or MRI rating experience. The inter-observer agreement varied from a kappa factor of 0.68 to one of 0.97 in these studies. In general, agreement about the number of CMBs is higher than that for presence of CMBs (data not shown). Because of the heterogeneity in these studies, the data cannot be easily compared and interpreted [20].

The presence and distribution of CMBs can potentially be assessed either using automated methods to detect various properties of CMBs (e.g. signal

Table 4.2 Variations in MRI specifications, brain microbleed size and results of inter- and intra-rater reliabilities in cohort studies published in 2009

Study number	Sample size	Demographics	MRI Parameters TE (ms)	TR (ms)	Magnet strength (T)	Slice thickness (mm)	Slice gap (mm)	Microbleeds Size (mm)	Raters	Agreement IE	IA	Characteristic
Lee et al. 2009 [9]	24	Warfarin users	15	500	1.5	6	2	<5	2 N	0.88	NR	Presence
Henneman et al. 2009 [21]	1138	Memory clinic	15–22	600–800	1.0/1.5	5	1	<10	3, trained	>0.90	>0.90	Number
Nandigam et al. 2009 [22]	20	CAA	24–25	750–763	1.5–3.0	1.5–5	0–1	NR	2 raters	0.97	0.8–0.9	Number
Igase et al. 2009 [23]	377	Healthy	NR	NR	3.0	NR	NR	<5	2 N	"very good"	NR	NR
Staekenborg et al. 2009 [24]	152	MCI	22	800	1.0	5	1.5	2–10	NRa	NR	NR	NR
Henskens et al. 2009 [25]	192	Hypertensive	23	736	1.5	5	0.5	<5	2 N	0.68	NR	Presence
Kirsch et al. 2009 [26]	73+33	MCI + healthy	18	500	1.5	4	NR	≤10	4 "readers"	NR	NR	NR
Tang et al. 2009 [15]	519	Acute IS	30	350	1.5	5	0.5	2–10	1 N	0.78	0.85	Presence + number
van Rooden et al. 2009 [27]	27	ICH with HCHWA-D	45–48	2593–3070	1.5	6	0.6	<5–10	1 NRa	NR	NR	NR
Nishikawa et al. 2009 [28]	698	No previous clinical event	23	889	1.5	6	1	<10	1 NRa, 1 NS	NR	NR	NR
Cho et al. 2009 [29]	152	Acute IS	20	700	1.5	5	2	<10	2 N	0.881	0.881	NR
Shima et al. 2010 [30]	162	Chronic kidney disease	NR	NR	1.5	5	1.5	NR	2 NRa	NR	NR	NR
Staals et al. 2009 [31]	123	First-ever lacunar stroke	23	shortest	1.5	5	0.5	<10	2 N	0.68	NR	Presence
Nishikawa et al. 2009 [32]	106	ICH	23	889	1.5	6	1	<10	1 Ra, 1 NS	NR	NR	NR
Lim et al. 2009 [33]	234	Primary ICH	20	425	3.0	5	2	<5	1 NRa	NR	NR	NR
Sun et al. 2009 [34]	998	Acute IS	30	300	1.5	5	0.5	2–10	NR	NR	NR	NR
Jeon et al. 2009 [35]	237	Acute IS	30	400	1.5	5	2	≤5	2 raters	NR	NR	NR
Klein et al. 2009 [36]	60	Infective endocarditis	17.3	750	1.5	5	0.5	≥5, >5 to ≤10	2 NRa	NR	NR	NR
Orken et al. 2009 [37]	141	IS on warfarin	15	640	1.5	NR	NR	<5	2 raters	NR	NR	NR
Goos et al. 2009 [38]	63	Alzheimer disease	22–25	415–800	1 + 1.5	5	1–1.5	≤10	NR	NR	NR	NR
Park et al. 2009 [39]	21	Mild TBI without ICH	26	800	1.5	5	2	<5	NR	NR	NR	NR

CAA, cerebral amyloid angiopathy; HCHWA-D, hereditary cerebral hemorrhage with amyloidosis-Dutch type; ICH, intracerebral hemorrhage; IA, intra-rater; IE, inter-rater; IS, ischemic stroke; MCI, mild cognitive impairment; N, neurologist; NR, not reported; NRa, neuroradiologist; NS, neurosurgeon; RA, radiologist; TBI, traumatic brain injury; TE echo time; TR, repetition time.

characteristics, size, shape) to distinguish them from other tissue types, or manual rating. Although automated methods potentially have major benefits in terms of reliability and speed, they may also require research-quality scans and sophisticated post-processing, and then may still require some observer intervention. By contrast, standardized CMB rating scales are simple and inexpensive to use, applicable to standard clinical images and can also be fast and reliable in the hands of an experienced observer. The CMB rating scales provide a uniform rating methodology (including clear definitions of CMB criteria and anatomical regions) and enable easy and reliable (reproducible) quantification and categorization of CMBs even when scales are used by observers from different backgrounds or experience. It is logical that a standardized scale will improve inter- and intra-rater reliability for classifying CMBs, and certainly the use of standardized definitions of anatomical regions (which are seldom fully reported in publications) should facilitate the pooling of data from different groups.

Standardized microbleed visual rating scales

To date, two CMB rating scales have been pusblished: the Microbleed Anatomical Rating Scale (MARS) [20] and the Brain Observer Micro Bleed Scale (BOMBS) (Figs. 4.1 and 4.2) [40]. Both scales provide guidance for use, definition criteria for CMBs and CMB mimics and a table for anatomical categorization of the CMBs. In the BOMBS study, pilot evaluations (not using a standardized scale) showed inter-rater agreement for "certain" microbleeds with a kappa value of 0.44, which improved with modifications and standardization as the BOMBS scale to one of 0.68, tested in a different population to the pilot study. The BOMBS approach did not improve agreement about total CMB counts (certain and uncertain). The BOMBS includes a subclassifcation of CMB size as >5 mm or 5–10 mm, although the value of this information in distinguishing CMBs remains unclear [5]. The main difference between BOMBS and MARS is that the latter classifies CMBs into individual lobar anatomical regions, as well as deep structures, with the hypothesis that the lobar location of CMBs is likely to be an important factor in how they might affect brain function (particularly cognition). Both MARS and BOMBS have good to very good intra- and inter-reliability for CMB presence and number in the

brain. The inter-rater reliability for the presence of ≥ 1 CMB reliability for BOMBS and MARS were generally very similar, though MARS had higher reliability for rating deep CMBs ($\kappa = 0.71$; 96% confidence interval [CI] 0.59–0.83 for MARS versus $\kappa = 0.54$; 95% CI, 0.25–0.83 for BOMBS), albeit with overlapping CIs. The MARS system was also shown to have very good intra-rater reliability over a 1-year interval ($\kappa = 0.85$ for presence of at least one CMB), and high reliability was found using two MRI sequences with different TE values. The testing of rating scales on images collected using different MRI sequences is important because these affect the conspicuity and size of CMBs, which have been shown to influence CMB identification [22].

In each of these scales, there are two steps: first to identify whether a given lesion is likely to be a CMB or not and, second, to record the distribution of CMBs in the brain according to an anatomical scheme. These scales give the option of including definite/certain CMBs, as well as "possible" or "uncertain" CMBs. The inclusion of less-certain lesions has been shown in both studies to lower the agreement between raters, so it is recommended that, at least for research studies, only "definite" CMBs are reported. Furthermore, the clinical relevance of having a single CMB compared with multiple CMBs is not yet determined, though it seems likely that a single CMB has less relevance for clinical impact on brain function or prognosis [38]. Consequently, in research studies, it is recommended that a distinction is made between patients with just one CMB and those with multiple (>1) CMBs. Furthermore, the classification of patients into those having single versus multiple CMBs may vary with the MRI technique used, since MRI acquisition characteristics (including field strength, slice thickness or SWI) have a great influence on CMB detection and identification [3].

Microbleed definition and mapping: future prospects

Although visual rating scales can improve the reliability of identifying and mapping CMBs, more sophisticated automated methods are under investigation[42]. These would have the advantage of being quick, reliable and not operator dependent, and they may allow the comparison of CMB anatomical distributions between patient groups using group overlap or probabilistic maps in standard stereotactic space. They

Microbleed Anatomical Rating Scale (MARS) Rating Form

Patient ID: _____ Date of Birth _ _/_ _/_ _ _ _   Date of MRI _ _/_ _/_ _ _ _

DEFINITE MICROBLEEDS: Small, round, well-defined, hypointense on GRE T2*; 2-10 mm; not well seen on T2

MICROBLEED MIMICS
- Vessels: linear / curvilinear lesions in subarachnoid space, usually cortical or juxta-cortical (visible on T2)
- Mineralization in globi pallidi or dentate nuclei: symmetrical hypointensities (may be bright flecks on CT)
- Haemorrhages within area of infarction (look at the T2, FLAIR or DWI sequences to identify infarction)
- Air-bone interfaces: frontal / temporal lobes (check adjacent GRE T2* slices to clarify)
- Partial volume artifact at the edges of the cerebellum (check adjacent GRE T2* to clarify)
- Small haemorrhages close to a large ICH (visible on GRE T2*) or to an infarct (visible on T2, FLAIR or DWI)

| Right | | Left |

		DEFINITE		POSSIBLE	
		R	L	R	L
Infratentorial TOTAL	Brainstem (B)				
	Cerebellum (C)				
	Basal Ganglia (Bg)*				
Deep TOTAL	Thalamus (Th)				
	Internal Capsule (Ic)				
	External Capsule (Ec)				
	Corpus Callosum (Cc)				
	Deep and periventricular WM (DPWM)				
	Frontal (F)				
	Parietal (P)				
Lobar TOTAL**	Temporal (T)				
	Occipital (O)				
	Insula (I)				
	TOTALS				

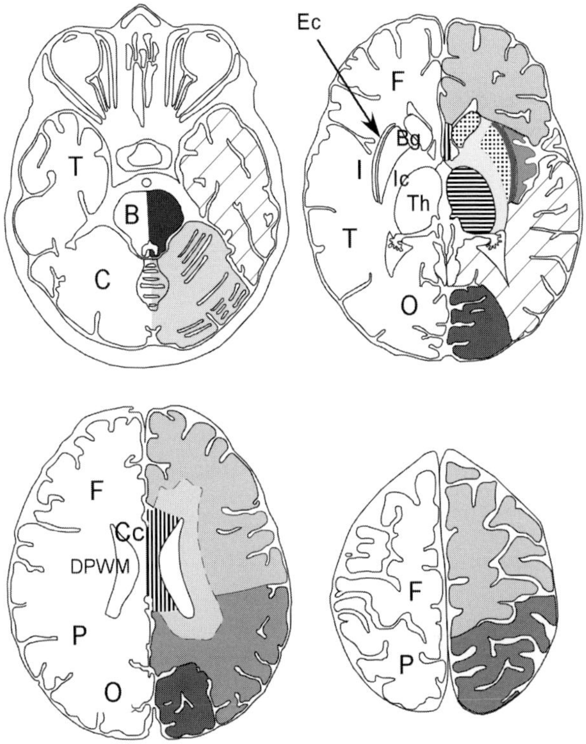

* (Caudate, Lentiform), **Lobar regions include cortex and subcortical white matter

Fig. 4.1 Rating form for the Microbleed Anatomical Rating Scale (MARS).

may also allow the automated quantification of microbleed size and volume. Developing an automated rating method for CMBs is challenging, because of the many CMB mimics with similar signal and morphological characteristics, and the widespread distribution of CMBs in the brain. Furthermore, more sophisticated approaches may require research-quality rather than standard clinical scans, and distinguishing CMBs

Brain Observer Micro Bleed Scale (BOMBS)

Date of MRI ___ / ___ / ___   Date of birth ___ / ___ / ___   Study ID_____

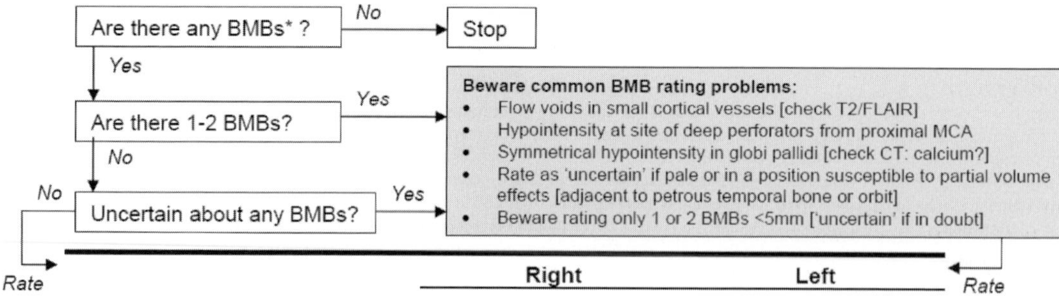

Are there any BMBs* ?   → No → Stop

Yes ↓

Are there 1-2 BMBs?   → Yes →

No ↓

Uncertain about any BMBs?   → Yes →

No ←

Beware common BMB rating problems:
- Flow voids in small cortical vessels [check T2/FLAIR]
- Hypointensity at site of deep perforators from proximal MCA
- Symmetrical hypointensity in globi pallidi [check CT: calcium?]
- Rate as 'uncertain' if pale or in a position susceptible to partial volume effects [adjacent to petrous temporal bone or orbit]
- Beware rating only 1 or 2 BMBs <5mm ['uncertain' if in doubt]

Rate →   ← Rate

	Right		Left	
	Certain	Uncertain	Certain	Uncertain
► Cortex / grey-white junction[1]				
Number of BMBs <5mm				
Number of BMBs 5-10mm				
► Subcortical white matter[2]				
Number of BMBs <5mm				
Number of BMBs 5-10mm				
► Basal ganglia grey matter[3]				
Number of BMBs <5mm				
Number of BMBs 5-10mm				
► Internal and external capsule				
Number of BMBs <5mm				
Number of BMBs 5-10mm				
► Thalamus				
Number of BMBs <5mm				
Number of BMBs 5-10mm				
► Brainstem				
Number of BMBs <5mm				
Number of BMBs 5-10mm				
► Cerebellum				
Number of BMBs <5mm				
Number of BMBs 5-10mm				

---

* Small, homogeneous, round foci of low signal intensity on T2*-weighted images of less than 10 mm in diameter. Low signal on T2* within infarcts or haemorrhagic strokes are not counted as BMBs.
[1] Includes subcortical BMBs that touch the grey-white matter junction.
[2] Includes periventricular white matter and deep portions of the centrum semiovale.
[3] Caudate and lentiform nuclei.

Fig. 4.2 Brain Observer Micro Bleed Scale (BOMBS).

from mimics is a complex process that will require sophisticated post-processing and probably at least some observer intervention. Additional opportunities and challenges arise with the increasing use of high-resolution techniques of CMB detection, including SWI [41]; although SWI increases the tissue contrast of CMBs [22], reveals more CMBs than conventional T_2^* GRE and can detect smaller lesions on the order of 1 mm in diameter [2], it also reveals many flow voids from small blood vessels, which may present a challenge for reliable CMB detection. Further studies are needed to establish whether the increase in sensitivity of SWI comes at the expense of some reduction in specificity. One proposed method for automated identification of CMBs on SWI is described in Ch. 3. For the moment, however, visual rating scales offer a simple and practical solution to assess the presence, number and distribution of brain CMBs on standard clinical-quality brain MR images without the need for sophisticated post-processing facilities.

Conclusions

To address the important questions relating to CMBs, it is essential to reliably map their presence and distribution in the brain. This chapter has considered some sources of observer variation and has discussed two standardized rating scales, which both have good reliability throughout the brain. Box 4.1 lists some suggestions for rating and mapping CMBs in research studies. In the end, the most appropriate type of rating scale used may well depend upon the particular clinical question(s) being addressed. For example, some studies may need to consider CMBs in specific arterial territories (e.g. investigations of arterial recanalization interventions); others may require classification into the cerebral lobes (e.g. cognitive correlations); still others will concentrate on deep versus lobar distributions of CMBs (e.g. diagnosis of CAA and other small vessel arteriopathies). The use of standardized rating scales in CMB studies should allow more informative cross-study comparisons, and if the rating method is fully standardized this may also help to identify other sources of variation in CMB evaluation, including MRI acquisition strategies. Standardized rating instruments and CMB definition criteria will be essential in determining the value of newer MRI acquisition techniques including SWI. It seems reasonable that CMB research studies wherever possible should use a standardized rating system with central rating by

a single observer. These, and as many other study factors as possible, should be kept constant where longitudinal CMB data are collected in prospective studies. In the coming years, more sophisticated automated or semiquantitative methods for detecting CMBs are likely to emerge, but there will remain a need for simple, practical rating scales that can be applied to routinely collected clinical datasets.

Box 4.1 Recommendations for mapping cerebral microbleeds in research studies

- Use standardized MRI parameters (field strength, spatial resolution, slice thickness, TE, post-processing, etc.) – particularly relevant if studies are carried out in multiple centers.
- Apply clear definition of CMBs and mimics (Table 4.1) – rigid size criteria are probably not needed.
- Use a standardized rating instrument with clearly defined anatomical regions, appropriate to the research question (e.g. deep versus lobar, or individual lobes).
- Scale should have good inter- and intra-rater reliability applied to sequences and used by the observers in the study.
- Use trained observers (ideally a single observer for all analysis in a study).
- Observers should be blinded to clinical details relevant to the study hypothesis.
- Images rated on diagnostic quality workstations in semi-dark conditions.

References

1. Fazekas F, Kleinert R, Roob G et al. Histopathologic analysis of foci of signal loss on gradient-echo T_2^*-weighted MR images in patients with spontaneous intracerebral hemorrhage: evidence of microangiopathy-related microbleeds. *AJNR Am J Neuroradiol* 1999;**20**:637–42.

2. Schrag M, McAuley G, Pomakian J et al. Correlation of hypointensities in susceptibility-weighted images to tissue histology in dementia patients with cerebral amyloid angiopathy: a postmortem MRI study. *Acta Neuropathol* 2010;**119**:291–302.

3. Greenberg SM, Vernooij MW, Cordonnier C, Viswanathan A, Al-Shahi SR, Warach S et al. Cerebral microbleeds: a guide to detection and interpretation. *Lancet Neurol* 2009;**8**:165–74.

4. Cordonnier C, Al-Shahi SR, Wardlaw J. Spontaneous brain microbleeds: systematic review, subgroup

analyses and standards for study design and reporting. *Brain* 2007;**130**:1988–2003.

5. Greenberg SM, Nandigam RN, Delgado P *et al.* Microbleeds versus macrobleeds: evidence for distinct entities. *Stroke* 2009;**40**:2382–6.

6. Vernooij MW, van der Lugt A, Ikram MA *et al.* Prevalence and risk factors of cerebral microbleeds: the Rotterdam Scan Study. *Neurology* 2008;**70**: 1208–14.

7. Knudsen KA, Rosand J, Karluk D, Greenberg SM. Clinical diagnosis of cerebral amyloid angiopathy: validation of the Boston criteria. *Neurology* 2001;**56**: 537–9.

8. Rosand J, Muzikansky A, Kumar A *et al.* Spatial clustering of hemorrhages in probable cerebral amyloid angiopathy. *Ann Neurol* 2005;**58**: 459–62.

9. Lee SH, Ryu WS, Roh JK. Cerebral microbleeds are a risk factor for warfarin-related intracerebral hemorrhage. *Neurology* 2009;**72**:171–6.

10. Rosand J, Hylek EM, O'Donnell HC, Greenberg SM. Warfarin-associated hemorrhage and cerebral amyloid angiopathy: a genetic and pathologic study. *Neurology* 2000;**55**:947–51.

11. Wong KS, Chan YL, Liu JY, Gao S, Lam WW. Asymptomatic microbleeds as a risk factor for aspirin-associated intracerebral hemorrhages. *Neurology* 2003;**60**:511–13.

12. Gregoire SM, Jager HR, Yousry TA *et al.* Brain microbleeds as a potential risk factor for antiplatelet-related intracerebral haemorrhage: hospital-based, case-control study. *J Neurol Neurosurg Psychiatry* 2010;**81**:679–84.

13. Biffi A, Halpin A, Towfighi A *et al.* Aspirin and recurrent intracerebral hemorrhage in cerebral amyloid angiopathy. *Neurology* 2010;**75**:693–8.

14. Werring DJ, Frazer DW, Coward LJ *et al.* Cognitive dysfunction in patients with cerebral microbleeds on T_2^*-weighted gradient-echo MRI. *Brain* 2004;**127**: 2265–75.

15. Tang WK, Chen YK, Lu JY *et al.* Microbleeds and post-stroke emotional lability. *J Neurol Neurosurg Psychiatry* 2009;**80**:1082–6.

16. Viswanathan A, Godin O, Jouvent E *et al.* Impact of MRI markers in subcortical vascular dementia: a multi-modal analysis in CADASIL. *Neurobiol Aging* 2010;**31**:1629–36.

17. Ayaz M, Boikov AS, Haacke EM, Kido DK, Kirsch WM. Imaging cerebral microbleeds using susceptibility weighted imaging: one step toward detecting vascular dementia. *J Magn Reson Imaging* 2010;**31**:142–8.

18. Hachinski VC, Potter P, Merskey H. Leuko-araiosis. *Arch Neurol* 1987;**44**:21–3.

19. Scheltens P, Erkinjunti T, Leys D *et al.* White matter changes on CT and MRI: an overview of visual rating scales. European Task Force on Age-Related White Matter Changes. *Eur Neurol* 1998;**39**:80–9.

20. Gregoire SM, Chaudhary UJ, Brown MM *et al.* The Microbleed Anatomical Rating Scale (MARS): reliability of a tool to map brain microbleeds. *Neurology* 2009;**73**:1759–66.

21. Henneman WJ, Sluimer JD, Cordonnier C *et al.* MRI biomarkers of vascular damage and atrophy predicting mortality in a memory clinic population. *Stroke* 2009; **40**:492–8.

22. Nandigam RN, Viswanathan A, Delgado P *et al.* MR imaging detection of cerebral microbleeds: effect of susceptibility-weighted imaging, section thickness, and field strength. *AJNR Am J Neuroradiol* 2009;**30**: 338–43.

23. Igase M, Tabara Y, Igase K *et al.* Asymptomatic cerebral microbleeds seen in healthy subjects have a strong association with asymptomatic lacunar infarction. *Circ J* 2009;**73**:530–3.

24. Staekenborg SS, Koedam EL, Henneman WJ *et al.* Progression of mild cognitive impairment to dementia: contribution of cerebrovascular disease compared with medial temporal lobe atrophy. *Stroke* 2009;**40**: 1269–74.

25. Henskens LH, van Oostenbrugge RJ, Kroon AA *et al.* Detection of silent cerebrovascular disease refines risk stratification of hypertensive patients. *J Hypertens* 2009;**27**:846–53.

26. Kirsch W, McAuley G, Holshouser B *et al.* Serial susceptibility weighted MRI measures brain iron and microbleeds in dementia. *J Alzheimer Dis* 2009;**17**: 599–609.

27. van Rooden S, van der Grond J, van den Boom R *et al.* Descriptive analysis of the Boston crtieria applied to a Dutch-type cerebral amyloid angiopathy population. *Stroke* 2009;**40**:3022–7.

28. Nishikawa T, Ueba T, Kajiwara M *et al.* Cerebral microbleeds predict first-ever symptomatic cerebrovascular events. *Clin Neurol Neurosurg* 2009; **111**:825–8.

29. Cho AH, Lee SB, Han SJ *et al.* Impaired kidney function and cerebral microbleeds in patients with acute ischemic stroke. *Neurology* 2009;**73**: 1645–8.

30. Shima H, Ishimura E, Naganuma T *et al.* Cerebral microbleeds in predialysis patients with chronic kidney disease. *Nephrol Dial Transplant* 2010;**25**:1554–59.

31. Staals J, van Oostenbrugge RJ, Knottnerus IL *et al.* Brain microbleeds relate to higher ambulatory blood pressure levels in first-ever lacunar stroke patients. *Stroke* 2009;**40**:3264–8.

32. Nishikawa T, Ueba T, Kajiwara M, Miyamatsu N, Yamashita K. Cerebral microbleeds in patients with intracerebral hemorrhage are associated with previous cerebrovascular diseases and white matter hyperintensity, but not with regular use of antiplatelet agents. *Neurol Med Chir (Tokyo)* 2009;**49**:333–9.

33. Lim JB, Kim E. Silent microbleeds and old hematomas in spontaneous cerebral hemorrhages. *J Korean Neurosurg Soc* 2009;**46**:38–44.

34. Sun J, Soo YO, Man Lam WW *et al.* Different distribution patterns of cerebral microbleeds in acute ischemic stroke patients with and without hypertension. *Eur Neurol* 2009;**62**:298–303.

35. Jeon SB, Kwon SU, Cho AH *et al.* Rapid appearance of new cerebral microbleeds after acute ischemic stroke. *Neurology* 2009;**73**:1638–44.

36. Klein I, Iung B, Labreuche J for the Image Study Group. Cerebral microbleeds are frequent in infective endocarditis. A case–control study. *Stroke* 2009;**40**:3461–5.

37. Orken DN, Kenangil G, Uysal E, Forta H. Cerebral microbleeds in ischemic stroke patients on warfarin treatment. *Stroke* 2009;**40**:3638–40.

38. Goos JD, Kester MI, Barkhof F *et al.* Patients with Alzheimer disease with multiple microbleeds. Relation with cerebrospinal fluid biomarkers and cognition. *Stroke* 2009;**40**:3455–60.

39. Park JH, Park SW, Kang SH *et al.* Detection of traumatic cerebral microbleeds by susceptibility-weighted image of MRI. *J Korean Neurosurg Soc* 2009;**46**:365–9.

40. Cordonnier C, Potter GM, Jackson CA *et al.* Improving interrater agreement about brain microbleeds: development of the Brain Observer MicroBleed Scale (BOMBS). *Stroke* 2009;**40**:94–9.

41. Sehgal V, Delproposto Z, Haacke EM *et al.* Clinical applications of neuroimaging with susceptibility-weighted imaging. *J Magn Reson Imaging* 2005;**22**:439–50.

42. Seghier ML, Kolanko MA, Leff AP *et al.* Microbleed detection using automated segmentation (MIDAS): a new method applicable to standard clinical MR images. PLoS One 2011;**6**:e0017547.

Chapter

5

Cerebral microbleed mimics

Neshika Samarasekera, Gillian Potter and Rustam Al-Shahi Salman

Introduction

An awareness of the abnormalities that mimic cerebral microbleeds (CMBs) on gradient-recalled echo (GRE) MRI is essential to investigations of their prognostic and therapeutic significance, as well as future implementation of the results of these investigations in clinical practice. These "microbleed mimics" have similar morphologies and signal properties to CMBs on T_1- and T_2-weighted spin echo and GRE MRI sequences [1]. The keys to the identification of CMB mimics are an awareness of their distinctive imaging hallmarks and the use of other investigations that might help to distinguish them from CMBs.

The CMB mimics form two types: those that contain blood products and those that do not (resembling CMBs because of shared signal intensity and morphology on GRE MRI). This chapter describes both types, outlines how these can be differentiated from true CMBs and suggests a topographical approach to the recognition of CMB mimics on brain imaging. Box 5.1 describes the search strategy used to select pertinent articles for this chapter.

Box 5.1   Search strategy

In February 2010, we searched Ovid Medline with an electronic strategy used in a prior systematic review [2] combining it with the textword "mimic;" we then selected articles for this chapter. We also used our personal bibliographies and experience of identifying microbleed mimics during the development of the Brain Observer Microbleed Scale (BOMBS) [3].

Cerebral microbleed mimics that do not contain blood products

Partial volume artefact

An image derived with MRI consists of a matrix of picture elements, or pixels, reflecting the content of volume elements, or voxels. Voxel and pixel size influence spatial resolution and thus contrast. All anatomical structures within one voxel add to its averaged signal intensity in the final image. The smaller the voxel size, the better the spatial resolution of the MR image; however, the bigger the voxel size, the better the signal (and signal-to-noise ratio). In general, the signal-to-noise ratio is the determining factor for the final voxel/pixel size. Averaging of signal intensities of different structures within voxels – with loss of contrast between different tissues – is known as the partial volume effect. In the brain, partial volume artefact occurring adjacent to the petrous temporal bones, paranasal sinuses, frontal bones, orbit [3] and occipital bones [4] can lead to small hypointense areas on GRE and T_2-weighted imaging that mimic CMBs (Fig. 5.1). Awareness of the anatomical sites predisposed to partial volume artefacts, and reviewing of adjacent slices in these areas, will reduce misinterpretatation of partial volume artefacts as CMBs.

Paramagnetic substances

The GRE sequences used in the detection of CMBs are sensitive not only to blood breakdown products (deoxyhemoglobin, methemoglobin, hemosiderin and

---

Cerebral Microbleeds, ed. David J. Werring. Published by Cambridge University Press. © Cambridge University Press 2011.

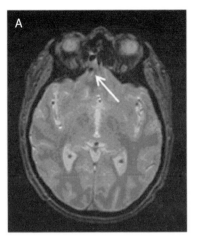 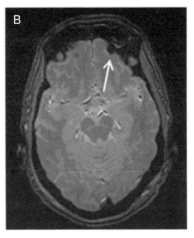 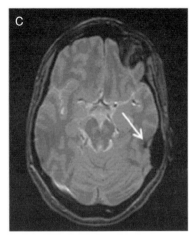

Fig. 5.1 Microbleed mimics resulting from partial volume artefact on axial gradient-recalled echo (GRE) MRI, occurring adjacent to the paranasal sinuses (A, arrow), orbit (B, arrow) and petrous temporal bone (C, arrow).

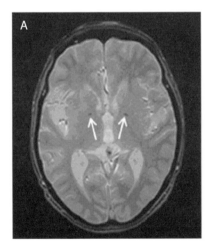 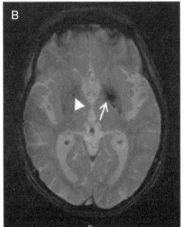 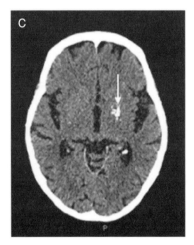

Fig. 5.2 Basal ganglia mineralization mimicking microbleeds. (A) Minor, symmetric basal ganglia mineralization, with small, solitary foci of low signal on axial gradient-recalled echo (GRE) MRI (arrows). (B) Asymmetric basal ganglia mineralization on axial gradient-recall echo MRI, demonstrating multiple hypointense foci on the right (arrow) and a solitary hypointense focus on the left (arrowhead). (C) Axial CT brain in the same patient confirms the presence of calcification in the left basal ganglia (arrow).

ferritin) but also to other paramagnetic substances such as calcium, manganese and iron, all of which may appear as foci of low signal. Basal ganglia mineralization is a frequent finding on brain imaging in older adults, and in some cases it is associated with disordered calcium metabolism, extrapyramidal syndromes or neuropsychiatric disorders [5]. Where basal ganglia mineralization is suspected, CT imaging of the brain may be helpful in identifying calcification (Fig. 5.2), although correlation of suspected basal ganglia calcification on MRI with CT was mentioned in only 14 of 53 studies identified by systematic review [2].

Air embolism, iatrogenic devices and metallic embolism

There has been a single case report of cerebral air emboli causing multiple, bilateral, small round foci of hypointensity on GRE imaging [6] and there are several descriptions of multifocal GRE hypointensities caused by embolization of metallic fragments from prosthetic heart valves [7]. Non-metallic ventricular shunt tubes in cross-section have also been reported as potential mimics of CMBs [8]. In such cases, correlation with the clinical history and review of all MRI sequences, as well as use of other types of

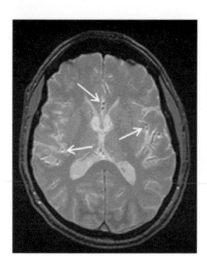 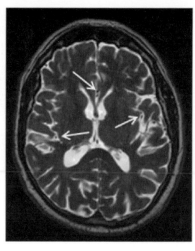

Fig. 5.3 Flow voids of leptomeningeal vessels imaged in cross-section, appearing as punctate foci of hypointensity (arrows) in the cortical sulci on axial gradient-recalled echo (GRE) (left) and T$_2$-weighted (right) brain MRI.

imaging (such as plain radiography and CT), should enable these CMB mimics to be correctly identified.

Blood vessels

On GRE imaging, foci of low signal representing vascular flow voids may be mistaken for CMBs (particularly when seen in cross-section). Most often, these are flow voids in pial and leptomeningeal vessels in the cerebral sulci, but flow voids in small, deep perforating (lenticulostriate) vessels supplying the deeper structures of the brain may also be mistaken for CMBs (Fig. 5.3) [3,9]. However, in contrast to true CMBs, flow voids do not demonstrate susceptibility ("blooming") artefact on GRE sequences. Furthermore, flow voids, but not CMBs, may be seen as linear structures on consecutive axial slices. Careful examination of lesion morphology on consecutive axial slices, and review of T$_2$-weighted imaging (on which vascular flow voids are seen more easily than with GRE), should help to correctly distinguish small vessel branches from CMBs situated close to blood vessels.

Cerebral microbleed mimics containing blood products

Traumatic microbleeds

Microbleeds are one imaging manifestation of diffuse axonal injury, a type of traumatic brain injury usually caused by rapid rotational acceleration and deceleration of the brain and leading to shearing of axons in susceptible areas such as the gray–white matter junction, splenium of the corpus callosum, intern-

al capsule and dorsolateral brainstem [10]. Multiple, small hypointensities on T$_2$-weighted imaging, fluid attenuated inversion recovery (FLAIR) and GRE MRI sequences may appear following diffuse axonal injury [11]. Although these lesions are likely to be neuropathologically similar to the spontaneous microbleeds discussed in most of this book, they are by definition presumed to be related to brain trauma rather than small vessel pathologies, and they are, therefore, considered here as a microbleed mimic. Traumatic microbleeds may be differentiated from spontaneous microbleeds on the basis of the clinical history as well as other associated imaging abnormalities (such as parenchymal contusions and skull fractures). Microbleeds in relation to brain trauma are discussed in detail in Ch. 14.

Cavernous malformations

Cavernous malformations are composed of clusters of thin-walled endothelial vessels, missing components of the blood–brain barrier, without intervening neural tissue [12]. On MRI, their hallmark is a hypointense rim of hemosiderin, within which there is a core of variable signal intensity [13]. On MRI, a mixed signal intensity core (representing hemorrhage in different stages of evolution) gives many cavernous malformations a distinctive "mulberry" or "popcorn-like" appearance (Fig. 5.4). This appearance is seen in type II of the four proposed subtypes of *familial* cavernous malformation: type I, subacute hemorrhage; type II, mixed subacute and chronic hemorrhage; type III, chronic hemorrhage; and type IV, punctate hypointensity [14]. In general, types I–III

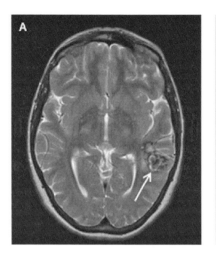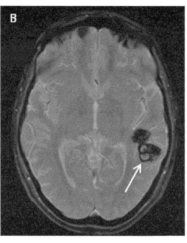

Fig. 5.4 Typical "popcorn-like" appearance of a cavernous malformation (arrows) on axial T_2-weighted (A) and axial gradient-recalled echo (B) brain MRI.

can usually be distinguished from CMBs by the presence of blood in various stages of evolution and a hemosiderin rim on T_1- and T_2-weighted imaging, but type IV cavernous malformations, appearing as punctuate hypointensities, exhibit similar signal characteristics to CMBs on MRI. Some type IV lesions evolve into type I–III lesions over time [15]. However, to what extent type IV lesions are distinct from CMBs is less clear, particularly when they are solitary or are unaccompanied by type I–III cavernous malformations, a family history or a relevant genetic mutation.

Hemorrhagic metastases

Diffuse hemorrhagic micrometastases (e.g. from renal cell carcinoma or melanoma) may lead to the appearance of multifocal CMBs [16]. Differentiation of these metastases from CMBs may be aided by clinical history and careful examination, as well as by the associated imaging findings such as perilesional edema (particularly after recent hemorrhage) and the typical signal characteristics of the lesions on other MRI sequences (e.g. T_1 hyperintensity in melanomatous deposits [16]).

Hemorrhagic transformation of a cerebral infarct

In hemorrhagic transformation of recent infarcts, small (petechial) areas of hemorrhage may be seen within, or along the margin of, the infarct. In most cases, identification of this particular CMB mimic should be possible from the clinical history and exam-

ination, and from associated imaging findings, particularly on diffusion-weighted imaging [4].

Suggested topographical approach to the interpretation of cerebral microbleed mimics

The approach outlined here to distinguishing CMBs from mimics on the basis of the presence of blood products may be further refined by considering the anatomical location of the abnormalities identified. In lobar regions of the brain (cortical gray matter, subcortical white matter and gray–white matter junction), common CMB mimics include vascular flow voids and hypointensities arising from partial volume artefact. In deep regions of the brain (basal ganglia, thalamus and internal and external capsule), mineralization of the basal ganglia and flow voids from perforating vessels should be considered. Other mimics tend not to be so easily distinguished on anatomical grounds. We have recently devised an online guide to aid the rating and interpretation of CMBs, which describes our approach to CMB mimic interpretation and also highlights difficulties that may be encountered in identifying potentially solitary CMBs. This is available at http://www.sbirc.ed.ac.uk/imageanalysis.html#bombs.

Future methods for identifying cerebral microbleed mimics

The development of susceptibility-weighted imaging (SWI; Ch. 4) has improved the detection of structures containing extravascular blood products, as well as those containing venous deoxygenated blood [17]. This approach may improve the detection of small vascular malformations such as telangiectasia, developmental venous anomalies and dural arteriovenous fistulae when compared with standard MRI sequences. It may also help to distinguish the diamagnetic and paramagnetic effects of calcium and blood, respectively [18]. However, whether the greater sensitivity of SWI diminishes or compounds the problem of CMB mimics in comparison with GRE MRI remains to be determined.

Acknowledgements

NS is funded by a Medical Research Council/Stroke Association clinical research training fellowship. RA-SS is funded by a Medical Research Council clinician scientist fellowship. GP was funded by HNS Lothian R&D and the Chief Scientist Office of the Scottish Health Department. The illustrations used in this chapter were obtained from the Scottish Funding Council's Brain Imaging Research Centre based at the Division of Clinical Neurosciences, University of Edinburgh, a core area of the Wellcome Trust Clinical Research Facility and part of the SINAPSE collaboration (Scottish Imaging Network – A Platform for Scientific Excellence), funded by the Scottish Funding Council and the Chief Scientist Office of the Scottish Government's Health Department.

References

1. Greenberg SM, Vernooji MW, Cordonnier C et al. Cerebral microbleeds: a guide to detection and interpretation. Lancet Neurol 2009;8:165–74.

2. Cordonnier C, Al-Shahi Salman R, Wardlaw JM. Spontaneous brain microbleeds: systematic review, subgroup analyses and standards for study design and reporting. Brain 2007;130: 1988–2003.

3. Cordonnier C, Potter GM, Jackson CA et al. Improving interrater agreement about brain microbleeds: development of the Brain Observer MicroBleed Scale (BOMBS). Stroke 2009;40: 94–9.

4. Gregoire SM, Chaudary UJ, Brown MM et al. The Microbleed Anatomical Rating Scale (MARS): reliability of a tool to map brain microbleeds. Neurology 2009;73:1759–66.

5. Casanova MF, Araque JM. Mineralization of the basal ganglia: implications for neuropsychiatry, pathology and neuroimaging. Psychiatry Res 2003;121:59–87.

6. Jeon SB, Kang DW. Cerebral air emboli on T_2-weighted gradient echo magnetic resonance imaging. J Neurol Neurosurg Psychiatry 2007;78:871.

7. Almansori M, Naik S, Ahmed SN. Magnetic susceptibility in a patient with a metallic heart valve. Pak J Neurol Sci 208;3:40–1.

8. Tsushima Y, Endo K. Hypointensities in the brain on T_2^*-weighted gradient echo magnetic resonance imaging. Curr Probl Diagn Radiol 2006;35:140–50.

9. Werring DJ. Cerebral microbleeds: clinical and pathophysiological significance. J Neuroimaging 2006;17:1–11.

10. Hortobagyi T, Al-Sarraj S. The significance of diffuse axonal injury: how to diagnose it and what does it tell us? Adv Clin Neurosci Rehabil 2008;8:16–18.

11. Scheid R, Preul C, Gruber O et al. Diffuse axonal injury associated with chronic traumatic brain injury: evidence from T_2^*-weighted gradient-echo imaging at 3 T. AJNR Am J Neuroradiol 2003;24:1049–56.

12. Clatterbuck RE, Eberhart CG, Crain BJ, Rigamonti D. Ultrastructural and immunocytochemical evidence that an incompetent blood–brain barrier is related to the pathophysiology of cavernous malformations. J Neurol Neurosurg Psychiatry 2001;71:188–92.

13. Rigamonti D, Drayer BP, Johnson PC et al. The MRI appearance of cavernous malformations (angiomas). J Neurosurgery 1987;67:518–24.

14. Zabramaski JM, Wascher TM, Spetzler RF. The natural history of familial cavernous malformations: results of an ongoing study. J Neurosurgery 1994;80:422–32.

15. Clatterbuck RE, Elmaci I, Rigamonti D. The nature and fate of punctate (type IV) cavernous malformations. Neurosurgery 2001;49:26–30.

16. Blitstein MK, Tung GA. MRI of cerebral microhaemorrhages. Am J Radiol 2007;189:720–5.

17. Haacke EM, Xu Y, Cheng YC, Reichenbach JR. Susceptibility- weighted imaging (SWI). Magn Reson Med 2004;52:612–18.

18. Thomas B, Somasundaram S, Thamburaj K et al. Clinical applications of susceptibility weighted MR imaging of the brain: a pictorial review. Neuroradiology 2008;50:105–16.

Chapter

6

Histopathology of cerebral microbleeds

Sebastian Brandner

Introduction

It will be clear from Chs. 1 to 4 that the term cerebral microbleed (CMB) was introduced by radiologists to describe hypointensities (small signal voids) thought to reflect small hemorrhages. Naturally, it has been hoped that the correlation of these MRI lesions with histopathological analysis will definitively establish the causes of CMBs. Indeed, MRI–pathology correlations have shown that the majority of radiologically detected CMBs result from the accumulation of blood or blood products in the vicinity of pathologically altered vessels, in the context of a widespread cerebral small vessel vasculopathy, typically cerebral amyloid angiopathy (CAA) or hypertensive vasculopathy. However, although MRI–pathology studies, as discussed in this chapter, are critical in fully understanding the causes of CMBs, such studies are limited by technical factors. The CMBs are small lesions (radiological generally <5 mm, and pathologically often considerably smaller than this) that may be present almost anywhere in the brain. They may, therefore, be easily missed by visual inspection of postmortem material but can be detected by conventional histology when specimens are carefully and systematically examined. Notwithstanding these challenges, this chapter will describe the vascular pathologies that underlie CMBs, concentrating on the two commonest disorders: hypertensive small vessel disease (SVD) and CAA. It will also describe the process of blood degradation, and the correlation of imaging with histological findings.

Vascular pathology underlying cerebral microbleeds

The most common pathological processes underlying CMBs are (1) arteriosclerosis in the context of chronic hypertension; and (2) amyloid angiopathies with intramural accumulation of beta-amyloid (Aβ). Rarer causes include: (3) CADASIL (cerebral autosomal dominant arteriopathy with subcortical infarcts and leukoencephalopathy); and (4) moyamoya disease. In addition there are a number of miscellaneous causes and these are covered in Ch. 16. This chapter will concentrate on hypertensive arteriopathy and CAA, which is usually diagnosed following symptomatic lobar intracerebral hemorrhage (ICH) but is a common pathological finding in Alzheimer's disease.

Chronic hypertension, atherosclerosis and arteriosclerosis

Vascular changes in the context of chronic hypertension affect arteries, arterioles of various sizes and capillaries in different ways. Arteriosclerosis describes a generalized hardening of the arterial vessel wall (most commonly termed fibrohyalinosis). Atherosclerosis is a form of arteriosclerosis with deposition of lipids (atheroma) in the endothelium. Arteriosclerosis and atherosclerosis are often combined. Sometimes the terms arteriosclerosis and atherosclerosis may be used interchangeably.

Hypertensive arteriopathy is thought to be caused by a forced dilation of resistance vessels: that is, those vessels that regulate the blood supply volume to the distal capillary bed. Loss of autoregulation of the arteries exposes smaller vessels and capillaries to excessive, unregulated blood pressure, disrupting the blood–brain barrier and causing vasogenic edema [1]. Chronic severe hypertension and blood pressure dysregulation leads to deposition of plasma proteins including fibrin in the vessel wall. This, in turn, causes structural alteration and damage to the smooth muscle cells in the media of small arteries. This chronic

Cerebral Microbleeds, ed. David J. Werring. Published by Cambridge University Press. © Cambridge University Press 2011.

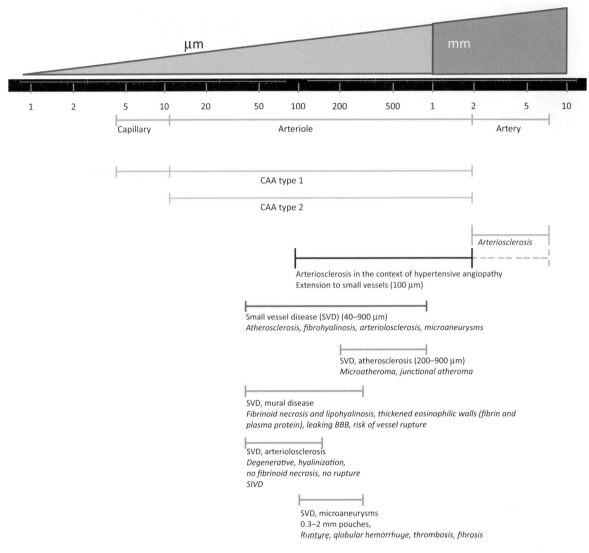

Fig. 6.1 Size distribution of vessels involved in cerebrovascular diseases. The upper plot represents a logarithmic scale of the vessel diameter. The green bar indicates the size range of capillaries, arterioles and arteries. The blue bar shows the vascular involvement of cerebral amyloid angiopathy (CAA) type 1 and type 2. Arteriosclerosis with atherosclerosis involves large vessels and extends to smaller vessels in the context of hypertension (dark brown bar). The range of vessels involved in small vessel disease (SVD) is indicated by the dark red bar and the different subpathologies within this group are indicated below in light red bars. SIVD, subcortical ischemic vascular dementia. See the color plate section.

endothelial damage, together with platelet activation and triggering of the coagulation cascade, gives rise to microthrombosis and ischemia. Overcompensatory vasoconstriction in an attempt to counteract the blood pressure peaks may also cause focal microischemia. Chronic hypertension augments arteriosclerotic changes in extracranial and intracranial arteries.

While arteriosclerotic or atherosclerotic changes per se are typically present in larger arteries (>2 mm), hypertension extends this effect to smaller arteries and arterioles (Fig. 6.1), down to a size of 100 mm. The pathophysiological effects of hypertension on cerebral vessels, and the relationship of these changes to CMBs, are considered further in Ch. 12.

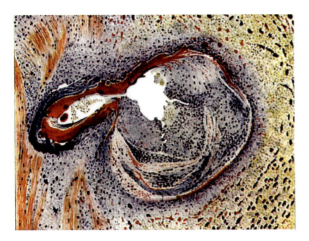

Fig. 1.3 Miliary aneurysm in the pons. There is partial thrombus in the aneurysmal sac, with red blood cells in its proximal portion. There is evidence of recent hemorrhage with deposition of pigment around the aneurysmal sac. These findings are relevant to our understanding of cerebral microbleeds. Hematoxylin and sudan III stain. (With permission from Green, 1930 [10].)

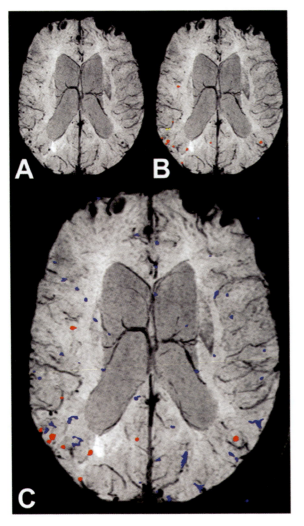

Fig. 3.13 (A) Minimum intensity projection (mIP) over 26 mm of susceptibilty-weighted image (SWI) data. (B) Manually marked true cerebral microbleeds (CMBs) identified using magnitude, phase, SWI and mIP images. (C) Automatically marked suspected CMBs. The yellow CMBs indicate the ones that were missed by the automated methods; the red indicate bleeds that were identified in both methods; and blue are the false positives from the automated methods. The bleeds that were missed by the automated methods (yellow) were erroneously merged with the vein they were adjacent to.

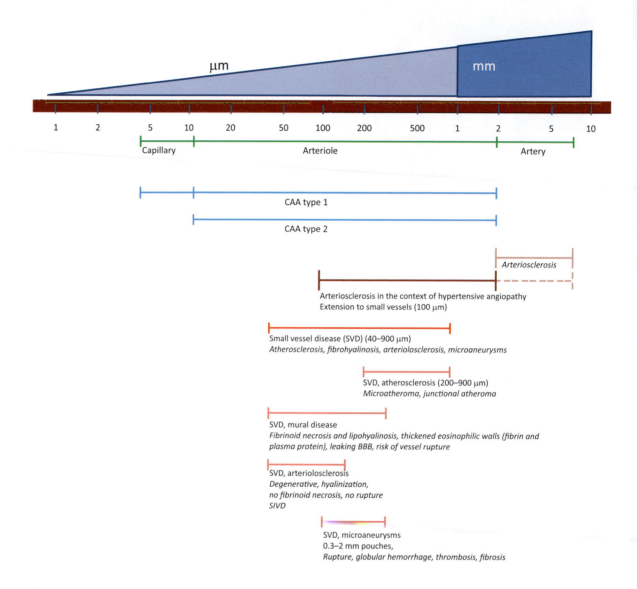

Fig. 6.1 Size distribution of vessels involved in cerebrovascular diseases. The upper plot represents a logarithmic scale of the vessel diameter. The green bar indicates the size range of capillaries, arterioles and arteries. The blue bar shows the vascular involvement of cerebral amyloid angiopathy (CAA) type 1 and type 2. Arteriosclerosis with atherosclerosis involves large vessels and extends to smaller vessels in the context of hypertension (dark brown bar). The range of vessels involved in small vessel disease (SVD) is indicated by the dark red bar and the different subpathologies within this group are indicated below in light red bars. SIVD, subcortical ischemic vascular dementia.

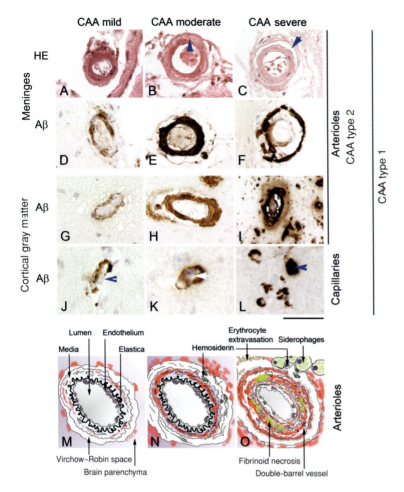

Fig. 6.2 Histological features and schematic representation of pathological features in cerebral amyloid angiopathy (CAA). Type 1 CAA is defined by involvement of meningeal vessels and cortical arterioles and capillaries. Type 2 includes only cortical and meningeal arterioles but excludes cortical capillaries (see right of the panel). (A–C) Morphology of CAA-related changes in vessel walls of meningeal vessels. (A,B) In CAA type 1 (A) and CAA type 2 (B), there are minimal structural changes, with microscopically detectable amyloid in the vessel wall in moderate CAA (B, arrowhead). (C) In severe CAA, there are significant structural alterations with detachment and delamination of the outer part of the tunica media, resulting in the formation of so-called double-barrel vessels (arrowhead). (D–F) Immunohistochemical detection of beta-amyloid (Aβ) in the wall of meningeal vessels. In mild CAA (D) there is a diffuse, fluffy deposition of amyloid in the vessel wall, often beginning in the basal lamina. The next stage (E) is characterized by a more dense deposition encompassing the entire wall. In severe CAA (F), the outer and inner detached media as well as the endothelium and surrounding brain parenchyma are heavily loaded with Aβ. (G–I) Manifestation of amyloid angiopathy in cortical arterioles. (G) Mild, diffuse accumulation in cortical arterioles, usually with relatively mild generalized Aβ deposition in the surrounding brain. (H) There is pan-mural deposition of Aβ. In this example there is also Aβ deposited in the surrounding brain parenchyma in immediate vicinity to the Virchow–Robin space. (I) In the severe form of CAA, there is formation of double-barrel vessels, which are generally less common than in meningeal vessels. There is a very heavy parenchymal Aβ accumulation, with a perivascular diffuse deposition. (J–L) Capillary CAA with the three images showing the stages of capillary CAA. (J) Diffuse, mild and often partly circumferential Aβ in the capillary wall (open area indicated by arrowhead). (K) In moderate capillary CAA, the Aβ encompasses the entire circumference but does not impede on the lumen (arrowhead). (L) Only in the most severe form is there luminal obstruction (arrowhead). (M–O) Schematic summary of the sequence of events and development of pathological features in the progression of CAA. (M) In mild CAA, there is an intact vessel wall structure with diffuse deposition of Aβ in the outer part of the wall. There are no structural alterations, particularly in the intact tunica media and elastica. (N) In moderate CAA, there is a relatively intense, pan-mural Aβ accumulation, leading to medial atrophy and hemosiderin deposition in the Virchow–Robin space or in the surrounding brain parenchyma. (O) The severe form of CAA shows severe impairment of the vessel wall integrity, with fibrinoid necrosis, splitting of the vessel, perivascular erythrocytes, hemosiderin and macrophages containing hemosiderin (siderophages) as evidence of microbleeds in the recent or distant past. HE, hematoxylin and eosin. Scale bar: 160 mm (A–F) and 80 mm (G–L).

Hypertension

CAA

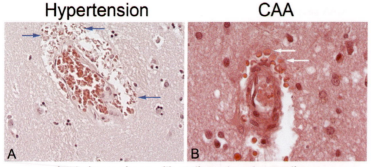

Acute hemorrhage with erythrocyte extravasation

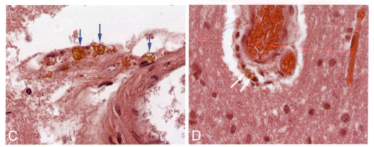

Chronic hemorrhage with hemosiderin deposits

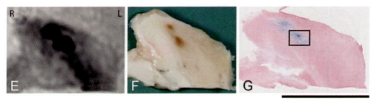

Correlation of imaging, macroscopy and histology

Fig. 6.4 Histological images of microbleeds in autopsy samples with chronic hypertension (A,C) or cerebral amyloid angiopathy (CAA) (B,D), and correlation of imaging with macroscopy and microscopy (E–G). (A,B) Histological correlate of acute erythrocyte extravasations into the perivascular (Virchow–Robin) space (blue arrows pointing to extravasated erythrocytes). (C,D) The same patients as in (A,B), with examples of chronic bleeds with formation of hematoidin. The arrows point to small deposits in the perivascular space. (E–G) Correlation of autopsy imaging (E), the corresponding formalin-fixed autopsy specimen and the corresponding histology after wax embedding and staining with Perl's Prussian blue stain to visualize iron (hemosiderin) deposition (blue dye). The lesion is located in the thalamus. Difference in size in the imaging scale bar: 160 mm (A), 80 mm (B–D), 17 mm (E,F) and 15 mm (G). (E–G adapted from Tatsumi *et al.* 2008 [41].)

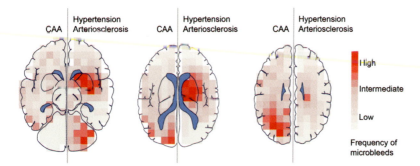

Fig. 6.5 Illustration of the relative frequency of microbleeds in cerebral amyloid angiopathy (CAA) and in hypertensive angiopathy. Colour-coded representation of the likelihood to encounter microbleeds in all brain regions with high likelihood (red) and low likelihood (white). The images represent different axial sections of the brain. Data were compiled from selected MRI studies of patients clinically diagnosed with hypertensive vasculopathy and CAA.

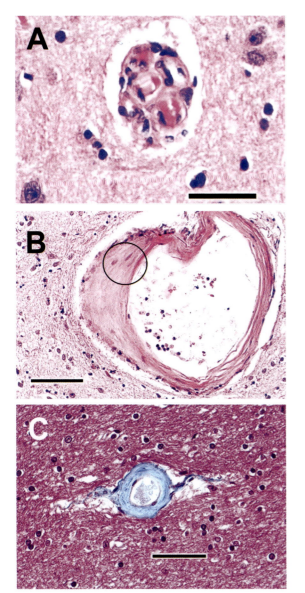

Fig. 11.1 Arteriolar changes caused by hypertension. (A) Tortuous hyperplastic arteriolar change, with six lumena visible in section. Abundant smooth muscle nuclei are seen, prior to the stage of medial cell death. Sections from a hypertensive male, aged 82, heart weight 660 g. Bar = 100 mm. (B) Loss of smooth muscle cells in tunica media, with only faint nuclear outlines seen (encircled). Bar = 100 mm. (C) Masson trichrome stain showing collagen (blue) to be a major part of the arteriolar change seen in hypertension. Although two endothelial cells are seen, the tunica media is acellular collagen. Bar = 100 mm.

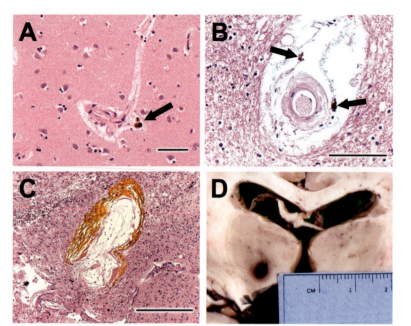

Fig. 11.2 Arteriolar bleeding. (A) Two brown macrophages containing iron (arrow) attest to microbleeding around a relatively normal arteriole (at a branch point). Such findings may relate to transient increases in blood pressure even in the absence of significant arteriolary pathology (see text). Bar = 150 mm. (B) Leakage of blood from acellular arterioles. The tunica media of a brain arteriole in hypertension (same patient as in Fig. 11.1) is acellular. Two brown-colored, iron-laden macrophages are seen (arrows), signifying previous microbleeding into the Virchow–Robin space. Bar = 200 mm. (C) Larger arteriole showing simultaneous leakage and dilatation. Leakage is seen as bright yellow-colored hematoidin (biliverdin) pigment, derived from blood. Hemorrhage approaches detectable size in current MR methodology (see text). Bar 500 mm. (D) Small ball hemorrhage in the thalamus in an asymptomatic patient, visible on gross pathology.

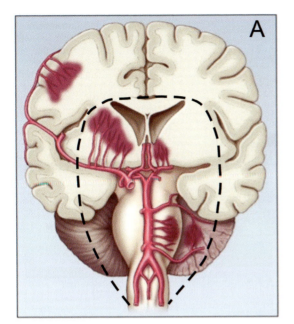

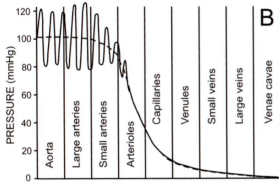

Fig. 11.3 Distribution of hypertensive microbleeds and macrobleeds to the centrencephalon (within dashed line in A). Hypertensive vascular changes are most severe in the centrencephalic arteries arising directly from the major branches of the Circle of Willis (A), where the pulse pressure and blood pressure in the vascular tree are highest (B). By contrast, the lobar arteries are exposed to lower pulse pressure and blood pressure and are less severely affected.

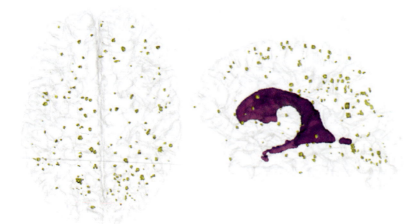

Fig. 12.1 Three-dimensional templates of hemorrhage distribution related to cerebral amyloid angiopathy. The axial (A) and sagittal (B) images display the composite locations of all identified hemorrhages in a subject imaged with T$_2$*-weighted MRI. Each dot represents a single bleed. Notice that most are located in the posterior part of the brain (occipital region).

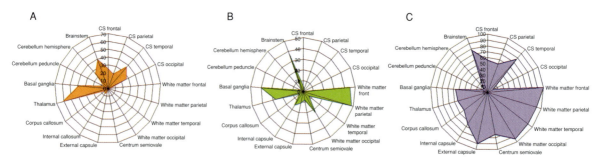

Fig. 15.2 Distribution of MRI lesions in 147 patients with CADASIL (cerebral autosomal dominant arteriopathy with subcortical infarcts and leukoencephalopathy). Radar plots show the frequency at each location of (A) cerebral microhemorrhages, (B) lacunar infarctions and (C) white matter hyperintensities. In each category, frequency is expressed as a percentage of the number of patients harboring a lesion at a given location divided by the total number of patients with that specific lesion. CS, cortical sulci. (Adapted from Viswanathan *et al.* 2006 [14].)

Pathology of small vessel disease

The vessels affected by SVD are between 40 and 900 mm in size (Fig. 6.1 and Table 6.1). The arteries affected are:

- *superficial perforating vessels*: pial branches of the anterior, middle and posterior cerebral arteries, which supply gray matter with short branches of three lengths, reaching cortical layer III, layer V and the gray–white matter junction and the depth of the subcortical white matter with longer branches
- *basal perforating vessels*: basal (deep) perforating vessels branch off the first segments of the anterior and middle cerebral arteries and form the lenticulostriatal arteries to supply the basal ganglia; there are also deep perforating branches from the PCA to supply the thalamus [2].

Four types of structural change have been described in SVD: each of the types affects vessels of different size ranges (Fig. 6.1).

Atherosclerosis affects distal vessels (200–800 mm) with atheromatous microplaques, which can occlude vessels before they reach the advanced stage that is typically required to occlude vessels with larger lumina. Hypertension appears to "drive" atherosclerosis into smaller, more distal reaches of the cerebrovascular bed. Fisher identified lacunae, particularly larger symptomatic lesions, which resulted from atherosclerotic plaques in vessels of diameter 200–800 mm. The plaques were either in the proximal perforating arteries (microatheroma), at their origin (junctional atheroma) or in the parent artery on the circle of Willis (mural atheroma) [1].

Lipohyalinosis (also referred to as "complex" SVD [3]) describes fibrinoid deposition in the walls of vessels of diameter 40–300 mm [4]. It is *commonly* but not always related to hypertension and preferentially affects small, long, scarcely branching arteries arising directly from large vessels in the basal ganglia, the hemispheric white matter, the brainstem and the cerebellum. The term lipohyalinosis is often incorrectly applied to almost any cerebral small vessel pathology. It is distinct from, and should not be confused with, the concentric, hyaline wall thickening that is a feature of most aged brains [3]. The pathogenic events start with proliferation of smooth muscle cells of the media, with thickening of the vessel wall and a reduction of the ratio of the lumen to the external diameter. Effusion of plasma proteins through damaged endothelium leads to thickening of the basal lamina and deposition of amorphous eosinophilic material (escaped plasma proteins). Because this plasma protein stains positive with fibrin stains, it has been mistaken for fibrin, and the pathogenesis of lipohyalinosis has been misinterpreted as necrosis, Finally, fibroblasts replace smooth muscle cells and collagen is deposited in the wall, the resulting unequal resistance to pressure resulting in irregular lumen diameter, and even in the formation of true microaneurysms [5,6].

Arteriolosclerosis with hyaline thickening of vessel walls (vessel diameter 50–150 mm) and concentric fibrohyalinosis is also referred to as "simple" SVD [3]. This condition is aggravated with increasing age. The microvascular degeneration is likely the cause of white matter lesions (leukoaraiosis) in elderly people [7]. Age-related microvascular wall pathology in the periventricular white matter appears in the form of fibrohyalinosis, which is in keeping with observations of vascular wall thickening in larger medullary arteries of patients with dementia, in periventricular veins in leukoaraiosis and in small vessels associated with diffuse white matter lesions. Thickening of the microvascular walls at the ultrastructural level corresponds to massive collagen deposits affecting the basement membrane. These structural changes share similar characteristics with those of cortical and white matter capillaries. Decreased cerebral blood flow induces the accumulation of fibrous collagen in the microvascular walls, including those within the white matter [8].

Microaneurysms occur at branching sites in vessels of 100–300 mm diameter. The aneurysmal walls contain hyaline connective material and show a destruction of the elastica interna of the smooth muscle cells [9]. Rupture of microaneurysms causes small globular hemorrhages (which may correspond to CMBs) followed by a repair process involving thrombosis and fibrosis, finally resulting in fibrocollagenous spheres. The existence of microaneurysms has been challenged, as

Table 6.1 Overview of the characteristics of common vasculopathies related to microbleeds

Characteristics	Atherosclerosis	Hypertensive angiopathy with arteriosclerosis	CAA	CADASIL	Moyamoya
Vessels and distribution	Large extracranial and intracranial vessels; decreases in distal vessels (down to 2 mm)	Large extracranial and intracranial vessels; extends the range to more distal vessels down to 100 mm; Small vessel disease: (90–400 µm) (Fig 5.1)	Type 1: arterioles in cortex and meninges and cortical capillaries Type 2: arterioles in cortex and meninges (Fig. 6.2)	Small and medium-sized arteries	Distal portions of the internal carotid arteries and proximal parts of the ACA and MCA; vessels branching off the posterior parts of the circle of Willis
Location	Subcortical, deep gray matter	Superficial perforating vessels (pial branches of ACA, MCA and PCA, supplying gray (short) and white matter (long) and basal areas) Deep perforating vessels: base of brain, PCA and lenticulostriatal Fig. 6.5)	Meningeal and cortical, particularly occipital (Fig. 6.5)	White matter of frontal, parietal and occipital lobes; basal ganglia and thalamus, mesencephalon and pons (longitudinal tracts)	Effects of bilateral stenosis of distal carotid artery/MCA and MCA; hemorrhages in basal ganglia, thalamus and lateral ventricle wall
Pathogenesis	Dysfunction of endothelium; accumulation of low density lipoprotein in the intima; disruption of endothelial barrier function	Breakdown of autoregulation; aggravation of arteriosclerotic effects; causes arteriosclerosis to extend more distally; focal disruption of blood–brain barrier	Deposition of Aβ$_{40}$ in the vessel wall	NOTCH3 mutation causative but pathogenesis not known	Not known; gene association (linkage) with chromosome 3p24 and 8q23
Pathological findings	Collagenization; lipohyalinosis; atheroma; proliferation of smooth muscle cells; monocyte and macrophage immigration; formation of fibrous plaques	Collagenization; lipohyalinosis; atheroma; deposition of brightly eosinophilic "fibrinoid" in vessel walls; reduplication of basal lamina under endothelial cells	Amyloid deposition; thickening of the media; splitting of vessel wall (double barrel)	Thickening and fibrosis of arterial walls with PAS-positive deposits in the tunica media; granular osmiophilic deposits in the smooth muscle cells of degenerating vessels	Excessive fibrous thickening of intima; duplication of elastica

CADASIL, cerebral autosomal dominant arteriopathy with subcortical infarcts and leukoencephalopathy; CAA, cerebral amyloid angiopathy; ACA, MCA and PCA, anterior, middle and posterior cerebral arteries, respectively; PAS, periodic acid–Schiff stain.

microaneurysms were not convincingly demonstrable in some recent studies. It has been suggested that the concept of microaneurysms more likely arose as a misinterpretation of the relatively crude original injection studies, and the lesions detected were, in fact, aneurysm mimics: complex arteriolar coils and perivascular clots [10], which caused micro-tortuosities rather than true aneurysms [11]. A fuller discussion of evolving concepts of these lesions is presented in Ch. 1. *Lacunes*, small cavities in the deep brain parenchyma, are closely associated with small vessels. They are histologically classified into three types. Type 1 lacunae are small old infarcts, typically occurring in the putamen, caudate, thalamus, pons, internal capsule and hemispheric white matter. These lesions are further subclassified into type 1a and 1b. Type 1a lacunae are deep infarcts consisting of a small cavity containing occasional small vessels and scattered astrocytes while type 1b lacunae are incomplete lacunar infarcts, with selective loss of neurons and oligodendrocytes but relative preservation of astrocytes, causing patchy astrogliosis. In contrast, type 2 lacunae are presumed small deep hemorrhages, in which the cavity contains numerous hemosiderin-laden macrophages [5]. It is unclear as to whether these type 2 lesions are old hemorrhages into small lacunar infarcts, or primary small hemorrhages. Type 3 lacunae are dilated perivascular spaces (enlarged Virchow–Robin space; status cribrosus) and are rarely clinically significant.

Pathology of cerebral amyloid angiopathy

Sporadic forms

Previously considered to be an uncommon entity in association with rare hereditary syndromes, vascular amyloid deposition (usually referred to as cerebral amyloid angiopathy [12]) is now recognized as a frequent, almost invariable component of the disease process in Alzheimer's disease, as well as being extremely common in normal aging. Outside the context of Alzheimer's disease, sporadic CAA is generally recognized in life by the occurrence of lobar cerebral hemorrhages [13], and it is considered to be a common and important cause of lobar cerebral hemorrhage and dementia in the elderly. It is also clear

that CAA is related to cerebral infarcts [14], and white matter pathology [15], but the clinical implications of these associations remains to be clarified. The CAA process involves primarily larger arteriolar vessels in the neocortical and leptomeningeal vessels (Fig. 6.2A–F,G–I), but can also involve capillaries (Fig. 6.2J–L). However, in Alzheimer's disease, there is no correlation between the formation of neurofibrillary tangles (containing hyperphosphorylated tau), the formation of neuritic plaques and the degree of CAA [16]. Importantly, vascular amyloid often occurs independently of plaque formation. Also, while plaques are predominantly composed of the 42 amino acid residue fragment ($A\beta_{42}$), CAA amyloid is composed of the shorter fragment ($A\beta_{40}$), suggesting different mechanisms for their processing, accumulation and clearance [17]. Analysis of the relationship between Braak stage of Alzheimer's disease progression [18], vascular amyloid and the clinical picture of Alzheimer's disease, vascular dementia and mixed dementia [17] showed no correlation between these parameters and disease groups. The description and staging of pathological features of CAA was initially based on their occurrence in larger vessels. The progression of the vascular involvement was described and staged by Vonsattel into three grades: (1) mild, with amyloid restricted to a congophilic rim around normal or atrophic smooth muscle fibers in the media of otherwise normal vessels (Fig. 6.2M); (2) moderate, with replacement of the media by amyloid, thickening but no evidence of remote or recent blood leakage (Fig. 6.2N); and (3) severe, characterized by extensive amyloid deposition with focal wall fragmentation and at least one focus of perivascular leakage with presence of erythrocytes, hemosiderin or both (Fig. 6.2O). Availability of an immunohistochemical detection method for $A\beta$ has led to a further refinement of the staging of CAA pathology (Fig. 6.2D–I): grade 1 (mild CAA), in which $A\beta$ deposition is primarily in a fine rim on the basement membrane; grade 2 (moderate CAA), in which disease extends to allocortical and cerebellar vessels and deposition of $A\beta$ among smooth muscle cells partially replacing the tunica media; and grade 3 (severe CAA), in which there is total replacement of arteriolar vascular smooth muscle.

Thal *et al.* [19] described two types of sporadic CAA: type 1, where they acknowledged the existence of capillary $A\beta$, and type 2, where capillaries are spared (Fig. 6.2). A genetic component to the pathogenesis

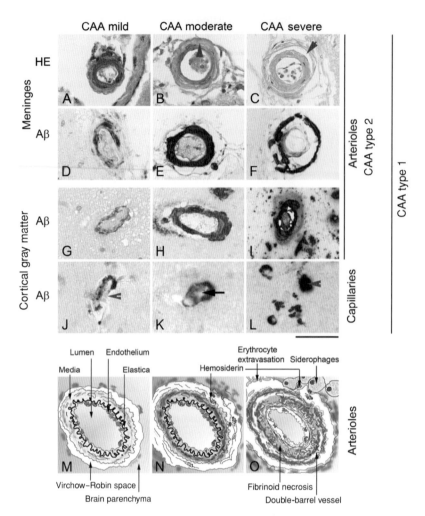

Fig. 6.2 Histological features and schematic representation of pathological features in cerebral amyloid angiopathy (CAA). Type 1 CAA is defined by involvement of meningeal vessels and cortical arterioles and capillaries. Type 2 includes only cortical and meningeal arterioles but excludes cortical capillaries (see right of the panel). (A–C) Morphology of CAA-related changes in vessel walls of meningeal vessels. (A,B) In CAA type 1 (A) and CAA type 2 (B), there are minimal structural changes, with microscopically detectable amyloid in the vessel wall in moderate CAA (B, arrowhead). (C) In severe CAA, there are significant structural alterations with detachment and delamination of the outer part of the tunica media, resulting in the formation of so-called double-barrel vessels (arrowhead). (D–F) Immunohistochemical detection of beta-amyloid (Aβ) in the wall of meningeal vessels. In mild CAA (D) there is a diffuse, fluffy deposition of amyloid in the vessel wall, often beginning in the basal lamina. The next stage (E) is characterized by a more dense deposition encompassing the entire wall. In severe CAA (F), the outer and inner detached media as well as the endothelium and surrounding brain parenchyma are heavily loaded with Aβ. (G–I) Manifestation of amyloid angiopathy in cortical arterioles. (G) Mild, diffuse accumulation in cortical arterioles, usually with relatively mild generalized Aβ deposition in the surrounding brain. (H) There is pan-mural deposition of Aβ. In this example there is also Aβ deposited in the surrounding brain parenchyma in immediate vicinity to the Virchow–Robin space. (I) In the severe form of CAA, there is formation of double-barrel vessels, which are generally less common than in meningeal vessels. There is a very heavy parenchymal Aβ accumulation, with a perivascular diffuse deposition. (J–L) Capillary CAA with the three images showing the stages of capillary CAA. (J) Diffuse, mild and often partly circumferential Aβ in the capillary wall (open area indicated by arrowhead). (K) In moderate capillary CAA, the Aβ encompasses the entire circumference but does not impede on the lumen (arrowhead). (L) Only in the most severe form is there luminal obstruction (arrowhead). (M–O) Schematic summary of the sequence of events and development of pathological features in the progression of CAA. (M) In mild CAA, there is an intact vessel wall structure with diffuse deposition of Aβ in the outer part of the wall. There are no structural alterations, particularly in the intact tunica media and elastica. (N) In moderate CAA, there is a relatively intense, pan-mural Aβ accumulation, leading to medial atrophy and hemosiderin deposition in the Virchow–Robin space or in the surrounding brain parenchyma. (O) The severe form of CAA shows severe impairment of the vessel wall integrity, with fibrinoid necrosis, splitting of the vessel, perivascular erythrocytes, hemosiderin and macrophages containing hemosiderin (siderophages) as evidence of microbleeds in the recent or distant past. HE, hematoxylin and eosin. Scale bar: 160 mm (A–F) and 80 mm (G–L). See the color plate section.

of these two types is likely, with an association of apolipoprotein E (*APOE*) *ε4* allele with CAA type 1, while the *APOE ε2* allele is associated with CAA type 2. Within capillaries, Aβ deposits often appear as "dysphoric amyloid angiopathy" (Fig. 6.2J–L) [20] and/or are located at the outer basement membrane close to the neuropil [21], whereas Aβ deposits in larger vessels occur in the media near smooth muscle cells [22]. In keeping with the known association of the *APOE ε4* genotype with Alzheimer's disease and CAA, these carriers have an overall high prevalence of CMBs and strictly lobar CMBs significantly more often than non-carriers [23], although this was not confirmed in an unbiased population study in Austria [24].

Cerebral microbleeds are increasingly recognized as an important way of detecting CAA in life, and are discussed in detail in Ch. 12.

Hereditory forms of cerebral amyloid angiopathy

The entity of CAA encompasses a number of highly diverse sporadic and genetic disorders that nevertheless share the same pathological hallmark of amyloid fibril deposition in small leptomeningeal and cortical vessels. The most common protein found in vivo in amyloid angiopathies is Aβ (including sporadic Alzheimer's disease or CAA, discussed in Chs. 13 and 12). Mutations in the gene *APP*, encoding the Aβ precursor protein, are associated with familial Alzheimer's disease and CAA and cause overproduction of Aβ by facilitated cleavage of APP. One of the autosomal dominant "hereditary cerebral hemorrhages with amyloidosis" is the Dutch type (HCHWA-D), caused by a single point mutation at codon 693 of *APP* (E220Q) in a limited number of families in the Netherlands [25]. The mutation does not affect total Aβ production but may alter the $A\beta_{42}:A\beta_{40}$ ratio, resulting in extensive amyloid deposition in meningocortical arterioles. Sporadic CAA and HCHWA-D are clinically characterized by recurrent strokes and cognitive impairment and radiologically present with CMBs, lobar ICH, superficial siderosis and white matter hyperintensities [26]. Different forms of amyloid may form in other rare hereditary amyloid disorders depending on the underlying molecular pathology. The proteins include ABri, ADan, cystatin C, transthyretins, prion proteins and gelsolin. A range of different phenotypes – often named by the geographical locations where the disorders were first identified – have been described. In some of these syndromes, CMBs have been iden-

tified on MRI; these disorders are briefly discussed in Ch. 16.

Rare vascular diseases
CADASIL

The CADASIL syndrome was first described by Bogaert in 1955 [1]. A mutation in the gene *NOTCH3* was identified in 1996 [27]; it results in N-terminal point mutations or small deletions in the epidermal growth factor (EGF)-like domains of the Notch-3 protein. Despite the identification of approximately 130 mutations and detailed work-up of the effect of the mutation in vitro and in mouse models, the pathogenesis has yet to be elucidated.

Macroscopically, brain lesions appear remarkably uniform, with multiple small cystic infarctions, particularly localized to the central gray and white matter and pons, as well as cortical and central brain atrophy. Periventricular white matter, basal ganglia, thalamus, mesencephalon and the pons are involved and an obvious ventricular dilatation is noted. The cerebral white matter is grayish-brown or granular, with multiple small cystic lacunae that may be extensive and confluent. Most often the subcortical white matter is better preserved [28,29]. Histological findings include a diffuse and focally myelin pallor throughout the white matter, partially preserving the subcortical U-fibers. In the deep areas of the white matter and in the internal and external capsules, there are multiple infarcts at different stages of development with typical reactions (macrophages, formation of lacunae and astrogliosis). Lesions are symmetrical in both hemispheres, and are most prevalent in the frontal, parietal and occipital lobes, and in basal ganglia and thalamus. Similar lesions are present in the mesencephalon and pons, with longitudinal tract myelin pallor and infarcts [30,31].

Vascular lesions are caused by an occlusive disease of leptomeningeal arteries and arterioles and of the intracerebral penetrating small and medium-sized arteries affecting the white matter. Microscopically, there is thickening and fibrosis of arterial walls with periodic acid–Schiff stain-positive deposits in the tunica media, resulting in a narrowing of the lumina, impaired circulation and in ischemic infarctions. Ultrastructurally, there are granular osmiophilic deposits in the smooth muscle cells of degenerating vessels, near the plasmalemmal indentations in the abluminal aspects [1]. However, to date it is not clear how the *NOTCH3* mutations are involved in the pathogenesis of CADASIL [1]. Most patients with clinically symptomatic CADASIL develop CMBs [32]. These CMBs manifest histologically as siderophages in the vicinity of small blood vessels (diameter, 100–300 mm) in the majority of brains at autopsy. Hemorrhages are found in white matter, basal ganglia, pons and optic nerve, ranging in size from 0.2 to 1.0 mm, and only seen at the microscopic level [33]. These CMBs are found in 25–69% of patients with CADASIL [32] and are discussed in more detail in Ch. 8.

Moyamoya disease

Moyamoya disease was first described in Japan, where it is common, but has increasingly been described in other countries and in all major ethnic groups [34].

The main pathological features are an occlusion of distal portions of the internal carotid arteries and proximal parts of the anterior and middle cerebral arteries and numerous dilated thin-walled collateral vessels branching off the posterior parts of the circle of Willis. Moyamoya syndrome is defined angiographically by spontaneous occlusion of the circle of Willis and the presence of an abnormal collateral vascular network in the brain. The outer diameter of the occluded vessels is often significantly reduced and histologically the intima shows excessive fibrous thickening but no atheromatous changes. The elastica is often duplicated or triplicated.

A higher frequency of asymptomatic CMBs has been reported in patients with moyamoya disease compared with normal controls [35,36]. In keeping with the histological findings in CMBs associated with other vasculopathies, moyamoya-associated CMBs show encapsulated hematoma and hemosiderin [37]. The occurrence of CMBs in moyamoya disease is discussed further in Ch. 16.

The natural history of hemorrhages: formation blood products and their degradation

The first event in a hemorrhage is the extravasation of all constituents of blood (i.e. erythrocytes) along with plasma. Extravasation may occur by rhexis (rupture of a vessel wall) or by diapedesis (when there is no discoverable lesion) affecting arterioles, veins or capillaries.

On a *molecular and biochemical level*, degradation of hemoglobin contained in erythrocytes results in the formation of hemosiderin, which is yellowish or brownish in color, amorphous, contains iron and is insoluble in water, alkaline, alcohol, ether, xylene and chloroform. It occurs in cells and intercellular tissues following recent hemorrhage and results from the slow degradation of erythrocytes. Hemosiderin is paramagnetic and is the key compound underlying magnetic susceptibility effects that allow CMBs to be detected (see Chs. 2 and 3). Further degradation of hemosiderin leads to the formation of hematoidin, which is chemically identical with bilirubin but is formed in cells or tissues from hemoglobin, particularly under conditions of reduced oxygen tension. Hematoidin crystals are composed of a core of empty clefts, consistent with dissolved lipids and suggestive of cholesterol crystals, surrounded by myelinoid membrane aggregates [38,39]. Hematoidin crystals then undergo degradation and are phagocytosed by macrophages under conditions of reduced oxygen tension, followed by removal of globin. The enzyme heme oxygenase-1, which is induced by the presence of hematoidin [39], is a pro-oxidative enzyme that catalyzes the degradation of heme into biliverdin, carbon monoxide and free iron [40].

Most relevant to CMBs, on the *cellular level* (Fig. 6.3), the sequence of events starts with the appearance of erythrocytes ($t = 0$ h) (see also Fig. 6.4A,B), which can preserve their normal biconcave configuration for a few days within a clot after a hemorrhage [42]; this is followed by the appearance of polymorph nuclear leukocytes ($t = 2$ h), scavenger cells (i.e. monocytes and macrophages containing erythrocytesleukocytes or fat) ($t = 14$ h), hemosiderophages (i.e. hemosiderin-containing macrophages) ($t = 71$ h), hematoidin (intracellular and extracellular) ($t = 12$ days) (Fig. 6.4C,D). These events have been meticulously demonstrated in a detailed study on the natural history of trauma-associated hemorrhages, where the sequence of events can be pinpointed more accurately than in CMBs [22]. Figure 6.3 shows the events recorded in this study and Fig. 6.4 illustrates the pathological correlates in chronic hypertension (Fig. 6.4A,C) or CAA (Fig. 6.4B,D).

Correlation of imaging findings with pathology: cerebral microbleeds

From the perspective of neuroimaging, CMBs are focal deposits of hemosiderin and can be visualized with MRI. The introduction of gradient-recall echo

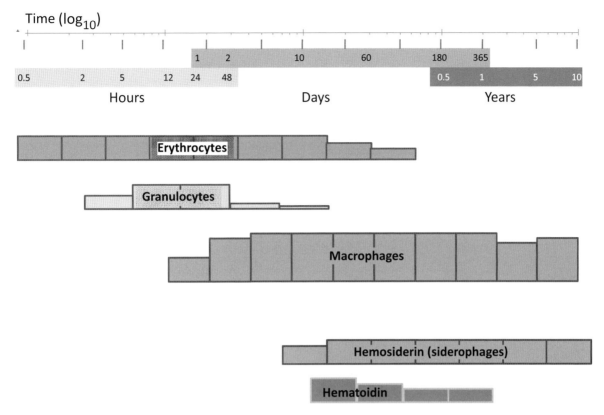

Fig. 6.3 Degradation of blood products in intracerebral hemorrhages over time. The time is shown in a logarithmic scale with hours, days and years overlapping. The height of the individual bars relate to the frequency observed in this study. Decreasing bar height indicates decreasing frequency of this finding in the study. (Data are adapted from Oehmichen and Raff, 1980 [22].)

(GRE) T_2^*-weighted and susceptibly-weighted (SWI) MRI detects hemosiderin degradation products as small rounded hypointense lesions. A number of studies have correlated radiological CMBs with their histopathological counterparts, and these are summarized in Table 6.2. The challenges involved in correlating MRI with histopathology for such small lesions with a widespread distribution in the brain have already been mentioned. Such technical aspects probably account for the small number of brains with CMBs that have been analyzed in this way. Notwithstanding these limitations, in the majority of cases, radiological CMBs did reflect old, small foci of hemorrhage composed of hemosiderin-containing macrophages, suggesting that CMBs are quite specific for pathological CMBs. However, CMBs have also been related to microaneurysms [39,41] or pseudoaneurysm [46]. A systematic appraisal of the development of ideas about microaneurysms, and their link with CMBs, is given in Ch. 1.

It seems likely, therefore, that CMBs most often relate to small foci of blood degradation products (Fig. 6.4C,D), but these may occasionally be related to aneurysmal or pseudoaneurysmal lesions rather than well-defined extramural bleeds. Although many CMB "mimics" are encountered radiologically (Ch. 5.), pathological studies have only rarely documented these (e.g. pseudocalcification was described by Tatsumi et al. [41]; see also Table 6.2).

Several studies carried out since 1999 have addressed the morphological correlates of CMBs. The findings of nine such studies of CMBs are summarized in Table 6.2: Hypertensive angiopathy was analyzed in four studies [41,46–48], CAA in two [39,43], CADASIL in two [33,44] and moyamoya disease in one study [37]. Older studies used tinctorial

Hypertension

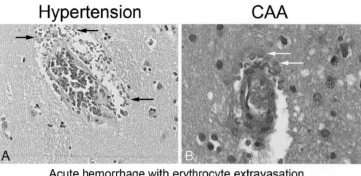

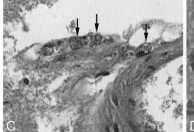

Acute hemorrhage with erythrocyte extravasation

CAA

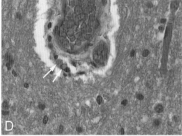

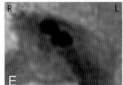

Chronic hemorrhage with hemosiderin deposits

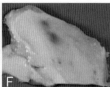

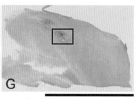

Correlation of imaging, macroscopy and histology

Fig. 6.4 Histological images of microbleeds in autopsy samples with chronic hypertension (A,C) or cerebral amyloid angiopathy (CAA) (B,D), and correlation of imaging with macroscopy and microscopy (E–G). (A,B) Histological correlate of acute erythrocyte extravasations into the perivascular (Virchow–Robin) space (blue arrows pointing to extravasated erythrocytes). (C,D) The same patients as in (A,B), with examples of chronic bleeds with formation of hematoidin. The arrows point to small deposits in the perivascular space. (E–G) Correlation of autopsy imaging (E), the corresponding formalin-fixed autopsy specimen and the corresponding histology after wax embedding and staining with Perl's Prussian blue stain to visualize iron (hemosiderin) deposition (blue dye). The lesion is located in the thalamus. Difference in size in the imaging scale bar: 160 mm (A), 80 mm (B–D), 17 mm (E,F) and 15 mm (G). See the color plate section. (E–G adapted from Tatsumi et al. 2008 [41].)

stainings to assess vessel morphology and myelin density, a classical iron stain (Perl's reaction) to assess hemosiderin deposits and Congo red to detect amyloid. Most of the more sophisticated markers for macrophages, inflammatory cells, vessel structure and gliosis have been available since the mid 1990s. However, only the most recent studies [39,43,44] have used advanced immunohistochemical markers to assess factor VII, basement membrane integrity (collagen IV) smooth muscle actin, macrophage and lymphocyte markers, and Aβ. The aim of all the studies has been to address the morphological correlate of MRI-recorded hypointensities (mostly GRE T_2^*). The consistent histological finding was that of hemosiderin deposits corresponding to MRI CMBs. More recent studies have systematically compared the size of MRI CMBs with the actual diameter of the deposit (assessed by histology) and found an

overestimation of size on MRI, termed the "blooming effect." An autopsy imaging study of 38 lesions in 10 brains showed a range of 0.5–5 mm lesional diameter [39]. However, the size estimated by GRE or SWI MRI appeared consistently larger than confirmed by subsequent histology of the imaged tissue block (blooming) [39,43]. Anatomically, the majority of the lesions appeared beneath the gray–white matter junction and at the penetration site of pial arterioles into the gray matter.

A limitation of most large studies published so far is the inclusion of MRI studies of living patents in one cohort and histopatholgoical analysis of postmortem brains in a separate cohort [33,43,47], while those studies that compared pre- and postmortem brains, followed by histology, only included small numbers or were case studies [37,41,44]. Schrag et al. [39] did compare postmortem brain MRI with histology

Table 6.2 Summary of publications correlating MRI findings and histology of microbleeds

Source	No. patient (MRI)	MRI Sequence	No. autopsy MRI	No. microbleeds	No. blocks (micro)	Histological techniques	Disease	Correlation/ hypothesis	Results and conclusions
Schrag et al. 2009 [39]	n/a	HR 3D GRE T_2^*; SWI (3 T)	10	38	13	H&E; $A\beta$; CD68; C6 IHC; CD3 + CD20; MAP2; HO1; iron	CAA (AD)	CAA and CMB correlation PM MRI–histology; size correlation MRI–histology	The vast majority of lesions located near the cortical ribbon: old hematomas in 16/38 cases with hemosiderin deposition; macrophages in all larger parenchymal lesions; two main areas: beneath the gray–white matter junction and in the superficial cortex where pial arterioles penetrate the gray matter. In several hemorrhages it was possible to determine which vessel ruptured. One hypointensity was caused by a microaneurysm. SWI consistently overestimated the diameter of small lesions (blooming effect)
Greenberg et al. 2009 [43]	46[a]	GRE (1.5 T)	6	181		H&E; $A\beta$; IHC	CAA	Comparison high and low CMB count in brains with macrobleeds; CAA pathology with CMB frequency	Increased wall thickness of amyloid-positive vessels in brains with high CMB count relative to low count; no other qualitative pathological differences (frequency or type of amyloid-positive vessels); no correlation with dysphoric amyloid deposits, double-barrel vessels. In vivo study: hemorrhage size in bimodal distribution (mixture of two separate populations); hemosiderin and macrophages not assessed
Yamamoto et al. 2009 [44]	9 + controls	T_2 FLAIR	9 + controls	n/a	> 9	H&E; CV; LFB; SMA; Coll IV; GLUT1	CADASIL	Pathological changes in white matter of temporal pole in CADASIL; correlation with histology	Small vessel arteriopathic and perivascular space widening; perivascular space significantly widened in CADASIL compared with subcortical vascular ischemic dementia; hemosiderin-laden macrophages in 6/7 brains
Tatsumi et al. 2008 [41]	1	GRE T_2^*; SWI (3 T)	1	9	9	H&E; iron	Hypertension	Correlation MRI–histology; case study	All CMBs were hemosiderin deposits and frequently associated with hypertensive microangiopathy; deposits usually associated with lipohyalinosis or microaneurysms; one CMB related to vascular pseudocalcification

(cont.)

Table 6.2 (cont.)

Source	No. patient (MRI)	MRI Sequence	No. autopsy MRI	No. microbleeds	No. blocks (micro)	Histological techniques	Disease	Correlation/ hypothesis	Results and conclusions
Kikuta et al. 2007 [37]	1	GRE T_2^*; SW (1.5 T)	n/a	1	1/1	H&E; EVG; factor VIII; IHC	Moyamoya	Hypointensity = CMB? case study	MRI-detected CMB confirmed by histology (small hematoma)
Dichgans et al. 2002 [33]; Messori and Salvolina 2003 [45]	16 (+16 controls)	GRE T_2^* (1.5 T)	7	94		H&E; iron	CADASIL	Compared in vivo and PM imaging; PM imaging and PM histology	All CADASIL individuals show hyperintense T_2-weighted abnormalities on brain MRI; focal accumulations of hemosiderin-containing macrophages in 6/7 brains (not imaged by MRI before PM, precluding direct correlation); significant correlation between age and number of CMB
Tanaka et al. 1999 [46]	89	FSE T_2; T_2^* (1 T)	3	108 (7 were patients)	3	H&E; MTC; KB	Hypertension	Compare in vivo and PM imaging; PM MRI–histology	Small hypointense lesions were foci of old hemorrhages caused by rupture of arteriosclerotic microvessels; incomplete ischemic necrosis in the surrounding areas Old hemorrhages were hemosiderin pigments One case of organized pseudoaneurysm
Roob et al. 1999 [47][a]	7	GRE T_2^* (1.5 T)	7	34	34	H&E; MTC; KB; iron; CR	Hypertension	Compared PM MRI–histology	Most CMBs were hemosiderin deposits and frequently associated with hypertensive microangiopathy; no detection of pathology in 13/34 regions
Fazekas et al. 1999 [48]	n/a	GRE T_2^* (1.5 T)	11	34	11	H&E; MTC; KB; iron; CR	Hypertension	Hypointensity = microbleed = histology?	All brains examined showed moderate to severe small vessel disease; areas of signal loss predominantly in basal ganglia, thalami, brainstem or cerebellum

AD, Alzheimer's disease; CAA, cerebral amyloid angiopathy; CADASIL, cerebral autosomal dominant arteriopathy with subcortical infarcts and leukoencephalopathy; CMB, cerebral microbleed; n/a, not available; PM, postmortem.

Imaging: 3D, three dimensional; FLAIR, fluid attenuated inversion recovery; FSE, fast spin echo; GRE, gradient-recalled echo; HR, high resolution; SWI, susceptibility-weighted imaging.

Histology: Aβ, beta-amyloid; C6 IHC, complemen; CD3 + CD20, lymphocytes; CD68, macrophages; Coll IV, basement membrane collagen (collagen IV); CR, Congo red (amyloid); CV, Cresyl violet (neurons); EVG, elastic Van Gieson (in ima elastic amina); GLUT1, glucose transporter 1; H&E, hematoxylin and eosin; HOI, hemoxygenase I; IHC, immunohistochemistry; KB, Klüver–Barrera (myelin); LFB, Luxol fast blue (myel n); MAP2, neurons; MTC, Masson trichrome (collagen); SMA, smooth muscle actin.
[a] PM brain scans (described here) unrelated to the in vivo study in the same publication.

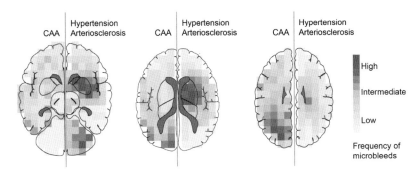

Fig. 6.5 Illustration of the relative frequency of microbleeds in cerebral amyloid angiopathy (CAA) and in hypertensive angiopathy. Colour-coded representation of the likelihood to encounter microbleeds in all brain regions with high likelihood (red) and low likelihood (white). The images represent different axial sections of the brain. Data were compiled from selected MRI studies of patients clinically diagnosed with hypertensive vasculopathy and CAA. See the color plate section.

in an Alzheimer's disease cohort. The ideal study of CMB pathophysiology and pathogenesis will be a prospective study with clinical and radiological follow-up of a mixed cohort, ideally including CAA, hypertensive vasculopathy and age-matched controls. The cohort size would ideally be large, to cover ethnic, socioeconomic and environmental variations and to ensure generalizability to different populations. Ideally multiple standardized premortem and at least one postmortem brain scan would be available, with subsequent histological analysis of carefully registered brain scans with a large panel of histological, morphometric and immunohistochemical assessments. The MRI results could then be systematically analyzed for CMBs and other imaging abnormalities, using validated tools, and directly correlated with a systematic histological work-up. Only such a study will allow a better understanding of the pathophysiology of CMBs and ICHs.

Cerebral microbleed distribution and underlying arteriopathy

It has been suggested that, in analogy with spontaneous ICH, the etiology of CMBs differs according to their location in the brain, with lobar CMBs being caused by CAA and deep or infratentorial CMBs resulting from hypertension and atherosclerosis/arteriosclerosis. In Fig. 6.5, a schematic version of the distribution of CMBs in clinically probable CAA and hypertensive arteriopathy is summarized. Although these data seem to support the hypothesis of different CMB distributions in CAA and hypertensive arteriopathy, it should be remembered that these data are based on clinical and imaging diagnoses, not

on pathological confirmation of the underlying arteriopathy.

These ideas about the distribution of hemorrhage predicting the underlying arteriopathy underlie current diagnostic criteria for CAA. The likelihood of the presence of CAA during life, with categories of probable and possible CAA based on the clinical presentation, pattern of hemorrhagic lesions on neuroimaging studies and histopathological findings, is described in the Boston criteria (Table 6.3) [26,49,50]. The Boston criteria grade the likelihood for CAA as *possible* (single lobar, cortical or cortico-subcortical hemorrhage, age 55+ years, absence of other cause of hemorrhage), *probable* (multiple hemorrhages restricted to lobar, cortical or cortico-subcortical regions, age 55+ years), *probable with supporting pathology* (pathological tissue available and detection of CAA) and *definite* (full autopsy examination with lobar, cortical or cortico-subcortical hemorrhage, severe CAA with vasculopathy and absence of other diagnostic lesions). The Boston criteria have been validated in several studies [26,51] but only in fairly small populations of patients who presented with clinically symptomatic ICH; it remains to be established whether these criteria have similar diagnostic value in asymptomatic individuals with hemorrhagic lesions, including only CMBs [26]. In a cohort of patients with CAA, the size of bleeds (macrobleeds versus CMBs) was found to form a bimodal distribution, indicating a possible distinction between different pathogenetic entities underlying small and large bleeds [43]. This study also showed that subjects with CAA and many CMBs had significantly thicker amyloid-positive vessels than those with few CMBs, suggesting that CMBs may be a biomarker not only for diagnosis but also for severity of CAA.

Table 6.3 Boston criteria for cerebral amyloid angiopathy

Criteria	Possible	Probable	Probable if supporting pathology	Definite
Pathological tissue required	No	No	Yes, hematoma and/or cortical brain biopsy; demonstration of severe CAA with vasculopathy	Yes, full brain autopsy; demonstration of severe CAA with vasculopathy
Imaging required	MRI or CT	MRI or CT	No, but likely in clinical practice	No, but likely in clinical practice
Age	55+ years	55+ years	Not specified	Not specified
Distribution of bleeding	Single lobar, cortical or cortico-subcortical hemorrhage	Multiple hemorrhages restricted to lobar, cortical or cortico-subcortical regions (cerebellar hemorrhage allowed)	Lobar, cortical or cortico-subcortical hemorrhage	Lobar, cortical, or cortico-subcortical hemorrhage
Other criteria	Absence of other cause of hemorrhage	Absence of other cause of hemorrhage	Absence of other diagnostic lesion	Absence of other diagnostic lesion

CAA, cerebral amyloid angiopathy.
Source: adapted from Knudsen et al., 2001 [51].

References

1. Ferrer I, Kaste M, Kalil J. Vascular diseases. In Love S, Louis D, Ellison D, (eds.) *Greenfield's Neuropathology*. London: Arnold, 2008, pp. 121–220.

2. Fisher CM. Pathological observations in hypertensive cerebral hemorrhage. *J Neuropathol Exp Neurol* 1971; **30**:536–50.

3. Lammie GA. Pathology of small vessel stroke. *Br Med Bull* 2000;**56**:296–306.

4. Fisher CM. Cerebral miliary aneurysms in hypertension. *Am J Pathol* 1972;**66**:313–30.

5. Lammie GA. Hypertensive cerebral small vessel disease and stroke. *Brain Pathol* 2002;**12**:358–70.

6. Munoz DG. Small vessel disease: neuropathology. *Int Psychogeriatr* 2003;**15**(Suppl. 1):67–9.

7. Takebayashi S, Kaneko M. Electron microscopic studies of ruptured arteries in hypertensive intracerebral hemorrhage. *Stroke* 1983;**14**:28–36.

8. Farkas E, de Vos RA, Donka G *et al.* Age-related microvascular degeneration in the human cerebral periventricular white matter. *Acta Neuropathol* 2006;**111**:150–7.

9. Spangler KM, Challa VR, Moody DM, Bell MA. Arteriolar tortuosity of the white matter in aging and hypertension. A microradiographic study. *J Neuropathol Exp Neurol* 1994;**53**:22–6.

10. Challa VR, Moody DM, Bell MA. The Charcot–Bouchard aneurysm controversy: impact of a new histologic technique. *J Neuropathol Exp Neurol* 1992;**51**:264–71.

11. Jellinger K. Cerebrovascular amyloidosis with cerebral hemorrhage. *J Neurol* 1977;**214**:195–206.

12. Cadavid D, Mena H, Koeller K, Frommelt RA. Cerebral beta amyloid angiopathy is a risk factor for cerebral ischemic infarction. A case control study in human brain biopsies. *J Neuropathol Exp Neurol* 2000; **59**:768–73.

13. Haglund M, Englund E. Cerebral amyloid angiopathy, white matter lesions and Alzheimer encephalopathy: a histopathological assessment. *Dement Geriatr Cogn Disord* 2002;**14**:161–6.

14. Jellinger KA. Alzheimer disease and cerebrovascular pathology: an update. *J Neural Transm* 2002;**109**: 813–36.

15. Gravina SA, Ho L, Eckman CB *et al.* Amyloid beta protein (Abeta) in Alzheimer's disease brain. Biochemical and immunocytochemical analysis with antibodies specific for forms ending at A beta 40 or A beta 42(43). *J Biol Chem* 1995;**270**:7013–16.

16. Haglund M, Kalaria R, Slade JY, Englund E. Differential deposition of amyloid beta peptides in cerebral amyloid angiopathy associated with Alzheimer's disease and vascular dementia. *Acta Neuropathol* 2006;**111**:430–5.

17. Vonsattel JP, Myers RH, Hedley-Whyte ET *et al.* Cerebral amyloid angiopathy without and with cerebral hemorrhages: a comparative histological study. *Ann Neurol* 1991;**30**:637–49.

18. Vinters HV, Wang ZZ, Secor DL. Brain parenchymal and microvascular amyloid in Alzheimer's disease. *Brain Pathol* 1996;**6**:179–95.

19. Thal DR, Ghebremedhin E, Rub U *et al.* Two types of sporadic cerebral amyloid angiopathy. *J Neuropathol Exp Neurol* 2002;**61**:282–93.

20. Tate J, Schumacher D. Interferometric pump-probe study of intense field excitation of sapphire. *Phys Rev Lett* 2001;**87**:053901.

21. Xi G, Fewel ME, Hua Y *et al.* Intracerebral hemorrhage: pathophysiology and therapy. *Neurocrit Care* 2004;**1**:5–18.

22. Oehmichen M, Raff G. Timing of cortical contusion. Correlation between histomorphologic alterations and post-traumatic interval. *Z Rechtsmed* 1980;**84**: 79–94.

23. Vernooij MW, van der Lugt A, Ikram MA *et al.* Prevalence and risk factors of cerebral microbleeds: the Rotterdam Scan Study. *Neurology* 2008;**70**:1208–14.

24. Seifert T, Lechner A, Flooh E *et al.* Lack of association of lobar intracerebral hemorrhage with apolipoprotein E genotype in an unselected population. *Cerebrovasc Dis* 2006;**21**:266–70.

25. Levy E, Carman MD, Fernandez-Madrid IJ *et al.* Mutation of the Alzheimer's disease amyloid gene in hereditary cerebral hemorrhage, Dutch type. *Science* 1990;**248**:1124–6.

26. van Rooden S, van der Grond J, van den Boom R *et al.* Descriptive analysis of the Boston criteria applied to a Dutch-type cerebral amyloid angiopathy population. *Stroke* 2009;**40**:3022–7.

27. Joutel A, Corpechot C, Ducros A *et al.* Notch3 mutations in CADASIL, a hereditary adult-onset condition causing stroke and dementia. *Nature* 1996;**383**:707–10.

28. Sourander P, Walinder J. Hereditary multi-infarct dementia. *Lancet* 1977;**i**:1015.

29. Sourander P, Walinder J. Hereditary multi-infarct dementia. Morphological and clinical studies of a new disease. *Acta Neuropathol* 1977;**39**:247–54.

30. Ruchoux MM, Maurage CA. CADASIL: cerebral autosomal dominant arteriopathy with subcortical infarcts and leukoencephalopathy. *J Neuropathol Exp Neurol* 1997;**56**:947–64.

31. Stevens DL, Hewlett RH, Brownell B. Chronic familial vascular encephalopathy. *Lancet* 1977;**i**: 1364–5.

32. Lesnik Oberstein SA, van den Boom R, van Buchem MA *et al*. Cerebral microbleeds in CADASIL. *Neurology* 2001;**57**:1066–70.

33. Dichgans M, Holtmannspotter M, Herzog J *et al*. Cerebral microbleeds in CADASIL: a gradient-echo magnetic resonance imaging and autopsy study. *Stroke* 2002;**33**:67–71.

34. Fukui M. Guidelines for the diagnosis and treatment of spontaneous occlusion of the circle of Willis ('moyamoya' disease). Research Committee on Spontaneous Occlusion of the Circle of Willis (Moyamoya Disease) of the Ministry of Health and Welfare, Japan. *Clin Neurol Neurosurg* 1997; **99**(Suppl. 2):S238–40.

35. Ishikawa T, Kuroda S, Nakayama N *et al*. Prevalence of asymptomatic microbleeds in patients with moyamoya disease. *Neurol Med Chir (Tokyo)* 2005;**45**:495–500; discussion 500.

36. Kikuta K, Takagi Y, Nozaki K *et al*. Asymptomatic microbleeds in moyamoya disease: T_2^*-weighted gradient-echo magnetic resonance imaging study. *J Neurosurg* 2005;**102**:470–5.

37. Kikuta K, Takagi Y, Nozaki K, Okada T, Hashimoto N. Histological analysis of microbleed after surgical resection in a patient with moyamoya disease. *Neurol Med Chir (Tokyo)* 2007;**47**:564–7.

38. Brenner DS, Drachenberg CB, Papadimitriou JC. Structural similarities between hematoidin crystals and asteroid bodies: evidence of lipid composition. *Exp Mol Pathol* 2001;**70**:37–42.

39. Schrag M, McAuley G, Pomakian J *et al*. Correlation of hypointensities in susceptibility-weighted images to tissue histology in dementia patients with cerebral amyloid angiopathy: a postmortem MRI study. *Acta Neuropathol* 2010,**119**:291–302.

40. Fazekas F, Chawluk JB, Alavi A, Hurtig HI, Zimmerman RA. MR signal abnormalities at 1.5 T in Alzheimer's dementia and normal aging. *AJR Am J Roentgenol* 1987;**149**:351–6.

41. Tatsumi S, Shinohara M, Yamamoto T. Direct comparison of histology of microbleeds with postmortem MR images: a case report. *Cerebrovasc Dis* 2008;**26**:142–6.

42. Salzman KL, Osborn AG, House P *et al*. Giant tumefactive perivascular spaces. *AJNR Am J Neuroradiol* 2005;**26**:298–305.

43. Greenberg SM, Nandigam RN, Delgado P *et al*. Microbleeds versus macrobleeds: evidence for distinct entities. *Stroke* 2009;**40**:2382–6.

44. Yamamoto Y, Ihara M, Tham C *et al*. Neuropathological correlates of temporal pole white matter hyperintensities in CADASIL. *Stroke* 2009; **40**:2004–11.

45. Messori A, Salvolini U. Postmortem MRI as a useful tool for investigation of cerebral microbleeds. *Stroke* 2003;**34**:376–7; author reply 377.

46. Tanaka A, Ueno Y, Nakayama Y, Takano K, Takebayashi S. Small chronic hemorrhages and ischemic lesions in association with spontaneous intracerebral hematomas. *Stroke* 1999;**30**:1637–42.

47. Roob G, Kleinert R, Seifert T *et al*. [Indications of cerebral micro-hemorrhage in MRI. Comparative histological findings and possible clinical significance.] *Nervenarzt* 1999;**70**:1082–7.

48. Fazekas F, Kleinert R, Roob G *et al*. Histopathologic analysis of foci of signal loss on gradient-echo T_2^*-weighted MR images in patients with spontaneous intracerebral hemorrhage: evidence of microangiopathy-related microbleeds. *AJNR Am J Neuroradiol* 1999;**20**:637–42.

49. Greenberg SM. Cerebral amyloid angiopathy: prospects for clinical diagnosis and treatment. *Neurology* 1998;**51**:690–4.

50. Greenberg SM, Briggs ME, Hyman BT *et al*. Apolipoprotein E epsilon 4 is associated with the presence and earlier onset of hemorrhage in cerebral amyloid angiopathy. *Stroke* 1996;**27**:1333–7.

51. Knudsen KA, Rosand J, Karluk D, Greenberg SM. Clinical diagnosis of cerebral amyloid angiopathy: validation of the Boston criteria. *Neurology* 2001;**56**, 537–9.

Risk factors for cerebral microbleeds

Lenore J. Launer

Introduction

As we have seen, cerebral microbleeds (CMBs) are small, rounded areas of low signal on MRI that signify hemosiderin deposits resulting from frank minor hemorrhages or blood leakage through small vessel walls [1]. Cerebral microbleeds reflect an underlying angiopathy currently thought to result mainly from hypertension or from the deposition of beta-amyloid in small and micro vessel walls. In this chapter the prevalence of, and risk factors for, CMBs are described, and methodological issues related to their study are discussed.

Prevalence

Cerebral microbleeds can be present in up to 80% of a clinical hemorrhagic stroke sample [2]. The prevalence of CMBs is lower in community-based studies, although a recent report based on more sensitive imaging sequences [3] has suggested that almost one-quarter of the population over 65 years have at least one CMB [4]. The wide range of reported CMB prevalence reflects the characteristics of the sample, such as age, stroke history and subtype, comorbidities and genetic susceptibility as well as variations in methodology. Prevalence data have been recently reviewed [2,5,6] and the reader is referred to these for a more comprehensive overview. Below, a few examples are given to highlight the variability in studies conducted in samples from those aged 60–70 years of age.

In 120 patients with intracerebral hematoma (ICH) as a first event (mean age 60 years; 56% with severe hypertension) [7], the prevalence of CMB, ascertained retrospectively, was 23%. In contrast, a Finnish sample of 45 patients with intraparenchymal hemorrhage (mean age 67 years; 71% hypertensive), the prevalence of CMBs was 64%, compared with 18%

in 45 controls with non-hemorrhagic stroke (mean age 67 years; 60% hypertensive) identified in the same hospital [8]. In Korean patients with first-ever supratentorial ICH (61% older than 60 years; 67.2% hypertensive), the prevalence was 65.6% [9]. The prevalence of any CMB was 64.7% in 102 hypertensive patients with acute stroke (mean age approximately 64 years), excluding those with known causes of CMB and cardiac disease influencing echocardiographic results [10]. A summary statistic estimated in a recent meta-analysis suggests the prevalence of CMBs in patients with ischemic stroke is 34% and is 60% in patients with non-traumatic ICH [2].

The reported prevalence of CMBs in community-based cohorts varies by age studied and MR sequence used. These studies are considered in more detail in Ch. 9 but are briefly summarized here. Among the Austrian Stroke Prevention Study (ASPS) of healthy community-dwelling subjects (mean age 60 years; 31.8% with severe hypertension) the prevalence of CMBs was 6.4% [11]. A prevalence of 4.6% was reported in the 472 subjects from the Framingham Offspring cohort (mean age 64.4 years; 28.9% hypertension) [12]. In the Rotterdam Scan Study (RSS; mean age 69.6 years; 20.4% hypertensive), using a comparably more sensitive MR sequence [3], CMB were detected in 23.5% of men and women, with 58.4% having strictly lobar bleeds [4].

Two studies using similar MR protocols have reported CMB prevalence in samples with mean ages older than 70 years: the Age Gene/Environment Susceptibility-Reykjavik study (AGES-RS; mean age 76 years; 78% hypertensive) [13] and the randomized Prospective Study of Pravastatin in the Elderly at Risk (PROSPER; mean age 77 years; 64.5% hypertension) trial [14]. In AGES-RS, a population-based study of aging, 11.3% had CMB; 70% of the CMBs were located in the cerebral lobes, 10% in the deep gray matter structures and 18.6% in the infratentorium [13]. In PROSPER, which included patients at high risk for cardiovascular events, 24.1% of subjects had CMB at baseline. Of the 282 CMBs detected, 52% were located in the cortico-subcortical junction, 14% in the deep white matter, 18% in the basal ganglia and 16% in the infratentorial region [14]. In the Sunnybrook study of 80 patients with probable Alzheimer's disease (78.3% over 75 years of age), 23 (29%) had evidence of any CMB [15]; 11 of these (48%) had multiple CMB; there was lobar (rather than centrencephalic) predominance in 92% of those with Alzheimer's disease.

Risk factors for cerebral microbleeds

Demographic factors

Studies based on specific diseases or clinical events provide much of the data on what factors, within the patient samples, increase the likelihood of CMBs. Most studies with a reasonable distribution of subject age and sample size show CMB prevalence increases with age. In AGES-RS [13], the prevalence of CMBs was 10% in 70–74-year-old men and 17% in men >85 years. The prevalence was 7% and 17% in women in the 70–74 year and 85+ year groups, respectively. In the RSS, the prevalence increased from 17.8% in persons aged 60–69 years to 38.3% in those >80 years [4]. A prevalence of 12% in those <75 years and 30% in those >75 years of age was reported in a Dutch Memory Clinic study [16]. Some studies suggest men have more CMB than women [12,13], while others do not [4]. In a recent review of CMB studies [2], it was noted that, in different stroke subpopulations, Asian samples tended to have a higher prevalence of CMB than those based on presumably similar cases who were not of Asian ancestry. However, such comparisons are difficult to interpret because of the variation in samples. A small pilot study suggested significant black–white racial differences in the frequency and topography of CMBs in patients with primary ICH [17]. However, in general, data on race/ethnic differences are scarce.

Hypertension and other vascular risk factors

There is robust evidence that high blood pressure, measured in different ways, is a risk factor for CMB. In a study of 123 patients with first-ever lacunar stroke (mean age 64 years; prevalence 29%) [18], the presence and number of CMBs was significantly asso-

ciated with higher ambulatory day and night systolic and diastolic blood pressure, independent of age, sex and use of antihypertensive medication. Associations were strongest for CMBs located in the deep structures (basal ganglia, thalamus and internal, external or extreme capsule) and there was a trend with increasing numbers of CMB. Among PROSPER trial participants, only age and the presence of hypertension distinguished those with CMB from those with no CMB [14]. The CMBs located in the basal ganglia were most consistently related to measures of blood pressure. However CMBs located in the cortico-subcortical lobar areas were also associated with an increased risk for hypertension. The risk factors that did not distinguish the groups included blood triglycerides, total cholesterol, low density lipoprotein (LDL) and high density lipoprotein (HDL) cholesterol, current smoking, diabetes and history of myocardial infarction.

Using a target organ approach, a study of patients with hypertension and acute stroke suggests that left ventricular wall thickness and mass as well as prior stroke increased the risk for CMB, although it is not clear whether the statistics were adjusted for potential confounders such as age. Left ventricular characteristics were similarly associated with CMB located in the infratentorial, basal ganglia and thalamus; bleeds located in the subcortical white matter (lobar) were associated with the left ventricular mass index after patients with cerebral amyloid angiopathy (CAA) were excluded from the analysis [10]. By comparison, in a sample of 167 patients referred for treatment of hypertension (mean age 51 years; 95% hypertensive), aortic stiffness, determined by aortic pulse wave velocity and central blood pressure, was not associated with presence of CMB but was associated with both white matter lesions and lacunar stroke, adjusting for age, sex, brain volume (in the case of white matter lesions), mean arterial pressure and heart rate [19]. In another study of 152 patients with acute ischemic stroke, there was a significantly increased likelihood of CMB as glomerular filtration rate, a measure of kidney function, decreased [20].

In patients with CADASIL (cerebral autosomal dominant arteriopathy with subcortical infarcts and leukoencephalopathy), hemoglobin A1c (≥5.6%; a measure of control in diabetes mellitus), increased LDL (≥3.1 mmol/l) and increasing systolic blood pressure were associated with a higher probability of having any CMB. An increased risk for having multiple CMBs was associated with systolic blood pressure and hypertension. However, the authors did not specify whether these associations were corrected for the 7 year age difference in those with and without CMB [21]. In a study of 107 patients with acute stroke (including 40.3% with ICH) and 65 patients with other neurological diseases, lesion load was scored into categories by number of CMB. Hypertension, low cholesterol (<4.27 mmol/l), and high HDL (>1.47 mmol/l) were associated with an increased lesion load, but it is not clear what these associations were adjusted for. The investigators also examined univariate associations of age, diabetes, smoking, LDL and triglycerides; none was significant [22].

Other than age and CAA, clinic-based studies of dementia, where Alzheimer's disease is the most common dementia, have not consistently identified other risk factors for CMBs. In the Dutch Memory Clinic study, there was no association of the *APOE ε4* allele or hypertension with CMB [16], a finding that has been reported in the smaller Sunnybrook study of subjects with probable Alzheimer's disease (mean age 71.3 years), who by definition have few cardiovascular risk factors [15].

Risk factors identified in community-based studies

Risk factors identified in studies based on community-dwelling subjects are similar to those identified in patient-based clinical samples. Participants in the ASPS were more likely to have any CMB with increasing age, higher systolic and diastolic blood pressure, and having hypertension; no differences were found by history of diabetes, cardiac disease, current smoking and fasting glucose levels [11]. In contrast, the Framingham Offspring study, after correcting for age and sex, found no association with CMB for measured systolic blood pressure, smoking, hypertension, diabetes and total or HDL cholesterol [12].

In the population-based RSS [4], adjusting for age, sex, and relevant medications, increased systolic and diastolic blood pressure and pulse pressure were associated with a raised risk for CMB, in particular those located in the deep or infratentorial regions. In addition, ever smoking, low total cholesterol (<4.42 mmol/l versus higher) and having an *APOE ε4* allele increased the likelihood of having CMB. The association with low total cholesterol was strongest with CMBs located in the lobar areas.

There was no association with CMB for alcohol use, diabetes and serum HDL. The RSS also examined whether any use of antithrombotic or platelet aggregation inhibitors increased the risk for CMB. They found a significantly increased likelihood that CMBs would be detected in users of any antithrombotic drug, with a slightly stronger association in those using platelet aggregation inhibitors than in those using anticoagulant drugs. The magnitude of the risk associated with taking these drugs (odds ratio [OR], 1.6) was similar to that for white matter lesions (OR, 1.7), and lower than the risk associated with the presence of infarct on MRI (OR, 2.7), controlling for age, sex and Framingham Risk Score. Risks were similar for strictly lobar CMBs or deep infratentorial bleeds. The study also suggests that aspirin use may increase the likelihood of CMBs [23]. Of interest is whether the likelihood of CMB in persons using these drugs is moderated by the presence or absence of other vascular risk factors [24].

In an analysis based on AGES-RS, there was a significant trend of increasing CMB with increasing age (years); correcting for age, there were also significant trends with increasing systolic and diastolic blood pressure (mmHg) and total cholesterol. There was a marginal trend with body mass index, presence of diabetes, use of antihypertensive drugs and use of anticoagulants/aspirin. There was no association of increasing CMB number with fasting blood glucose, smoking or education [25]. In a subsample of the cohort, *APOE ε4* homozygosity was associated with a greater likelihood of having CMB ($p = 0.01$) [13]. Investigators in the AGES-RS have approached the study of CMB as one measure of microvascular disease, to be combined with others. They have shown that, in particular, people having diabetes together with retinal arteriovenous nicking or microaneurysms/hemorrhages were more likely to have multiple CMBs. The association was independent of major potential confounders, including high blood pressure, ischemic brain lesions and other vascular factors [25]. These findings suggest that CMBs are indicative of more systemic microvascular disease related to common mechanisms.

Most genetic diseases with increased susceptibility to CMBs are rare. Mutations identified in cerebral amyloid angiopathies are characterized by misfolding of proteins, including beta-amyloid, cystatin C, transthyretin and prions [26]. CADASIL, a disease of cerebral angiopathy leading to subcortical ischemic strokes and pure vascular dementia, is caused by mutations in *NOTCH3* [27]. Moyamoya disease, characterized by abnormal collateral development and premature ischemic strokes, may be a manifestation of mutations affecting proteins in smooth muscle cells [28].

The only candidate susceptibility gene identified as risk modifying is *APOE*, studied on the basis of CMB associations with CAA. Although not a consistent finding [16], several studies suggest the *APOE ε4* allele increases the risk for CMB [13], particularly those located in lobar areas [4], which is consistent with a CAA association. It is expected many more single nucleotide polymorphisms will be identified as more advanced technologies make it economically and technically feasible to study the genetic and epigenetic contributions to disease.

Risk factors from longitudinal data

There are a few small longitudinal studies looking for the appearance of new CMBs. One study followed 21 patients for 5 years after ischemic stroke and found that having CMBs at baseline predicted new CMBs, as did baseline systolic blood pressure [29]. Similarly in patients with CAA, the development of CMBs was related to baseline CMB number [30] and, in another study, to white matter changes [31].

Improving methodology in risk factor studies

Most studies of risk factor for CMB are based on clinical samples of patients at particularly high risk for CMBs. These studies by definition include a group that is more homogeneous with regard to disease severity and associated risk factors. To be eligible for recruitment, these populations had to have sought and obtained health services; factors associated with this health-seeking behavior may confound the association of risk factors with CMB. Further, several clinical studies use a case–control design whereby the control group is recruited from different settings than the cases. Controls determine the baseline rate against which the cases are evaluated, and so the choice of controls is just as much a determinant of study validity as choice of cases. Controls should come from the same source population as the cases: that is, if the control had been a case, the individual would have followed the same trajectory to hospital care as a sampled case did. Without appropriate controls, findings can be confounded by factors that differ between cases and controls [32].

Studies based on unselected community-dwelling subjects are generally accepted to show lower risk than clinic-based studies of selective participation. Subjects are recruited independently of existing disease and regardless of whether or not they seek healthcare for prevalent or incident conditions. Further, these studies include subjects with a wide range of disease severity, who may be more likely to have multiple morbidities associated with CMBs.

Regardless of design, the study of CMB risk factors is complicated by the high likelihood of co-morbid cerebrovascular lesions, such as ischemic and hemorrhagic stroke, as well as white matter lesions. This comorbidity may arise from similar risk factors as for CMBs, making it difficult to estimate the independence of a risk factor for CMBs. Statistically controlling for other lesions can reduce this confounding. However, the comorbidity also raises the question about the extent to which CMBs are a primary event, or whether they are secondary to other lesions. As reviewed, there are almost no longitudinal studies describing risk factors for new CMB. Cross-sectional studies, regardless of setting, cannot be used to assess the temporal sequence of when lesions develop relative to each other, and they cannot address questions such as whether CMBs result from a particular risk factor or whether CMBs lead to a clinical event, which, in turn, results from a risk factor. These questions can be addressed in prospective studies that follow the emergence of new lesions.

There are several other methodological issues that need to be kept in mind when interpreting the literature on CMBs. The MR techniques to detect and characterize these lesions are evolving toward a higher sensitivity for CMBs [3]. As discussed in Chs. 2 and 3, the detection of CMBs is dependent on the MR field strength and sequences, which ultimately determines the prevalence of lesions detected as well as group differences. Following from this, clinical and epidemiological studies conducted since the late 1990s have not been based on similar MR protocols. This may introduce imprecision in the measures, affecting statistical power. In addition, the technological differences may introduce confounding if CMBs have some risk factor specificity, for example for CAA, and they are differentially detected by MRI because of size or location.

Understanding the pathophysiology of CMBs is also an important component to designing appropriate analytical statistical approaches. As detailed in Ch. 12, studies suggest CMBs in lobar (cortico-subcortical junction) regions reflect CAA, and those in infratentorial, thalamic and basal ganglion regions reflect hypertensive processes. As discussed in Chs. 11–13, the extent to which location can reliably be used to distinguish the underlying pathology of CMBs [5] is under study. Currently, criteria are based on hospital series, which most likely represent the most severe and homogeneous presentation of the underlying pathology, making it easier to diagnose a primary cause of the bleed. This specificity of the location–pathology correlation is important for analysis and interpretation of studies on risk factors. If there are clear differences in the pathology, it is useful to present data analyzed by CMB location. Another issue related to analysis strategy is whether there are differences in risk factors between persons with a single bleed and those with a multiple bleeds, as suggested by studies of individuals with genetic susceptibilities to CMBs [27]. In both cases, the decision to stratify or not, will have an impact on the power of the statistical tests.

Comprehensive reviews published in 2006 [5] and 2007 [2] discussed several other methodological issues and factors that vary across studies. These include differences in the definition of CMB, such as lesion size and location criteria, and completeness of reporting study methods. Further, there is variability in whether location is reported relative to the total number of lesions or relative to the number of patients. However, progress has been made in standardizing methodology across studies. In addition to published guidelines for reporting [2], advances have been made in standardizing CAA diagnostic criteria with the publication and validation of the Boston criteria [33] and in developing CMB rating instruments, such as the Microbleed Anatomical Rating Scale [34]. In addition, recent publications have proposed standardized acquisition protocols [6].

Conclusions

Cerebral microbleeds, like other markers of cerebrovascular disease, increase with increasing age. High blood pressure is most consistently reported as a risk factor for CMBs. Other frequently reported risk factors include diabetes, cholesterol and antithrombotic drug use, which have been shown in some, but not all, studies to increase the likelihood of CMBs. Possibly

CMBs reflect a generalized microangiopathy, present in other organs. As the field moves forwards, research on risk factors for CMBs will bring into better focus issues related to comorbidity with other vascular and neurodegenerative lesions and location and number of lesions. Currently, most studies are cross-sectional and with this study design it is not possible to disentangle whether the lesions arise from a similar third factor, whether their co-occurrence is coincidence, or whether one lesion increases the risk for other lesions. Few studies control for comorbid lesions, and, in general, control for confounding is not adequate. Prospective studies, community-based studies and standardization in methods and reporting are needed. Effect sizes of risk across studies are hard to compare because of the wide variability in statistical analyses and reporting.

References

1. Fazekas F, Kleinert R, Roob G et al. Histopathologic analysis of foci of signal loss on gradient-echo T_2^*-weighted MR images in patients with spontaneous intracerebral hemorrhage: evidence of microangiopathy-related microbleeds. AJNR Am J Neuroradiol 1999;20:637–42.

2. Cordonnier C, Al-Shahi Salman R, Wardlaw J. Spontaneous brain microbleeds: systematic review, subgroup analyses and standards for study design and reporting. Brain 2007;130:1988–2003.

3. Vernooij MW, Ikram MA, Wielopolski PA et al. Cerebral microbleeds: accelerated 3D T_2^*-weighted GRE MR imaging versus conventional 2D T_2^*-weighted GRE MR imaging for detection. Radiology 2008;248:272–7.

4. Vernooij MW, van der Lugt A, Ikram MA et al. Prevalence and risk factors of cerebral microbleeds: the Rotterdam Scan Study. Neurology 2008;70: 1208–1214.

5. Koennecke HC. Cerebral microbleeds on MRI: prevalence, associations, and potential clinical implications. Neurology 2006;66:165–71.

6. Greenberg SM, Vernooij MW, Cordonnier C et al. Cerebral microbleeds: a guide to detection and interpretation. Lancet Neurol 2009;8:165–74.

7. Offenbacher H, Fazekas F, Schmidt R et al. MR of cerebral abnormalities concomitant with primary intracerebral hematomas. AJNR Am J Neuroradiol 1996;17:573–8.

8. Alemany M, Stenborg A, Terent A, Sonninen P, Raininko R. Coexistence of microhemorrhages and acute spontaneous brain hemorrhage: correlation with

signs of microangiopathy and clinical data. *Radiology* 2006;**238**:240–7.

9. Lee SH, Kim BJ, Roh JK. Silent microbleeds are associated with volume of primary intracerebral hemorrhage. *Neurology* 2006;**66**:430–2.

10. Lee SH, Park JM, Kwon SJ *et al.* Left ventricular hypertrophy is associated with cerebral microbleeds in hypertensive patients. *Neurology* 2004;**63**:16–21.

11. Roob G, Schmidt R, Kapeller P *et al.* MRI evidence of past cerebral microbleeds in a healthy elderly population. *Neurology* 1999;**52**:991–4.

12. Jeerakathil T, Wolf PA, Beiser A *et al.* Cerebral microbleeds: prevalence and associations with cardiovascular risk factors in the Framingham Study. *Stroke* 2004;**35**:1831–5.

13. Sveinbjornsdottir S, Sigurdsson S, Aspelund T *et al.* Cerebral microbleeds in the population based AGES–Reykjavik study: prevalence and location. *J Neurol Neurosurg Psychiatry* 2008;**79**:1002–6.

14. van Es AC, van der Grond J, de Craen AJ *et al.* Risk factors for cerebral microbleeds in the elderly. *Cerebrovasc Dis* 2008;**26**:397–403.

15. Pettersen JA, Sathiyamoorthy G, Gao FQ *et al.* Microbleed topography, leukoaraiosis, and cognition in probable Alzheimer disease from the Sunnybrook dementia study. *Arch Neurol* 2008;**65**:790–5.

16. Cordonnier C, van der Flier WM, Sluimer JD *et al.* Prevalence and severity of microbleeds in a memory clinic setting. *Neurology* 2006;**66**:1356–60.

17. Copenhaver BR, Hsia AW, Merino JG *et al.* Racial differences in microbleed prevalence in primary intracerebral hemorrhage. *Neurology* 2008;**71**:1176–82.

18. Staals J, van Oostenbrugge RJ, Knottnerus IL *et al.* Brain microbleeds relate to higher ambulatory blood pressure levels in first-ever lacunar stroke patients. *Stroke* 2009;**40**:3264–8.

19. Henskens LH, Kroon AA, van Oostenbrugge RJ *et al.* Increased aortic pulse wave velocity is associated with silent cerebral small-vessel disease in hypertensive patients. *Hypertension* 2008;**52**:1120–6.

20. Cho AH, Lee SB, Han SJ *et al.* Impaired kidney function and cerebral microbleeds in patients with acute ischemic stroke. *Neurology* 2009;**73**:1645–8.

21. Viswanathan A, Guichard JP, Gschwendtner A *et al.* Blood pressure and haemoglobin A1c are associated with microhaemorrhage in CADASIL: a two-centre cohort study. *Brain* 2006;**129**:2375–83.

22. Lee SH, Bae HJ, Yoon BW *et al.* Low concentration of serum total cholesterol is associated with multifocal signal loss lesions on gradient-echo magnetic resonance imaging: analysis of risk factors for multifocal signal loss lesions. *Stroke* 2002;**33**:2845–9.

23. Vernooij MW, Haag MD, van der Lugt A *et al.* Use of antithrombotic drugs and the presence of cerebral microbleeds: the Rotterdam Scan Study. *Arch Neurol* 2009;**66**:714–720.

24. Rosand J, Eckman MH, Knudsen KA, Singer DE, Greenberg SM. The effect of warfarin and intensity of anticoagulation on outcome of intracerebral hemorrhage. *Arch Intern Med* 2004;**164**:880–4.

25. Qiu C, Cotch MF, Sigurdsson S *et al.* Retinal and cerebral microvascular signs and diabetes: the Age, Gene/Environment Susceptibility–Reykjavik study. *Diabetes* 2008;**57**:1645–50.

26. Revesz T, Holton JL, Lashley T *et al.* Genetics and molecular pathogenesis of sporadic and hereditary cerebral amyloid angiopathies. *Acta Neuropathol* 2009;**118**:115–30.

27. Chabriat H, Joutel A, Dichgans M *et al.* Cadasil. *Lancet Neurol* 2009;**8**:643–53.

28. Guo DC, Papke CL, Tran-Fadulu V *et al.* Mutations in smooth muscle alpha-actin (ACTA2) cause coronary artery disease, stroke, and moyamoya disease, along with thoracic aortic disease. *Am J Hum Genet* 2009;**84**:617–27.

29. Gregoire SM, Brown MM, Kallis C *et al.* MRI detection of new microbleeds in patients with ischemic stroke: five-year cohort follow-up study. *Stroke*; **41**:184–6.

30. Greenberg SM, O'Donnell HC, Schaefer PW, Kraft E. MRI detection of new hemorrhages: potential marker of progression in cerebral amyloid angiopathy. *Neurology* 1999;**53**:1135–8.

31. Chen YW, Gurol ME, Rosand J *et al.* Progression of white matter lesions and hemorrhages in cerebral amyloid angiopathy. *Neurology* 2006;**67**:83–7.

32. Rothman KJ (ed.). *Modern Epidemiology.* Philadelphia, PA: Lippincott, Williams & Williams, 2008.

33. Knudsen KA, Rosand J, Karluk D, Greenberg SM. Clinical diagnosis of cerebral amyloid angiopathy: validation of the Boston criteria. *Neurology* 2001;**56**:537–9.

34. Gregoire SM, Chaudhary UJ, Brown MM *et al.* The Microbleed Anatomical Rating Scale (MARS): reliability of a tool to map brain microbleeds. *Neurology* 2009;**73**:1759–66.

Relationship of cerebral microbleeds to other imaging findings

Eric E. Smith, David J. Werring and Cheryl R. McCreary

Introduction

Cerebral microbleeds (CMBs) often do not occur in isolation. Rather, they are frequently accompanied by other brain structural changes that can also be detected by neuroimaging. Cerebral microbleeds are generally considered a marker of an underlying hemorrhage-prone small vessel vasculopathy. The brain changes that accompany CMB may be a direct consequence of the CMB, of an underlying vasculopathy (e.g. ischemic lesions in hypertensive arteriopathy), or of risk factors associated with CMB or the underlying vasculopathies that cause CMB (e.g. hypertension). A thorough understanding of the relationships between CMBs and other neuroimaging findings would enhance our knowledge of cerebral small vessel disease and its relationship to brain structure and function. Furthermore, integrating CMB and other neuroimaging information could increase our ability to detect or monitor small vessel disease and predict clinical risk.

This chapter will review data associating CMBs with other neuroimaging findings. The relationships between CMBs and brain infarcts, hemorrhage and brain atrophy will be discussed in general and in the context of specific small vessel diseases.

Brain infarcts

Studies in the general population and in persons with stroke show a strong association between CMBs and radiological evidence of brain infarction. In the population-based Austrian Stoke Prevention Study, 56% of the subjects with CMBs also had chronic lacunar infarcts, while only 5% of subjects without CMBs had lacunar infarcts [1]. Similarly, CMBs were associated with an increased prevalence of silent lacunar infarcts in the population-based Rotterdam Scan Study [2]. There was little or no association between CMB and non-lacunar cortical infarcts [1,2].

Cerebral microbleeds are common in patients with clinical and neuroimaging evidence of acute ischemic stroke [3,4]. The prevalence of CMB in patients with ischemic stroke is approximately 20–30% [5–19]. Differences in population selection, mean age and vascular risk factors, as well as differences in MR acquisition parameters (e.g. slice thickness, interslice gap and field strength), could all contribute to the wide ranges of reported prevalence [20].

Ischemic stroke can be further subclassified based on neuroimaging and clinical criteria, for example using the Trial of Orgaran in Acute Ischemic Stroke criteria or the Oxfordshire Community Stroke Project criteria [21,22]. There is evidence that CMBs are more frequent in lacunar stroke compared with other stroke subtypes. Acute lacunar infarction can be defined radiographically as a subcortical lesion with maximum diameter <1.5 cm that has the characteristics of infarction. Acute lacunar infarcts appear on MRI as T_2-hyperintense lesions with evidence of restricted diffusion on diffusion-weighted imaging (DWI), including hyperintensity on the DWI sequence and hypointensity on the apparent diffusion coefficient (ADC) sequence. They may be seen as hypodense lesions on CT but frequently cannot be visualized in the acute stage. Chronic lacunar infarcts undergo cavitation and, therefore, have MRI and CT characteristics similar to cerebrospinal fluid, with hyperintensity on T_2-weighted and ADC sequences, hypointensity on the T_1-weighted sequence or hypodensity on CT. On fluid attenuated inversion recovery (FLAIR) sequence, a rim of T_2 hyperintensity surrounding the central cavitation can usually be distinguished (Fig. 8.1).

The prevalence of CMBs in patients with an acute lacunar stroke syndrome is 35–60%, in contrast to

Cerebral Microbleeds, ed. David J. Werring. Published by Cambridge University Press. © Cambridge University Press 2011.

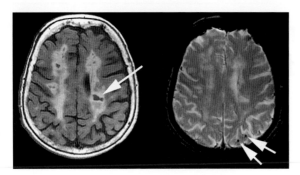

Fig. 8.1 An 81-year-old woman with a past history of ischemic stroke. (A) Fluid attenuated inversion recovery sequence demonstrating cortical atrophy, severe white matter hyperintensities and multiple cavitated white matter lacunar infarcts (an example is indicated by the arrow). (B) Gradient-recalled echo sequence shows two lobar microbleeds (arrows).

12–26% in stroke caused by large artery disease and 4–30% in stroke caused by cardioembolism [13,19,23]. Another study that discriminated ischemic stroke type based solely on radiological characteristics found that CMBs were present in 26% of patients with acute lacunar infarction on MRI compared with only 13% of patients with acute cortical infarction on MRI [24].

Additionally, CMBs are associated with an increased prevalence and number of past silent brain infarcts, mostly lacunar, in persons with stroke. Associations between CMBs and previous silent infarcts have been reported in patients scanned for acute ischemic stroke and acute intracerebral hemorrhage (ICH) [15,19,25]. Furthermore there is a "dose" effect, such that there is a moderate correlation between the number of CMBs and the number of lacunar infarcts, with correlation coefficients in the range 0.40–0.50 [15,19]. Patients with CMBs are more likely to have imaging evidence of previous lacunar infarcts rather than previous non-lacunar infarcts. This is probably because non-lacunar infarcts are caused by mechanisms other than small vessel disease, such as large artery atherosclerotic disease or cardiac disease. These observations are consistent with a disease model whereby CMBs and lacunar infarction are both manifestations of an underlying small vessel disease with common risk factors such as hypertension.

Limited data suggest a correlation between CMB pattern and the risk of accompanying silent lacunar infarcts. A population-based study found that the relationship between CMBs and lacunar infarction was restricted to subjects with deep hemispheric CMBs and was not present in the subjects with purely

lobar CMBs [2]. This may be because patients with purely lobar CMBs are likely to have cerebral amyloid angiopathy (CAA) as the cause of their CMBs, rather than hypertensive arteriopathy. A purely lobar pattern of CMBs, without CMBs in deep hemispheric structures such as the basal ganglia or thalamus, suggests the presence of CAA in the absence of evidence of another underlying cause of hemorrhage such as multiple cavernous malformations [26]. (However, pathological verification of this relationship between purely lobar CMBs and CAA has been restricted to patients with symptomatic macrobleeds.) Although CAA may cause small infarcts in the cortex and adjacent subcortical white matter [27,28], pathological studies show that vascular amyloid does not significantly involve the penetrating arteries at the base of the brain and, therefore, does not cause deep lacunar infarcts in the basal ganglia and thalamus. Consequently, relationships between CMBs and lacunar infarcts may well be different depending on whether CAA is the underlying cause of the CMBs.

Intracerebral hemorrhages

CMBs are thought to result to represent microhemorrhages from bleeding-prone small vessels [29], so naturally one would expect an association with larger parenchymal hemorrhages. The literature confirms that CMB are most highly prevalent in ICH, more so than other stroke types [3,6,7,12,14,19,30–33]. The prevalence of any CMB in ICH ranges from approximately 50 to 70%. The literature is conflicting regarding whether there is a relationship between parenchymal hematoma size and the number of microbleeds: one study found that larger hematomas were associated with more CMB [34] while another did not [35]. The reasons for the different results are not entirely clear. One difference between the studies is that the first investigated lobar and putaminal hemorrhages, while the second considered only deep hematomas. A potential confounding factor is that very large hematomas may obscure any CMB that were previously present, creating a bias toward fewer observable CMB for larger hematomas.

White matter lesions

White matter lesions (WML), also termed leukoaraiosis, appear on T_2-weighted FLAIR MRI sequences as regions of hyperintensity in the periventricular or subcortical white matter (Fig. 8.1B) and are associated with cognitive dysfunction and cognitive decline [36]. The lesions appear on CT as areas of relative hypoattenuation in the same regions. Although the exact pathogenesis of the lesions is unknown, there is abundant evidence that they are related to vascular disease. Epidemiological studies show strong relationships between WML and vascular risk factors, ischemic stroke and ICH. Furthermore, it is clear that small vessel arterial disease is sufficient to cause WML, as patients with the hereditary vascular diseases CADASIL (cerebral autosomal dominant arteriopathy with subcortical infarcts and leukoencephalopathy) and familial CAA present with extensive WML at a relatively early age, when conventional risk factors and aging are unlikely to make a major contribution.

Many studies have shown a significant moderate correlation between the number of CMBs and the amount of WML, as measured by either qualitative visual rating scales or quantitative lesion volume measurements [3]. This relationship has been consistently and repeatedly demonstrated in stroke-free healthy persons [1,2,37,38], ischemic stroke [5,10,11,15,19,23,39], ICH [30–32,40], CAA [41,42], CADASIL [43,44] and cognitive impairment [45–47]. There appears to be a relatively high burden of WML in persons with CMBs regardless of the underlying pattern of CMBs. A single study of patients with ICH found a similarly high burden of WML regardless of CMB pattern: lobar only (suggesting CAA), deep hemispheric only and mixed lobar and deep hemispheric [31]. A cohort study of vascular risk found an association between higher WML volume and the presence of CMBs regardless of whether the CMBs were purely lobar or included deep hemispheric CMBs [48].

The uniformly consistent relationship between CMBs and WML is in accordance with data that show that each is a marker of small vessel disease. Even so, it is noteworthy that the correlations between CMBs and WML, while highly statistically significant, are only moderate. Variation in WML measurement methods make between-study comparisons difficult; nonetheless, most studies report that correlations between CMB number and WML severity are in the range 0.40–0.60, which can be described as moderate, not strong. Put another way, there are a substantial number of patients with many CMBs but low WML volume or the converse, with few or no CMBs despite extensive WMLs. Consequently, both CMBs and WML seem to carry some independent information regarding the nature of the underlying small vessel disease.

Atrophy

There are only a few studies that have determined the relationship between CMBs and brain volumes. Interpreting and analyzing these data is challenging because CMBs are known to be associated with advanced age and WML, both of which are associated with lower brain volumes themselves.

Two population-based studies have investigated the relationship between CMBs and brain volumes. In the Framingham Study, CMBs were associated with lower brain volume in univariate unadjusted analysis. After controlling for age and sex, however, the association was no longer significant [37]. Similarly, in the Age Gene/Environment Susceptibility (AGES)-Reykjavik study, CMBs were associated with lower brain volumes in unadjusted analysis but not after controlling for age [38]. A cohort study of persons with vascular risk factors or cardiovascular disease failed to find an association between CMBs and brain volume [48]. A cohort study of persons with Alzheimer's disease failed to find a difference in brain atrophy in persons with or without CMBs [47]. Studies in CAA [41] and CADASIL [49] also failed to find an independent relationship between CMBs and brain atrophy in those diseases.

These data suggest that associations between CMBs and brain volume are driven by the relationship between CMBs and increased age. The CMBs do not appear to have an effect on brain volume independent of age, infarction and WMLs. This is in accordance with our understanding of the pathological basis of CMBs. The microscopic perivascular hemosiderin deposition that identifies CMBs may not be sufficient to cause enough damage to the neuropil to result in overall loss of brain volume, although whether it causes more restricted Wallerian degeneration awaits further study.

Other neuroimaging measurements

There are limited data on the relationship between CMBs and other neuroimaging measures. This section will highlight several imaging measures that may be of interest in the investigation of cerebral small vessel disease, but for which there are either only preliminary data or no data on their relationship with CMBs.

Diffusion-weighted imaging

The DWI technique allows measurement of the diffusivity of water protons. Restricted diffusion is recognized as a consequence of acute ischemic stroke. In general, other cerebral pathologies tend to disrupt the tissue microstructure, reducing the overall tissue organization, with a consequent increase in water proton diffusivity [50]. Diffusion tensor imaging provides other measures of not only the magnitude of water diffusivity but also the directionality of water diffusion, which may be particularly relevant to measuring microstructural disruption of white matter [51].

Emerging data suggest that increased water proton diffusion in regions of interest, or the whole brain, may be a consequence of small vessel disease. Increased diffusion can be detected in WML but can also be detected in white matter tissue that appears normal to the eye on conventional T_2-weighted sequences [52]. Therefore, increases in diffusion may be a sensitive MRI marker of cerebral injury from small vessel disease, and it offers additional information to that obtained with conventional T_2-weighted sequences.

Currently, there are limited data on the association between MRI diffusion measures and CMBs. One might expect a relationship because CMBs are associated with higher WML volume, and higher WML volume is, in turn, associated with increased diffusion. However, a small study of patients with CAA found no relationship between the number of CMBs and mean whole brain ADC [53]. Further studies are needed to investigate the relationship between CMBs and increased MRI diffusion in the general population and in persons with arteriosclerotic ischemic small vessel disease related to conventional vascular risk factors.

Cerebral blood flow and tissue perfusion

There are a number of imaging modalities for quantifying absolute or relative cerebral blood flow or tissue perfusion, including MRI perfusion-weighted imaging, CT perfusion-weighted imaging, MRI arterial spin label imaging, positron emission tomography (PET) and single photon emission computed tomography (SPECT). Cerebral perfusion is reduced in persons with extensive MRI evidence of small vessel disease such as high WML volume.

Few studies have looked at the relationship between cerebral blood flow and CMB. A cohort study of patients with cardiovascular disease or cardiovascular risk factors found no relationship between CMBs and cerebral blood flow [48]. Disrupted vascular integrity, leading to CMBs, may not, therefore, be either a consequence of, or causative of, reduced blood flow.

Altered vascular permeability

Pilot studies by several research groups have suggested that subtle leakage of radiological contrast, presumably reflecting a loss of vascular integrity with dysfunction of the blood–brain barrier, is associated with cerebral small vessel disease [54–56]. Because CMBs also presumably reflect a loss of vascular integrity, it will be of great interest to compare measures of vascular permeability in those with and without CMBs.

Retinal vascular imaging

A frustrating limitation of research on cerebral small vessel disease is that the vessels themselves cannot be directly imaged in humans in vivo using neuroimaging. Visualization of these small vessels along a significant portion of their course is even challenging in neuropathological studies, unless very thin sections are used. Retinal vascular imaging, however, allows visualization of small arteries and veins along a long portion of their course.

The retina contains layers of neural cells that process information and functionally and neuroanatomically can be considered similar to cerebral tissue. It is possible that the vasculature of the retina may share some characteristics with the vasculature of the brain. Research studies support this, by showing that retinal vascular abnormalities are associated with cerebral lesions attributed to cerebral small vessel disease, such as WML and lacunar infarcts. To our knowledge, only the population-based AGES-Reykjavik study has investigated the relationship between retinal vascular changes and the likelihood of CMBs [57]. Retinal focal arteriolar narrowing, arteriovenous nicking and microaneurysms or microhemorrhages were associated with an increased prevalence of multiple CMBs, with adjusted odds ratios ranging from 1.5 to 1.8. These data suggest that the eye is a window through which we can directly observe a vascular bed that may be undergoing similar changes as the cerebral vasculature.

Molecular imaging

Molecular imaging is a promising technique by which the tissue distribution of molecules of interest may be imaged using high-affinity tagged ligands for that molecule. The development of high-affinity ligands that cross the blood–brain barrier has, however, been a challenge. One exception where molecular brain imaging has already impacted neurological research, if not yet clinical practice, is cerebral beta-amyloid imaging. Pittsburgh compound B (PIB) has been shown to bind to fibrillar beta-amyloid deposits in both the brain and the vascular media in pathology studies, and this is also shown when radiolabeled PIB is imaged using PET [58,59]. In vivo studies confirm that patients with clinical probable CAA, based on validated research criteria, show evidence of PIB retention on PET [60,61]. Additional larger studies will be needed to investigate the global and regional relationship between PIB retention and the presence and number of CMBs in CAA.

Conclusions and directions for future study

Cerebral microbleeds are more frequent in patients with neuroimaging findings of WML and lacunar infarctions. By contrast, CMBs are not independently associated with brain atrophy, probably because the actual tissue damage directly caused by CMBs is minimal. These observations are consistent with the concept that CMBs are one of several neuroimaging markers of small vessel arterial disease. Because the presence and number of CMBs cannot be entirely predicted by other markers, it seems likely that CMBs represent a dimension of arterial disease that is not entirely captured by other markers. Cerebral microbleeds must represent some loss of vascular integrity, because pathology studies show that CMBs represent perivascular hemosiderin deposits, presumably resulting from leakage of red blood cells through the vessel wall. A tempting hypothesis is that CMBs are a marker of vascular integrity, conferring increased risk of subsequent bleeding, while WML and lacunar infarcts are a marker of vascular stenosis, occlusion or smooth muscle cell dysfunction, resulting in ischemia. However, this idea is likely to be an oversimplification, since smooth muscle disruption is also a major mechanism for microhemorrhage or microaneurysm formation (see Ch. 1). Moreover, microbleed burden in CAA seems to increase the risk of small silent ischemic lesions [28]. Additional larger MRI–pathology correlation studies are clearly needed to better understand the relationship between these neuroimaging findings and specific features of the vessel wall pathology. Molecular neuroimaging could eventually be another means of investigating the molecular changes in the vessel wall that are associated with small vessel disease and CMBs, if relevant compounds can be developed. For molecules that are expressed on the extracerebral side of the blood–brain barrier, the chemical challenge of engineering a compound that crosses the blood–brain barrier can be avoided.

The "neuroimaging toolkit" for investigation of cerebral small vessel disease seems likely to expand in the future. Diffusion, perfusion and vascular permeability imaging all show promise but have not yet been widely incorporated into clinical and research practice. As the most promising of these modalities enter clinical and research practice, it will be important to investigate correlations between them and CMBs, particularly using the most sensitive methods for microbleed detection.

There is a need for more studies that incorporate multimodality information and longitudinal changes over time. As noted throughout this chapter, CMBs represent only one of several neuroimaging findings in small vessel disease. Yet many previous studies have investigated the relationship between isolated single imaging measurements, such as CMBs, and clinical events, without simultaneously considering the relationship with other neuroimaging findings. The clinical utility of identifying CMBs rests largely on whether CMBs offer additional predictive information for clinical events beyond that which can be obtained from other neuroimaging markers.

To guide medical care it will be important to understand whether CMBs predict future clinical events including brain macrohemorrhages. If CMBs predict future events, then there is an opportunity to select patients at high risk and offer therapies that might prevent future events. In addition to longitudinal follow-up for clinical events, there is a need for studies with longitudinal follow-up for changes in neuroimaging markers. It is possible that change in the number of CMBs over time is more predictive of subsequent clinical events than a one-time measurement [62]. Additionally, longitudinal studies may inform our understanding of cause and effect relationships between multiple neuroimaging markers including CMBs, WML and brain atrophy.

Finally, there is a need for more comprehensive analysis of neuroimaging markers of small vessel disease across the whole brain, including the investigation of within-patient regional correlations between different markers. As an example, a study in CAA showed that CMBs are non-randomly distributed throughout the brain and tend to cluster in brain regions where intraparenchymal hematomas are subsequently more likely to occur [63]. There is also a need to investigate the within-patient regional relationships between CMB and other markers of small vessel disease in order to improve our understanding of the biological relationships between different aspects of small vessel disease.

References

1. Roob G, Schmidt R, Kapeller P et al. MRI evidence of past cerebral microbleeds in a healthy elderly population. *Neurology* 1999;**52**:991–4.

2. Vernooij MW, van der Lugt A, Ikram MA et al. Prevalence and risk factors of cerebral microbleeds: the Rotterdam Scan Study. *Neurology* 2008;**70**:1208–14.

3. Cordonnier C, Al-Shahi Salman R, Wardlaw J. Spontaneous brain microbleeds: systematic review, subgroup analyses and standards for study design and reporting. *Brain* 2007;**130**:1988–2003.

4. Viswanathan A, Chabriat H. Cerebral microhemorrhage. *Stroke* 2006;**37**:550–5.

5. Fan YH, Mok VC, Lam WW et al. Cerebral microbleeds and white matter changes in patients hospitalized with lacunar infarcts. *J Neurol* 2004;**251**:537–41.

6. Imaizumi T, Horita Y, Chiba M et al. Dot-like hemosiderin spots on gradient echo T_2*-weighted magnetic resonance imaging are associated with past history of small vessel disease in patients with intracerebral hemorrhage. *J Neuroimaging* 2004;**14**:251–7.

7. Lee SH, Bae HJ, Kwon SJ et al. Cerebral microbleeds are regionally associated with intracerebral hemorrhage. *Neurology* 2004;**62**:72–6.

8. Lee SH, Kwon SJ, Kim KS et al. Cerebral microbleeds in patients with hypertensive stroke. Topographical distribution in the supratentorial area. *J Neurol* 2004;**251**:1183–9.

9. Imaizumi T, Honma T, Horita Y et al. Dot-like hemosiderin spots are associated with past hemorrhagic strokes in patients with lacunar infarcts. *J Neuroimaging* 2005;**15**:157–63.

10. Werring DJ, Coward LJ, Losseff NA et al. Cerebral microbleeds are common in ischemic stroke but rare in TIA. *Neurology* 2005;**65**:1914–18.

11. Cho AH, Lee SB, Han SJ et al. Impaired kidney function and cerebral microbleeds in patients with acute ischemic stroke. *Neurology* 2009;**73**:1645–8.

12. Alemany M, Stenborg A, Terent A et al. Coexistence of microhemorrhages and acute spontaneous brain hemorrhage: correlation with signs of microangiopathy and clinical data. *Radiology* 2006;**238**:240–7.

13. Ovbiagele B, Saver JL, Sanossian N et al. Predictors of cerebral microbleeds in acute ischemic stroke and TIA patients. *Cerebrovasc Dis* 2006;**22**:378–83.

14. Jeon SB, Kang DW, Cho AH et al. Initial microbleeds at MR imaging can predict recurrent intracerebral hemorrhage. *J Neurol* 2007;**254**:508–12.

15. Han J, Gao P, Lin Y et al. Three-tesla magnetic resonance imaging study of cerebral microbleeds in patients with ischemic stroke. *Neurolog Res* 2009;**31**:900–3.

16. Orken DN, Kenangil G, Uysal E et al. Cerebral microbleeds in ischemic stroke patients on warfarin treatment. *Stroke* 2009;**40**:3638–40.

17. Staals J, van Oostenbrugge RJ, Knottnerus IL et al. Brain microbleeds relate to higher ambulatory blood pressure levels in first-ever lacunar stroke patients. *Stroke* 2009;**40**:3264–8.

18. Sun J, Soo YO, Lam WW et al. Different distribution patterns of cerebral microbleeds in acute ischemic stroke patients with and without hypertension. *Eur Neurol* 2009;**62**:298–303.

19. Kato H, Izumiyama M, Izumiyama K et al. Silent cerebral microbleeds on T_2*-weighted MRI: correlation with stroke subtype, stroke recurrence, and leukoaraiosis. *Stroke* 2002;**33**:1536–40.

20. Greenberg SM, Vernooij MW, Cordonnier C et al. Cerebral microbleeds: a guide to detection and interpretation. *Lancet Neurol* 2009;**8**:165–74.

21. Adams HP, Jr., Bendixen BH, Kappelle LJ et al. Classification of subtype of acute ischemic stroke. Definitions for use in a multicenter clinical trial. TOAST. Trial of Org 10172 in Acute Stroke Treatment. *Stroke* 1993;**24**:35–41.

22. Bamford J, Sandercock P, Dennis M et al. Classification and natural history of clinically identifiable subtypes of cerebral infarction. *Lancet* 1991;**337**:1521–6.

23. Gao T, Wang Y, Zhang Z. Silent cerebral microbleeds on susceptibility-weighted imaging of patients with ischemic stroke and leukoaraiosis. *Neurolog Res* 2008;**30**:272–6.

24. Wardlaw JM, Lewis SC, Keir SL *et al.* Cerebral microbleeds are associated with lacunar stroke defined clinically and radiologically, independently of white matter lesions. *Stroke* 2006;**37**:2633–6.

25. Lee SH, Bae HJ, Ko SB *et al.* Comparative analysis of the spatial distribution and severity of cerebral microbleeds and old lacunes. *J Neurol Neurosurg Psychiatry* 2004;**75**:423–7.

26. Knudsen KA, Rosand J, Karluk D *et al.* Clinical diagnosis of cerebral amyloid angiopathy: validation of the Boston criteria. *Neurology* 2001;**56**:537–9.

27. Haglund M, Passant U, Sjobeck M *et al.* Cerebral amyloid angiopathy and cortical microinfarcts as putative substrates of vascular dementia. *Int J Geriatr Psychiatry* 2006;**21**:681–7.

28. Kimberly WT, Gilson A, Rost NS *et al.* Silent ischemic infarcts are associated with hemorrhage burden in cerebral amyloid angiopathy. *Neurology* 2009;**72**:1230–5.

29. Fazekas F, Kleinert R, Roob G *et al.* Histopathologic analysis of foci of signal loss on gradient-echo T_2*-weighted MR images in patients with spontaneous intracerebral hemorrhage: evidence of microangiopathy-related microbleeds. *AJNR Am J Neuroradiol* 1999;**20**:637–42.

30. Roob G, Lechner A, Schmidt R *et al.* Frequency and location of microbleeds in patients with primary intracerebral hemorrhage. *Stroke* 2000;**31**:2665–9.

31. Smith EE, Nandigam KRN, Chen Y-W *et al.* MRI markers of small vessel disease in lobar and deep hemispheric intracerebral hemorrhage. *Stroke* 2010:**41**:1933–8.

32. Lim JB, Kim E. Silent microbleeds and old hematomas in spontaneous cerebral hemorrhages. *J Korean Neurosurg Soc* 2009;**46**:38–44.

33. Copenhaver BR, Hsia AW, Merino JG *et al.* Racial differences in microbleed prevalence in primary intracerebral hemorrhage. *Neurology* 2008;**71**:1176–82.

34. Lee SH, Kim BJ, Roh JK. Silent microbleeds are associated with volume of primary intracerebral hemorrhage. *Neurology* 2006;**66**:430–2.

35. Imaizumi T, Honma T, Horita Y *et al.* Hematoma size in deep intracerebral hemorrhage and its correlation with dot-like hemosiderin spots on gradient echo T_2*-weighted MRI. *J Neuroimaging* 2006;**16**:236–42.

36. Schmahmann JD, Smith EE, Eichler FS *et al.* Cerebral white matter: neuroanatomy, clinical neurology, and neurobehavioral correlates. *Ann N Y Acad Sci* 2008; **1142**:266–309.

37. Jeerakathil T, Wolf PA, Beiser A *et al.* Cerebral microbleeds: prevalence and associations with cardiovascular risk factors in the Framingham Study. *Stroke* 2004;**35**:1831–5.

38. Sveinbjornsdottir S, Sigurdsson S, Aspelund T *et al.* Cerebral microbleeds in the population based AGES–Reykjavik study: prevalence and location. *J Neurol Neurosurg Psychiatry* 2008;**79**:1002–6.

39. Jeon SB, Kwon SU, Cho AH *et al.* Rapid appearance of new cerebral microbleeds after acute ischemic stroke. *Neurology* 2009;**73**:1638–44.

40. Jeong SW, Jung KH, Chu K *et al.* Clinical and radiologic differences between primary intracerebral hemorrhage with and without microbleeds on gradient-echo magnetic resonance images. *Arch Neurol* 2004;**61**:905–9.

41. Smith EE, Gurol ME, Eng JA *et al.* White matter lesions, cognition, and recurrent hemorrhage in lobar intracerebral hemorrhage. *Neurology* 2004;**63**: 1606–12.

42. Maia LF, Vasconcelos C, Seixas S *et al.* Lobar brain hemorrhages and white matter changes: clinical, radiological and laboratorial profiles. *Cerebrovasc Dis* 2006;**22**:155–61.

43. Viswanathan A, Guichard JP, Gschwendtner A *et al.* Blood pressure and haemoglobin A1c are associated with microhaemorrhage in CADASIL: a two-centre cohort study. *Brain* 2006;**129**:2375–83.

44. Dichgans M, Holtmannspotter M, Herzog J *et al.* Cerebral microbleeds in CADASIL: a gradient-echo magnetic resonance imaging and autopsy study. *Stroke* 2002;**33**:67–71.

45. Cordonnier C, van der Flier WM, Sluimer JD *et al.* Prevalence and severity of microbleeds in a memory clinic setting. *Neurology* 2006;**66**:1356–60.

46. Pettersen JA, Sathiyamoorthy G, Gao FQ *et al.* Microbleed topography, leukoaraiosis, and cognition in probable Alzheimer disease from the Sunnybrook dementia study. *Arch Neurol* 2008;**65**:790–5.

47. Goos JD, Kester MI, Barkhof F *et al.* Patients with Alzheimer disease with multiple microbleeds: relation with cerebrospinal fluid biomarkers and cognition. *Stroke* 2009;**40**:3455–60.

48. van Es AC, van der Grond J, de Craen AJ *et al.* Risk factors for cerebral microbleeds in the elderly. *Cerebrovasc Dis* 2008;**26**:397–403.

49. Jouvent E, Viswanathan A, Mangin JF *et al.* Brain atrophy is related to lacunar lesions and tissue microstructural changes in CADASIL. *Stroke* 2007; **38**:1786–90.

50. Romero JM, Schaefer PW, Grant PE *et al.* Diffusion MR imaging of acute ischemic stroke. *Neuroimaging Clin North Am* 2002;**12**:35–53.

51. Pierpaoli C, Jezzard P, Basser PJ *et al.* Diffusion tensor MR imaging of the human brain. *Radiology* 1996;**201**: 637–48.

52. O'Sullivan M, Summers PE, Jones DK *et al.* Normal-appearing white matter in ischemic leukoaraiosis: a diffusion tensor MRI study. *Neurology* 2001;**57**:2307–10.

53. Viswanathan A, Patel P, Rahman R *et al.* Tissue microstructural changes are independently associated with cognitive impairment in cerebral amyloid angiopathy. *Stroke* 2008;**39**:1988–92.

54. Wardlaw JM, Farrall A, Armitage PA *et al.* Changes in background blood–brain barrier integrity between lacunar and cortical ischemic stroke subtypes. *Stroke* 2008;**39**:1327–32.

55. Topakian R, Barrick TR, Howe FA *et al.* Blood–brain barrier permeability is increased in normal-appearing white matter in patients with lacunar stroke and leucoaraiosis. *J Neurol Neurosurg Psychiatry* 2010;**81**: 192–7.

56. Huynh TJ, Murphy B, Pettersen JA *et al.* CT perfusion quantification of small-vessel ischemic severity. *AJNR Am J Neuroradiol* 2008;**29**:1831–6.

57. Qiu C, Cotch MF, Sigurdsson S *et al.* Retinal and cerebral microvascular signs and diabetes: the Age Gene/Environment Susceptibility–Reykjavik study. *Diabetes* 2008;**57**:1645–50.

58. Johnson KA. Amyloid imaging of Alzheimer's disease using Pittsburgh Compound B. *Curr Neurol Neurosci Rep* 2006;**6**:496–503.

59. Lockhart A, Lamb JR, Osredkar T *et al.* PIB is a non-specific imaging marker of amyloid-beta (Abeta) peptide-related cerebral amyloidosis. *Brain* 2007;**130**: 2607–15.

60. Johnson KA, Gregas M, Becker JA *et al.* Imaging of amyloid burden and distribution in cerebral amyloid angiopathy. *Ann Neurol* 2007;**62**: 229–34.

61. Ly JV, Donnan GA, Villemagne VL *et al.* 11C-PIB binding is increased in patients with cerebral amyloid angiopathy-related hemorrhage. *Neurology* 2010;**74**: 487–93.

62. Greenberg SM, Eng JA, Ning M *et al.* Hemorrhage burden predicts recurrent intracerebral hemorrhage after lobar hemorrhage. *Stroke* 2004; **35**:1415–20.

63. Rosand J, Muzikansky A, Kumar A *et al.* Spatial clustering of hemorrhages in probable cerebral amyloid angiopathy. *Ann Neurol* 2005;**58**: 459–62.

Chapter

9

Cerebral microbleeds in healthy populations

Bo Norrving

Introduction

In order to prevent and treat non-communicable diseases adequately, it is important to understand the full spectrum of stages from the earliest asymptomatic phases, detectable only by special techniques, to early signs and more advanced stages of the disease. For cerebrovascular diseases, knowledge on this spectrum has advanced considerably during the last few decades. It was previously thought that the majority of vascular lesions in the brain presented with acute focal neurological symptoms and that patients were usually diagnosed in emergency wards. Although silent brain infarcts had been previously described by neuropathologists, it nevertheless came as a surprise finding that they were at least fivefold more common in the general population than brain lesions presenting as acute transient ischemic attacks (TIAs) or strokes [1,2]. During the last few decades the discovery of high prevalence of white matter ischemic abnormalities in the general population and the associations of such findings with risks of vascular events have also added importantly to the spectrum of vascular diseases [2].

The latest addition to this spectrum of vascular disease is the discovery of cerebral microbleeds (CMBs) through the advent of gradient-recalled echo (GRE) T_2*-weighted MRI. Although first described as bystanders in patients presenting with acute intraparenchymal brain hemorrhages [3,4], it soon became apparent that CMBs were present also in the general population [5–8]. Other chapters in this section will review features of CMBs in patients with symptomatic cerebrovascular disease and in various other clinical settings.

This chapter summarizes the current knowledge on prevalence and characteristics of CMBs in nor-

mal individuals. The most solid current knowledge comes from reports from four population-based studies, although several other studies have reported findings in persons recruited in other ways, for example hospital-based selections and through screening programmes for asymptomatic brain diseases. Findings from all of these types of study are summarized below. The chapter does not include reports on small lesions in normal individuals included as control groups in studies focusing on CMBs in patients with stroke or dementia [9–12], patients without stroke but with other neurological disorders or symptoms [13], mix of patients with stroke and patients with other diseases [14], and patients with cognitive symptoms [15].

Population-based studies on prevalence of cerebral microbleeds in normal individuals

The four population-based studies with reported findings on CMBs in normal individuals are the Austrian Stroke Prevention Study (ASPS; [16]), the Framingham Study [17], the Age Gene/Environment Susceptibility (AGES)-Reykjavik study (AGES-R; [18]) and the Rotterdam Scan Study [19]. The principal features and findings in the studies are summarized in Table 9.1; the MRI methods and definitions of microbleeds used are summarized in Table 9.2.

The Austrian Stroke Prevention Study

The first population-based study to report on prevalence of CMBs in normal individuals was the

---

Cerebral Microbleeds, ed. David J. Werring. Published by Cambridge University Press. © Cambridge University Press 2011.

Table 9.1 Prevalence of cerebral microbleeds in normal individuals

Cohort	No.	Mean age (years)	Prevalence of CMB (No. [%])	Associations with risk factors and other conditions
Population-based studies				
Austrian Stroke Prevention Study [16]	280	60	18 (6.4)	Association with age and chronic hypertension
Framingham Study [17]	472	64.4	22 (4.7)	Strong association with age, male sex
AGES-Reykjavik study [18]	1962	76	218 (11.1)	Association with age, sex, *APOE ε4*
Rotterdam Scan Study [19]	1062	69.6	250 (23.5)	Associations with several risk factors, *APOE*, genotype and localization of CMBs
Other study types				
Annual medical check-up at hospital [20]	450	52.9	14 (3.1)	Association with hypertension, smoking
Self-paid screen for asymptomatic brain diseases [14]	1718	NA	64 (3.7)	Not specifically reported for non-stroke subgroup
"Healthy volunteers" [21]	209	56	16 (7.7)	Associated with age and hypertension
Persons wishing to undergo health screening (MRI) [22]	518	56.7	35 (6.8)	Association with mmT
Hypertensives evaluated with 24 h blood pressure monitoring [23]	218	52.5	35 (16.1)	Association with higher day-time and night-time blood pressure

CMB, cerebral microbleed; NA, not available.

Table 9.2 Protocols for MRI, inter-rater agreement and definitions of cerebral microbleeds used in population-based studies in normal individuals

Study	MRI	Inter-rater agreement (kappa value)	Definition of CMB
Austrian Stroke Prevention Study [16]	1.5 T, TR 600–800 ms, TE 16–20 ms, flip angle 20°, slice thickness 5 mm, interslice gap 10%	0.4–0.65	2–5 mm
Framingham Study [17]	1.0 T, TR 760 ms, TE 26 ms, flip angle 30°, slice thickness 5 mm, interslice gap 0.5 mm	0.33–0.57	<10 mm
AGES-Reykjavik study [18]	1.5 T, TR 3050 ms, TE 50 ms, flip angle 90°, slice thickness 3 mm, matrix 256 × 256, FOV 220 mm	0.71–0.73	No size limit
Rotterdam Scan Study [19]	1.5 T, high-resolution 3-dimensional T_2*-weighted GRE sequence; TR 45 ms; TE 31 ms, flip angle 13°, slice thickness 1.6 mm, matrix size 320 × 224	0.85–0.87	<10 mm

CMB, cerebral microbleed; TR, repetition time; TE, echo time; GRE, gradient recalled echo; FOV, field of view.

ASPS [16], a prospective study from a single center (Graz) in which individuals with no history of neuropsychiatric diseases (including any type of cerebrovascular disease) were randomly selected from the official population registry. Subjects underwent a structured clinical interview, physical and neurological examination, blood pressure recordings, electrocardiography, echocardiography and laboratory testing. Out of 1998 persons who initially entered the study, every fourth person was invited to a second phase that included MRI and neuropsychiatric testing. Imaging was performed in 458 persons, 89% of those invited. Three years later, these persons were invited for a second MRI (1.5 T), which this time also included a GRE T_2*-weighted sequence. The study finally included 280 individuals (149 men, 131 women) with a mean age of 60 years (range, 44–79).

Cerebral microbleeds were found in 18 (6.4%) of the 280 individuals. The frequency of CMBs ranged from 1 to 5 with a mean of 2.5. The locations of CMBs were cortico-subcortical in ten subjects, basal ganglia/thalamic in six and infratentorial in three.

More severe white matter hyperintensities and silent lacunar infarcts were found in those with CMBs who also were older and more often hypertensive. Overall, 72% of those with CMBs had chronic hypertension, which appeared to be related to CMB location; all seven individuals with CMBs in the basal ganglia had hypertension whereas only five of ten with cortico-subcortical CMBs had hypertension.

The Framingham Study

The Framingham Study of prevalence of CMBs in normal individuals [17] was based on participants in the original cohort and the offspring cohort, who were invited for a follow-up visit that included detailed risk factor surveillance, MRI at 1.0 T and determination of *APOE* genotype. Data on CMBs were available for 472 persons, which constituted 10.7% of the total Framingham cohort. The mean age of the study sample of 472 subjects was 64.4 years; 213 were men and 259 were women.

The prevalence of CMBs in the entire cohort was 4.7% (22 of 472). However, the prevalence was strongly related to age: among subjects >75 years, prevalence was 12.6% compared with only 2.2% among those <75 years. There was also a difference in CMB prevalence between men and women: 7.0% in men and 2.7% in women. Sixteen patients (73%) had lesions in the cerebral cortex or subcortical white matter, five had lesions in the basal ganglia or thalamus, and three had posterior fossa lesions. Eighteen of those with CMBs had single lesions whereas four had multiple CMBs, ranging from three to seven.

With respect to risk factors, those with CMBs had significantly higher mean age, systolic blood pressure and were mainly male in univariate comparisons. In logistic regression, age and male sex remained significantly related to CMBs after adjustment for each other, but systolic blood pressure was no longer significant after age and sex adjustments. There were no relations found between CMBs and other risk factors.

This study also analyzed the relationship with CMBs and *APOE* because a link between cerebral amyloid angiopathy (CAA) and CMBs had been established from previous studies. However, no significant associations between *APOE* status and CMBs were found, even if analyses were restricted to subjects with cortico-subcortical lesions only; however, the authors acknowledged the possibility of type II errors in these analyses.

Total cerebral brain volume was lower in persons with CMBs in crude analyses, but not after adjusted analyses. The quantity of white matter hyperintensities was higher in subjects with CMBs but no differences remained after adjustment for age and sex.

In summary, the prevalence of CMBs was similar to that found in the ASPS [16], but the Framingham Study showed a striking increase in the prevalence after the age of 75 years and also a higher prevalence in men.

The AGES-Reykjavik study

The AGES-R study [18] resulted from the Reykjavik Study, which was initiated in 1967 by the Icelandic Heart Association to study cardiovascular disease and risk factors. The cohort included men and women born between 1907 and 1935. Re-examination of surviving members of the cohort was initiated in 2002. The report included data on 1962 subjects out of a total of 2300 invited, who were examined with a questionnaire, clinical examination, laboratory testing and MRI acquired on 1.5 T equipment. The MRI data were missing for 14.7% of the sample, mainly through contraindications or barriers for examination of a practical cause. The study included a small proportion (169 subjects, 8.7% of the cohort) with self-reported history of stroke or TIA. The mean age of the cohort was 76 years (range, 66–93).

Cerebral microbleeds were detected in 218 (11.1%) of the 1962 subjects. The prevalence of CMBs significantly increased with age in both sexes. However, the prevalence of CMBs was significantly higher in men (14.4%) than in women (8.8%). Median size of the CMBs was 6 mm; 9% were larger than 10 mm in diameter. Microbleed size did not correlate with sex, age or location, neither in analyses including all CMBs nor in analyses confined to CMBs ≤10 mm. The size of the bleed was positively associated with hyperpertension, but this significance dropped when bleeds >10 mm were removed.

Associations with the presence of CMBs were borderline significant for diabetes and hypertension (and significant for previous TIA or stroke); adjusting for these variables did not change the strong associations found with age and sex. The presence of CMB was significantly associated with homozygote *APOE ε4* genotype.

Among subjects with CMBs, 61% had one CMB, 18% had two, 9% had four, 12% had 4–22, and 1.4% had ≥30. Among the 87% of subjects who had <30 CMBs, 61% of the lesions were localized to the cortical or subcortical cerebral hemispheres; 6% had lesions in the basal ganglia, and 19% had infratentorial lesions. In 10% of subjects, CMBs occurred in two regions of the brain and in 3% they occurred in three regions. Over one-third of all lesions were located in the parietal–occipital lobes and 24% were in the frontal lobes; 15.7% of all lesions were cerebellar and 10.4% were localized to the basal ganglia.

In summary, the AGES-R study showed a significant association of CMBs with age, and a higher prevalence in men. An association with homozygosity for *APOE ε4* allele was also found. The AGES-R study was four to six times larger than the Framingham Study or the ASPS [16,17], and an important difference was that subjects were much older, with a mean age 11–16 years higher than in those two studies. Rates of CMBs in AGES-R compared with those found in persons >75 years of age in the Framingham Study [17].

The Rotterdam Scan Study

The report from the Rotterdam Study [19] is based on subjects randomly selected from the Rotterdam Study Plus cohort, who were invited to the Rotterdam Scan Study as an addition to subjects who had undergone MRI (without sequences for detection of CMBs) in a previous round of the Rotterdam Scan Study. Of 1229 eligible persons, 1114 (91%) participated; complete MRI data were available for 1062 of these. Mean age was 69.6 years and 51% were women. Imaging was performed with a 1.5 T scanner with a sequence optimized to increase the conspicuity of CMBs.

The overall prevalence of CMBs was 23.5% and increased with age from 17.8% in persons aged 60–69 years to 38.3% in those >80 years. No difference in the prevalence between men and women was noted.

Of 250 patients with CMBs, 146 had strictly lobar CMBs, which were multiple in 44 subjects. In 104, the CMBs were located in a deep or intratentorial position and 58 of these also had one or more lobar CMBs.

High systolic blood pressure, high pulse pressure and smoking were associated with presence of CMBs in a deep or infratentorial location; this association was even stronger after exclusion of persons who also had lobar CMBs. The prevalence of CMBs decreased with increasing serum total cholesterol, and the study also reported a strong correlation with very low cholesterol (defined as the 10% lowest percentile) and strictly lobar CMBs.

Lacunar infarcts and white matter lesions volume were strongly associated with CMBs in a deep or infratentorial location but not with CMBs with a lobar location.

The Rotterdam Study found that carriers of the *APOE ε4* allele had CMBs significantly more often in a lobar location, and this finding was even more pronounced for persons with strictly lobar CMBs. They did not find an association with *ε2/ε2* genotype overall, but this association was present in subjects with strictly lobar CMBs, although based on few observations.

In summary, the prevalence of CMBs found in the Rotterdam Study is markedly higher than in previous studies, presumably because it used optimized MRI sequence to detect CMBs. Although the number of subjects was only half that in the AGES-R study [18], the absolute number of subjects with CMBs was higher, increasing the statistical power for correlative analyses. The Rotterdam Study demonstrated stronger associations between localization of CMBs and presumed etiologies than previous studies.

An interesting secondary analysis from the Rotterdam Study examined the relationship between use of antithrombotic drugs and the presence of CMBs [24]. Use of antithrombotic drugs was determined by cross-linking the population of the Rotterdam Study with pharmacy databases 14–15 years back in time. Prescriptions of antiplatelet drugs (aspirin and carbasalate calcium) were analyzed with respect to dosage suggesting use for treatment of pain or prevention of cerebrovascular and cardiac events. The authors were careful in considering confounding by indication (i.e. that findings were related to the underlying vascular diseases for which antithrombotics were prescribed, rather than to the drugs per se). The study showed that the presence of CMBs was more frequent among users of antiplatelet drugs than among non-users (odds ratio, 1.71), whereas a significant association between use of anticoagulants and CMBs was not detected. Strictly lobar CMBs were more prevalent among aspirin users than among persons using carbasalate calcium. This study is the first to suggest that use of antiplatelet drugs, in particular aspirin, may promote CMBs, in particular lobar CMBs, and contribute to an increased risk for symptomatic intracerebral hemorrhage. The possible relations between presence of CMBs and the use of antithrombotic drugs for secondary preventive purposes are discussed in Ch. 19.

Other studies on prevalence of cerebral microbleeds in normal individuals

A pioneering study from Japan (chronologically the second report in normal individuals) studied the prevalence of CMBs in 450 neurologically healthy Japanese adults with a mean age of 52.9 years [20]. The overall incidence was 3.1% (14/450), and lesions detected were closely related to hypertension and heavy cigarette smoking.

Another very large study from this group in Japan reviewed GRE MRI of more than 2000 patients aged from <1 to 96 years, 1718 of these had no history of stroke according to their medical report [14]. The recruitment of younger subjects might account for the overall low prevalence of CMBs in this study (3.7%) since almost no CMBs were detected in subjects under age 40. However, no separate studies on relations with age and hypertension were reported among the proportion free from previous stroke.

A further Japanese study (reported in Japanese only but with an English abstract) reported the prevalence of CMBs among 209 healthy volunteers (mean age 56 years) examined by MRI as part of a self-paid screening to detect asymptomatic brain diseases [21]. Cerebral microbleeds were detected in 7.7% of the cohort, and their presence was related to age, hypertension and headache.

Finally, another Japanese study reported associations between CMBs and global cognitive function in adults without a neurological disorder who had undergone health screening tests of the brain at their own expense [22]. The prevalence of CMBs among 518 subjects with a mean age of 56.7 years was 6.8% (35 subjects). The study suggested a relationship between presence and number of CMBs and global cognitive function as assessed by the Mini-Mental State Examination.

In a Dutch study of patients referred for 24-hour ambulatory blood pressure monitoring as part of evaluation of hypertension, CMBs were detected in 35 of 218 participants (16.1%), with a mean age of 52.5 years [23].

Comments

Summary of findings on cerebral microbleeds in normal individuals

The first studies on prevalence of CMBs in normal individuals indicated that the prevalence was quite low, for example 6.4% in the ASPS [16] and 4.7% in the Framingham Study [17]. However, one major reason for these relatively low proportions was the quite young age groups included. Later population-based studies have shown a higher prevalence in higher age groups; 11.1% in the AGES-R study [18] with a mean age of 76 years. Almost twice as high values were reported from the Rotterdam Study [19], which most likely reflects the MRI characteristics used (see below). Overall, the prevalence pattern of CMBs is quite similar to the general prevalence pattern of cerebrovascular disease with respect to age and sex.

Relations to vascular risk factors also largely fit into the pattern of cerebrovascular disease in general, with most studies showing associations with age, male sex and elevated blood pressure. However, the risk factor pattern appears to be related to localization of the CMBs.

It has been suggested that, in analogy to CMBs in the cerebral lobes being an indication of underlying CAA, CMBs located in the basal ganglia may reflect hypertensive or atherosclerotic disease. Overall the patterns and associations found in studies in the normal population support these hypotheses, which mainly have been derived from studies in patients with intracerebral hemorrhage. This issue is further discussed in Chs. 12 and 15.

Carriage of *APOE ε4* allele is presumed to lead to hemorrhage by increased vascular deposition of beta-amyloid. There are also thoughts that *APOE ε2* may accelerate the development of vasculopathies leading to hemorrhage of amyloid-laden vessels in CAA. Among studies in normal individuals, a relationship with *APOE* status has only been demonstrated in the Rotterdam Study [19], which may reflect the fact that this study had a much higher absolute number of subjects with CMBs and hence an increased statistical power to detect an association.

Generalizability of findings from currently available studies

The most solid knowledge on CMBs comes from the population-based studies, in particular those that have included also higher age groups and have used a sensitive technique to detect CMBs. For several studies that are not population based, the external validity is uncertain: several studies are based on those examined with MRI at their own expense as part of screening for asymptomatic brain disease, which inevitably creates a selection bias from socioeconomical aspects.

Because of the differences in methodology, comparisons between the population-based studies and studies using other sampling methods are difficult. All the population-based cohorts were restricted to a predominantly white, middle-class population with little ethnic diversity, whereas in Asian populations, other sampling methods were used. Therefore, currently available data on possible differences between regions is limited, and no firm conclusions can be made. Epidemiology of stroke incidence, stroke mortality and time trends is highly varied between geographical regions [25]. Patterns of risk factors and comorbidities are also different between regions, and one can assume that such factors should also affect prevalence rates of CMBs.

Method issues in detecting microbleeds

Recent studies have also highlighted the importance of hardware and software used in the sensitivity to detect CMBs, which needs to be considered as a background in all comparative analyses between studies [4]. As can be seen in Table 9.2, highly variable MRI techniques have been used in different studies. Technical issues of imaging are further discussed in Chs. 2–5.

With respect to lesion size, a diameter of 2–5 mm was applied in some studies; other studies set the upper limit to 10 mm, and yet other studies lacked a specific definition of CMB by size (Table 9.2). It should be noted that size of the lesion on MRI does not reflect the actual lesion size but rather the distortion of the magnetic field by the hemosiderin deposit.

Another methodological issue is the degree of subjectivity in the interpretation of CMBs, demonstrated in different levels of kappa values between raters in different studies. Use of a specified rating scale is an additional means to improve inter-rater agreement on CMBs [26,27].

Cerebral microbleeds: part of the spectrum of small vessel disease in the brain

Recent studies have changed our concepts of symptomatic and silent small vessel disease in the brain and CMBs should be regarded as part of the spectrum of covert small vessel brain disease, in which each component has somewhat different implications. The presence of CMBs may be a direct marker of bleeding-prone small vessel disease.

Recent studies have highlighted the importance of the total burden of small vessel disease in the brain as an important prognostic determinant. Cerebral small vessel disease is a much more active, dynamic process

than the simplistic commonly held stroke paradigm of risk factors → infarct → disability. There is a growing body of evidence that vascular risk factors and extent of asymptomatic small vessel disease (silent infarcts and white matter ischemic abnormalities) at the time of the index stroke have significant prognostic implications for almost all outcomes [28]. The role of CMBs in these aspects is discussed in other chapters of this book.

Conclusions and directions for further studies

Studies on CMBs in different settings have added important new knowledge to our understanding of the full picture of silent cerebrovascular disease in the brain. Although data are now available from quite large population-based studies, several aspects on the importance of CMBs are still incomplete.

Cerebral microbleeds are snap shots of the brain of something that has happened in the past. They appear to be the effect of small old hemorrhages, but the published reports on pathological studies of CMBs from autopsy specimens is limited to less than 20 persons [8,29]. Further autopsy studies are clearly warranted. Hemosiderin deposits remain visible in the brain for an undetermined period and there is little information on when the bleeds actually occurred. There is an urgent need for longitudinal data to answer a number of questions. How do CMBs evolve with time? In what way are CMBs a risk factor for later strokes (in particular brain hemorrhage), other types of vascular event or cognitive decline/dementia? Similar data have become available on silent brain infarcts [2,30] and have provided important new insights into the importance of this type of silent small vessel disease: corresponding data for CMBs are urgently needed. Studies on associations with other types which target organ damage elsewhere in the body are also warranted [31].

Further studies are currently underway regarding the genetics of CMBs, besides the associations with *APOE* detected in some studies.

Another important aspect is whether CMBs in the general population (as well as in specific patient groups) can be prevented. Despite the knowledge on silent brain infarcts and leukoaraiosis that has accumulated since the 1970s, very little is known on this issue. Studies on preventive aspects of CMBs should likely include also effects on progression of silent infarcts and leukoaraiosis, along with robust clinical outcome events to support progress in this area [32].

References

1. Vermeer SE, Longstreth WT, Jr., Koudstaal PJ. Silent brain infarcts: a systematic review. *Lancet Neurol* 2007;**6**:611–19.

2. Norrving B. Chapter 33, "Silent" cerebral infarcts and microbleeds. *Handb Clin Neurol* 2008;**93**:667–81.

3. Offenbacher H, Fazekas F, Schmidt R *et al*. MR of cerebral abnormalities concomitant with primary intracerebral hematomas. *AJNR Am J Neuroradiol* 1996;**17**:573–8.

4. Greenberg SM, Vernooij MW, Cordonnier C *et al*. Cerebral microbleeds: a guide to detection and interpretation. *Lancet Neurol* 2009;**8**:165–74.

5. Koennecke HC. Cerebral microbleeds on MRI: prevalence, associations, and potential clinical implications. *Neurology* 2006;**66**:165–71.

6. Viswanathan A, Chabriat H. Cerebral microhemorrhage. *Stroke* 2006;**37**:550–5.

7. Fiehler J. Cerebral microbleeds: old leaks and new haemorrhages. *Int J Stroke* 2006;**1**:122–30.

8. Cordonnier C, Al-Shahi Salman R, Wardlaw J. Spontaneous brain microbleeds: systematic review, subgroup analyses and standards for study design and reporting. *Brain* 2007;**130**:1988–2003.

9. Kinoshita T, Okudera T, Tamura H, Ogawa T, Hatazawa J. Assessment of lacunar hemorrhage associated with hypertensive stroke by echo-planar gradient-echo T_2*-weighted MRI. *Stroke* 2000;**31**:1646–50.

10. Kato H, Izumiyama M, Izumiyama K, Takahashi A, Itoyama Y. Silent cerebral microbleeds on T_2*-weighted MRI: correlation with stroke subtype, stroke recurrence, and leukoaraiosis. *Stroke* 2002;**33**:1536–40.

11. Hanyu H, Tanaka Y, Shimizu S, Takasaki M, Abe K. Cerebral microbleeds in Alzheimer's disease. *J Neurol* 2003;**250**:1496–7.

12. Lee SH, Bae HJ, Ko SB *et al*. Comparative analysis of the spatial distribution and severity of cerebral microbleeds and old lacunes. *J Neurol Neurosurg Psychiatry* 2004;**75**:423–7.

13. Lee SH, Bae HJ, Yoon BW *et al*. Low concentration of serum total cholesterol is associated with multifocal signal loss lesions on gradient-echo magnetic resonance imaging: analysis of risk factors for multifocal signal loss lesions. *Stroke* 2002;**33**:2845–9.

14. Tsushima Y, Aoki J, Endo K. Brain microhemorrhages detected on T_2*-weighted gradient-echo MR images. *AJNR Am J Neuroradiol* 2003;**24**:88–96.

15. Cordonnier C, van der Flier WM, Sluimer JD *et al*. Prevalence and severity of microbleeds in a memory clinic setting. *Neurology* 2006;**66**:1356–60.

16. Roob G, Schmidt R, Kapeller P *et al*. MRI evidence of past cerebral microbleeds in a healthy elderly population. *Neurology* 1999;**52**:991–4.

17. Jeerakathil T, Wolf PA, Beiser A *et al*. Cerebral microbleeds: prevalence and associations with cardiovascular risk factors in the Framingham Study. *Stroke* 2004;**35**:1831–5.

18. Sveinbjornsdottir S, Sigurdsson S, Aspelund T *et al*. Cerebral microbleeds in the population based AGES–Reykjavik study: prevalence and location. *J Neurol Neurosurg Psychiatry* 2008;**79**:1002–6.

19. Vernooij MW, van der Lugt A, Ikram MA *et al*. Prevalence and risk factors of cerebral microbleeds: the Rotterdam Scan Study. *Neurology* 2008;**70**:1208–14.

20. Tsushima Y, Tanizaki Y, Aoki J, Endo K. MR detection of microhemorrhages in neurologically healthy adults. *Neuroradiology* 2002;**44**:31–6.

21. Horita Y, Imaizumi T, Niwa J *et al*. [Analysis of dot-like hemosiderin spots using brain dock system.] *No Shinkei Geka* 2003;**31**:263–7.

22. Yakushiji Y, Nishiyama M, Yakushiji S *et al*. Brain microbleeds and global cognitive function in adults without neurological disorder. *Stroke* 2008;**39**:3323–8.

23. Henskens LH, van Oostenbrugge RJ, Kroon AA, de Leeuw PW, Lodder J. Brain microbleeds are associated with ambulatory blood pressure levels in a hypertensive population. *Hypertension* 2008;**51**:62–8.

24. Vernooij MW, Haag MD, van der Lugt A *et al*. Use of antithrombotic drugs and the presence of cerebral microbleeds: the Rotterdam Scan Study. *Arch Neurol* 2009;**66**:714–20.

25. Feigin VL, Lawes CM, Bennett DA, Barker-Collo SL, Parag V. Worldwide stroke incidence and early case fatality reported in 56 population-based studies: a systematic review. *Lancet Neurol* 2009;**8**:355–69.

26. Cordonnier C, Potter GM, Jackson CA *et al*. improving interrater agreement about brain microbleeds: development of the Brain Observer MicroBleed Scale (BOMBS). *Stroke* 2009;**40**:94–9.

27. Gregoire SM, Chaudhary UJ, Brown MM *et al*. The Microbleed Anatomical Rating Scale (MARS):

reliability of a tool to map brain microbleeds. *Neurology* 2009;**73**:1759–66.

28. Norrving B. Lacunar infarcts: no black holes in the brain are benign. *Pract Neurol* 2008;**8**:222–8.

29. Fazekas F, Kleinert R, Roob G *et al.* Histopathologic analysis of foci of signal loss on gradient-echo T_2^*-weighted MR images in patients with spontaneous intracerebral hemorrhage: evidence of microangiopathy-related microbleeds. *AJNR Am J Neuroradiol* 1999;**20**:637–42.

30. Vermeer SE, Prins ND, den Heijer T *et al.* Silent brain infarcts and the risk of dementia and cognitive decline. *N Engl J Med* 2003;**348**:1215–22.

31. Thompson CS, Hakim AM. Living beyond our physiological means: small vessel disease of the brain is an expression of a systemic failure in arteriolar function: a unifying hypothesis. *Stroke* 2009;**40**:e322–30.

32. Norrving B. Leucoaraiosis and silent subcortical infarcts. *Rev Neurol (Paris)* 2008;**164**:801–4.

Cerebral microbleeds in relation to cerebrovascular disease

Seung-Hoon Lee and Jae-Kyu Roh

Introduction

Although the history of cerebral microbleeds (CMBs) goes back little more than a decade, interest in CMBs has increased dramatically over the last few years. With a growing body of reports investigating their characteristics and significance, CMBs are now widely recognized to be associated with many types of cerebrovascular disease, including ischemic stroke, intracerebral hemorrhage (ICH), cerebral microangiopathy related to chronic hypertension and cerebral amyloid angiopathy (CAA). A major clinical question is whether CMBs are a marker for an increased risk of subsequent hemorrhagic stroke, particularly in relation to antithrombotic treatments. This chapter provides an overview of the prevalence and associations, temporal evolution and prognostic significance of CMBs in patients with cerebrovascular diseases. Detailed discussions on the specific topics of CMBs in the context of hypertensive arteriopathy and in CAA are presented in Chs. 11 and 12, respectively. The occurrence of CMBs and antithrombotic or thrombolytic treatments are considered further in Chs. 19 and 20.

Prevalence of cerebral microbleeds in cerebrovascular disease cohorts

Although the primary topic of this chapter is CMBs in cerebrovascular diseases, it is helpful to briefly review data on their prevalence in healthy populations for comparison. In healthy populations, CMBs were found in 5.7% of individuals in four studies involving participants in health screening programmes [1–5]. In these studies, the mean age of the participants was around 60

years and the prevalence of hypertension was relatively lower than that in established stroke cohorts. Recently, the result of population-based Rotterdam Scan Study was published, and CMBs were demonstrated in 17.8% of those aged 60–69 years, 31.3% of those aged 70–79 years and 38.3% of those aged 80–97 years [6]. In the Rotterdam Scan Study, a few subjects with MRI-proven infarct were included and the mean age of participants was 69.6 years ($\pm$7.2). Noteworthy in this study was the dose–response relationship between the rate of having multiple CMBs and aging, although such dose dependency was not so prominent in having single or multiple CMBs. Further detailed information on CMBs in normal populations is given in Ch. 9.

As shown in Table 10.1, the prevalence of CMBs in patients with ischemic stroke varies widely, suggestive of heterogeneity of pathology–etiology mechanisms in ischemic stroke, as well as differences in the cohorts studied. Koennecke *et al.* suggested a possible differential role of ethnicity in CMB prevalence, indicating higher prevalence of CMBs among subjects of Asian origin (43%) compared with Caucasian subjects (25%) [1]. However, recently, two publications from East Asia provided relatively lower figures, 29% and 22%, respectively [21,22], so the issue of ethnic difference should be investigated further. Another interesting issue is the association between subtype of ischemic stroke and prevalence of CMBs. Currently, three studies have provided data on detection rate of CMBs according to the subtype of stroke [7,13,18]. In spite of substantial heterogeneity in these three studies, the rate of CMBs in each subtype was as follows; 20% in atherothrombotic stroke, 23% in cardioembolic stroke and 53% in small vessel occlusion. Moreover, it was consistently demonstrated from various studies that the frequency

Table 10.1 Prevalence of cerebral microbleeds in patients with ischemic cerebrovascular diseases

Source	Patient characteristics	No. included patients	Age (years)	Prevalence of CMBs (%)	Associated findings
Kinoshita et al. 2000 [3]	Multiple lacunar infarction with hypertension	68	68.8 (range, 55–88)	65	5% in non-stroke controls
Kato et al. 2002 [7]	Ischemic stroke with variable time point of MRI:	113			Correlation between number of CMBs and severity of white matter hyperintensities
	atherothrombotic stroke	24	74 ± 10	21	
	cardioembolic stroke	23	77 ± 6	30	
	lacunar stroke	66	74 ± 9	62	
Tsushima et al. 2003 [8]	History of ischemic stroke	232	NR	18	71% in hemorrhagic stroke and 3.7% in non-stroke controls
Hanyu et al. 2003 [9]	Multiple lacunar stroke	51	75 ± 7	51	Higher CMB prevalence in so-called Binswanger's disease
Fan et al. 2003 [10]	Consecutive subjects; acute ischemic stroke within 7 days after onset	121	68 ± 11	36	CMBs as a risk factor of subsequent hemorrhagic stroke in survivors
Lee et al. 2004 [11]	Consecutive subjects (admitted 2000–2001); ischemic stroke	113	65 ± 9	65	CMB distribution being quite similar to alleged regional predilection of ICH
Lee et al. 2004 [12]	Consecutive subjects (admitted 1998–1999); acute ischemic stroke	144	65 ± 9	35	Regional association between CMBs and ICH
Naka et al. 2004 [13]	First ever ischemic stroke:	22	69 ± 13	23	CMBs associated with recurrent stroke and leukoaraiosis
	atherothrombotic stroke	13		0	
	cardioembolic stroke	31		23	
	lacunar stroke				
Imaizumi et al. 2004 [14]	Consecutive subjects; lacunar infarction	138	66 ± 9	51	Multiple CMBs (≥3) associated with recurrent events
Schoenwille et al. 2005 [15]	Consecutive subjects; lacunar infarction, MRI within 7 days after onset	68	NR	46	
Werring et al. 2005 [16]	Consecutive subjects; ischemic stroke	86	62 ± 16	23	
	Consecutive subjects; TIA	43	67 ± 9	2	
Boulanger et al. 2006 [17]	Ischemic stroke or TIA	236	NA	19	CMBs being associated with subsequent fatal or disabling stroke
Ovbiagele et al. 2006 [18]	Consecutive subjects with ischemic stroke or TIA:	164	78 (with CMB), 73 (without CMB)	35	
	large vessel disease	40		18	
	small vessel disease	44		61	
	cardioembolism	39		26	
Wardlaw et al. 2006 [19]	Mild stroke (partial anterior, lacunar and posterior circulation syndrome)	241	66 (19–89)	20	CMBs being associated with the clinicoradiological syndrome of lacunar ischemic stroke
Fiehler et al. 2007 [20]	Acute ischemic stroke; MRI within 6 h of onset	570	69 (IQR, 59–77)	15	No incremental symptomatic ICH after thrombolysis in presence of CMBs
Lee et al. 2008 [21]	Acute ischemic stroke with large artery atherosclerosis or cardioembolic stroke	377	66 ± 12	29	No incremental hemorrhagic transformation in presence of CMBs

(cont.)

Table 10.1 (*cont.*)

Source	Patient characteristics	No. included patients	Age (years)	Prevalence of CMBs (%)	Associated findings
Seo *et al.* 2008 [22]	Acute ischemic stroke or TIA	255	64 ± 12	22	CMBs being associated with pulse wave velocity
Cho *et al.* 2009 [23]	Consecutive subjects; acute ischemic stroke	152	67 ± 12	30	CMBs being associated with impaired kidney function
Jeon *et al.* 2009 [24]	Consecutive subjects; acute ischemic stroke, MRI within 24 h of onset	237	64 ± 13	32	Newly appeared CMBs after acute ischemic stroke

CMB, cerbral microbleed; ICH, intracerebral hemorrhage; IQR, interquartile range; NA, not available; TIA, transient ischemic attack.

and extent of CMBs were associated with the severity of white matter hyperintensities [7,13,25–28]. Therefore, available data so far indicate that the development of CMBs is in close relation to the severity of cerebral angiopathy, particularly in small arteries or arterioles. Histopathological investigations also support this hypothesis [29,30].

The overall prevalence of CMBs in patients with ICH ranges from 47% through 97%, as shown in Table 10.2, which is considerably higher than ischemic stroke cohorts in general. In parallel with the higher proportion of ICH in stroke in Asian populations, the detection rate of CMBs is also elevated in Asian cohorts [1]. Although the majority of articles dealt with "spontaneous" parenchymal ICH, an interesting article was recently published that documented cortical or deep CMBs in 7 of 29 patients with convexity subarachnoid hemorrhage [33]. Subarachnoid hemorrhage has been discussed in relation to CAA [34], and the association of lobar CMBs to CAA is also widely recognized (see Ch. 12).

Spatial distribution of cerebral microbleeds in intracerebral hemorrhage

The spatial distribution of microbleeds – as markers of small vessel microhemorrhagic or microaneurysmal lesions – may be of particular interest in attempts to understand the causes of macroscopic ICH in life. Only a few studies have investigated the spatial distribution of CMBs in relation to the locations of ICH. The first investigation was by Roob *et al.* in 2000 [25]. In a cohort of patients with both deep and lobar ICH, they reported that CMBs were equally found in the cortico-

subcortical (39%) and basal ganglia–thalami areas (38%). In 2004, Lee *et al.* analyzed the regional distribution of 2193 CMBs in 98 patients with hypertensive stroke using gradient-recalled echo (GRE) sequence images [11]. Lobar CMBs were detected in 67 patients and the total count of lobar CMBs was 991. The majority of lobar CMBs were observed at the cortico-medullary junction, and more CMBs were found in the temporo-occipital subcortex than in the fronto-parietal subcortex (Fig. 10.1). Deep-seated structures also had frequent CMBs. A total of 61 patients had 341 CMBs in the basal ganglia or putamen, and 61 patients were found to have 487 CMBs in the thalamus. In the caudate nucleus and putamen, more CMBs were observed in the posterolateral and upper parts of this region. In the thalamus, more CMBs were observed in the lateral and middle part of the region (Fig. 10.2). Lee *et al.* also analyzed the spatial distribution of pontocerebellar CMBs in 46 patients with hypertensive stroke [35]. More CMBs were observed in the middle and medial parts of pons and the middle–inferior–medial parts of the cerebellum (Figs. 10.3 and 10.4). This spatial analysis was based on 197 pontine CMBs from 40 patients and 177 cerebellar CMBs from 29 patients. Overall, no noticeable difference in the laterality of CMBs was observed in either supratentorial or infratentorial areas. Independently to the study by Lee *et al.*, Jeong *et al.* analyzed the location of pontine CMBs and observed almost identical distribution in 27 patients with vascular cognitive impairment [36].

Cerebral amyloid angiopathy is another important cause of primary ICH, particularly of lobar location. Greenberg *et al.* [37] and van den Boom *et al.* [38] independently reported an increased frequency of lobar CMBs in patients with CAA. In a study of 414 consecutive stroke patients, the odds of

Table 10.2 Prevalence of cerbral microbleeds in patients with hemorrhagic cerebrovascular diseases

Source	Patient characteristics	No. included patients	Age	Prevalence of CMBs (%)	Associated findings
Tanaka et al. 1999 [30]	ICH	30	60 (range, 43–77)	57	Providing pathological correlation data
Roob et al. 2000 [25]	Consecutive primary ICH	109	65 (range, 22–91)	54	CMBs associated with white matter hyperintensities and lacunar infarctions
Kinoshita et al. 2000 [3]	ICH proved by CT within 2 days after onset	130	64 (range 24–86)	71	5% in non-stroke controls
Kato et al. 2002 [7]	Hemorrhagic stroke with variable time point of MRI	35	72 ± 11	71	Correlation between number of CMBs and number of ICH
Tsushima et al. 2003 [8]	History of hemorrhagic stroke	69	63 ± 10	71	Increased distribution of lobar CMBs in those with lobar ICH compared with those with deep ICH
Jeong et al. 2004 [26]	Consecutive primary ICH	107	62 ± 13	70	CMBs associated with white matter hyperintensities and lacunar infarctions
Lee et al. 2004 [11]	Consecutive subjects (admitted 2000–2001); ICH with hypertension	51	65 ± 9	73	CMBs distribution being quite similar to the regional predilection of ICH
Lee et al. 2004 [12]	Consecutive subjects (admitted 1998–1999); acute hemorrhagic stroke	83	66 ± 11	80	Regional association between CMBs and ICH
Greenberg et al. 2004 [31]	Consecutive subjects; primary lobar ICH	94	≥55	59	New CMBs in follow-up imaging associated with recurrent ICH
Naka et al. 2004 [13]	First ever hemorrhagic stroke	36	69 ± 13	47	CMBs associated with recurrent stroke and leukoaraiosis
Imaizumi et al. 2004 [14]	Consecutive subjects; deep ICH	199	66 ± 11	77	Multiple CMBs (≥3) associated with recurrent events
Lee et al. 2005 [27]	Consecutive subjects (admitted 2002–2003); primary ICH	70	70 ± 10	97	CMBs in basal ganglia and thalamus having higher predictive value for ICH
Jeon et al. 2007 [32]	Primary ICH with follow-up	63	59 ± 9	60	Number of CMBs being associated with recurrent ICH

CMB, cerbral microbleed; ICH, intracerebral hemorrhage.

having lobar CMBs or non-lobar CMBs were different according to the genotype for apolipoprotein E [39], which suggests a different pathogenesis between lobar and deep CMBs. Moreover, analysis of hypertensive ICH and CAA-related ICH also reported that cortico-subcortical CMBs are more frequent in the CAA group [40], and the usual location of cerebral hemorrhage in CAA patients is lobar [41]. Differential location of lobar CMBs and lacunar infarctions have been reported in an analysis of 129 patients with hypertensive stroke [42].

Consequently, it can be hypothesized that CMBs may have two distinct patterns of pathogenic mech-

anisms: one as lobar CMBs in close association with CAA, and the other as deep-seated CMBs in association with lipohyalinosis and chronic hypertensive microangiopathy. Substantial overlap between the two patterns should certainly exist, as amyloid angiopathy may develop in relation to vascular aging and classical vascular risk factors, without full-blown manifestations of CAA (e.g. ICH). Such a distinction in CMB etiology may be supported by recent findings by Staals et al., who showed that elevated ambulatory blood pressure measured over 24 hours or as daytime or night-time values was associated with deep CMBs but not with lobar CMBs [43]. However, further

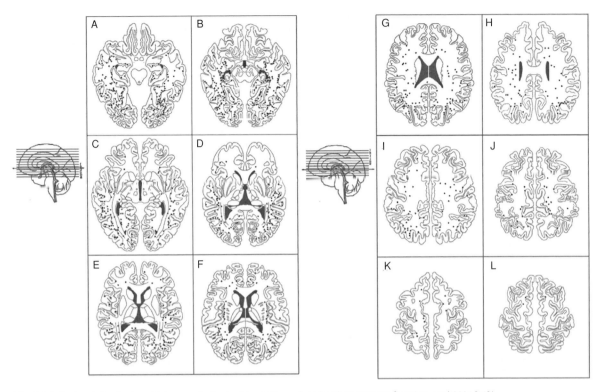

Fig. 10.1 Regional distribution of lobar cerebral microbleed. (Reproduced with permission from Lee *et al.* 2004 [11].)

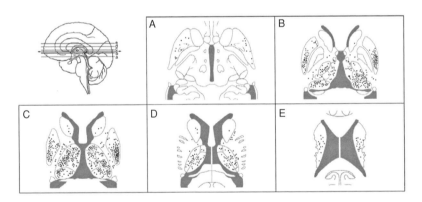

Fig. 10.2 Regional distribution of cerebral microbleeds in caudate nucleus, putamen, internal capsule and thalamus. (Reproduced with permission from Lee *et al.* 2004 [11].)

studies of larger sample size in well-phenotyped clinical cohorts are required to definitively answer the question as to whether lobar or non-lobar CMBs are predictive of underlying vascular pathologies.

As CMBs may suggest a hemorrhage-prone microangiopathy, regional association with macroscopic ICH has been sought [12]. In a study of 265 consecutive patients with stroke, Lee *et al.* observed that the severity of CMBs was associated with hemorrhagic stroke and significant association of CMBs in the cortico-subcortical area or deep gray matter with macroscopic ICH in the corresponding area. The spatial clustering of ICH and CMBs in deep structures was also documented in an independent study by Chen *et al.* [44]. Such regional association was also found in analysis of patients with infratentorial ICH [35]. Generally, these results show that the distribution of CMBs is similar to that of macroscopic ICH, suggesting that the pathophysiological origins are linked.

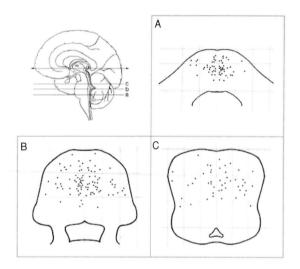

Fig. 10.3 Regional distribution of pontine cerebral microbleeds. (Reproduced with permission from Lee *et al.* 2004 [35].)

Risk factors for cerebral microbleeds in cerebrovascular disease

The topic of risk factors for CMBs is considered in detail in Ch. 7, together with a discussion of relevant methodological issues. Here, we briefly discuss risk factors for CMBs in cohorts of participants with cerebrovascular disease. Chronic hypertension has been repeatedly identified as a strong influence on the frequency and extent of CMBs, in patients with established stroke as well as in healthy subjects without stroke [25,30,45]. However, in a study of 472 subjects from the Framingham Study offspring cohort, Jeerakathil *et al.* did not confirm such effects of chronic hypertension or systolic blood pressure [5]. A couple

of sporadic reports also dissented from such associations [10,26]. Nevertheless, overall, hypertension does seem to be an important risk factor for CMBs. Strong associations have consistently been reported between CMBs and white matter hyperintensities or lacunar infarction, which also implies a strong influence of chronic hypertension [8,27,42]. The majority of CMB studies observed increased prevalence of CMBs in hypertensive patients [1,46]. Moreover, a dose dependency of CMBs and markers of chronic hypertension has been suggested. Left ventricular mass index (LVMI) is an accepted marker of ventricular hypertrophy and can be used to quantify the persistent hypertensive burden [45]. In a series of 102 patients with acute stroke (72 ischemic stroke and 30 hemorrhagic stroke), LVMI was significantly correlated with the severity of CMB prevalence. What may be noteworthy in this research is that the positive correlation of LVMI was only observed with CMBs in central gray matter, not with those in cortico-subcortical areas. As already discussed above, this regional discrepancy may support the concept of a differential underlying microvasculopathy between lobar and deep CMBs. Moreover, among various blood pressure parameters, studies monitoring 24-hour ambulatory blood pressure found that nocturnal hypertension, as well as elevated blood pressure across the 24-hour period, was strongly associated with CMBs [38,39]. Therefore, in spite of a few contradicting reports, chronic hypertension is accepted to have strong association with development of CMBs, more evidently with CMBs in deep gray matter.

Low cholesterol is known to increase the incidence of cerebral hemorrhage, possibly through unstable integrity of endothelial cells in cerebral small vessels

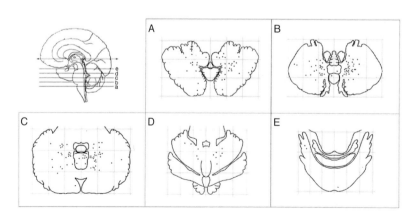

Fig. 10.4 Regional distribution of cerebellar cerebral microbleed. (Reproduced with permission from Lee *et al.* 2004 [35].)

[47,48]. Risk of hemorrhagic stroke after cholesterol-lowering treatment such as statin is still controversial [49,50]. It has been suggested that this risk might be explained by lower cholesterol levels being associated with an increased incidence of hemorrhagic transformation after atherothrombotic stroke [51]. In this context, patients having CMBs were reported to have low levels of serum cholesterol, and patients with serum cholesterol of <1.65 mg/l have an 11-fold increased risk of having CMBs [52]. This suggestion was also supported by the results of the Rotterdam Scan Study for a large cohort population [53].

Old age, a well-known but unmodifiable vascular risk factor, is also associated with the frequency and extent of CMBs [5,6]. The association between diabetes and CMBs is also controversial. In a case series of 100 patients with ischemic stroke, those who were diabetic had increased odds of having CMBs compared with their non-diabetic counterparts [54]. However, such an association was not replicated in a recent publication that analyzed data from 639 patients with acute stroke. In this study, neither diabetes itself nor hemoglobin A1c, a measure of glucose control, were correlated with CMBs [55].

Recently, much interest has been generated by the investigation of CMBs in patients with chronic kidney disease. These patients on hemodialysis are at heightened risk of experiencing stroke [56], and cerebral and renal small vasculatures share similar microvascular structures. Small arteries or arterioles in each organ are diverted from major middle-to-large sized arteries. As undamped elevated systolic blood pressure or wider pulse pressure is directly transmitted to the vascular walls, microvasculatures in both organs may suffer from similar pathological stress [57]. Earlier studies reported frequent CMBs in patients with chronic kidney disease on hemodialysis and in patients with established chronic kidney disease but without hemodialysis [58–60]. The pathological linkage between CMBs and renal dysfunction was further investigated in patients with stroke without established chronic kidney disease in an analysis of 236 consecutive patients with ischemic stroke or transient ischemic attack [61]. The results indicated that proteinuria of more than 300 mg/l on a spot urine test was strongly associated with the frequency and number of CMBs [61]. However, only urine protein excretion was analyzed in this study, and the renal impairment per se was not investigated. Estimated glomerular filtration rate, a reliable and practical indicator of kidney function,

was analyzed in conjunction with CMBs in a recently published study investigating 150 patients with acute ischemic stroke [23]. Patients with decreased kidney function, defined in this study as having an estimated glomerular filtration rate <60 ml/min per 1.73m^2, were found to have 3.8 times increased odds of CMB frequency. These reports provided valuable insights into development of CMBs and vascular pathology under chronic hypertension.

Temporal changes of cerebral microbleeds

The dynamic temporal course of CMBs has not been investigated in detail. Jeon *et al.* analyzed 237 consecutive patients with acute ischemic stroke who underwent GRE imaging within 24 hours and follow-up GRE imaging during the week after stroke onset [24]. At initial MRI scanning, 32% of these patients were observed to have baseline CMBs. At follow-up imaging approximately 4 days later (range, 1–7), 56 new CMBs were identified in 13% of patients. Baseline CMBs disappeared in seven patients at follow-up scanning. Factors associated with the development of new CMBs included the number of baseline CMBs, severity of white matter hyperintensities and increased body temperature. Although registration of spatial difference of CMBs between the two MRI scans seems not to have been performed, and the long-term fates of newly developed CMBs were not documented, these results suggested that CMBs may develop in close relation to certain critical events such as acute stroke. The clinical implication of acute CMB development during the critical ischemic event needs to be clarified by further research.

In 2010, Gregoire *et al.* analyzed 21 survivors of ischemic stroke or transient ischemic attack and compared two MRI scans obtained with a mean interval between them of 5.6 years [62]. At follow-up imaging, five patients (23%) developed 56 new lobar CMBs and no deep CMBs. New CMBs had developed in 50% of subjects with baseline CMBs and in only 8% of those who were free of CMBs at baseline. The development of new CMBs was strongly associated with elevated baseline or mean systolic blood pressure, and with the presence of CMBs at initial imaging. However, the limited sample size and new CMBs restricted in lobar locations prevent generalization of their results. We have performed baseline and follow-up MRI scanning in 224 survivors of acute ischemic stroke, with a mean interval of 27 months between scans [63]. Among 76 patients with CMBs at baseline, the numbers of CMBs decreased in 11 (14.5%) and increased in 41 (53.9%) patients. The numbers of CMBs in 24 (31.6%) patients did not change during the follow-up. The estimated annual change rates of CMB numbers correlated with the baseline count of CMBs. Multivariable analyses showed that severe white matter hyperintensities (adjusted odds ratio [OR], 2.39; 95% confidence interval [CI], 1.27–4.53), small vessel occlusion (adjusted OR, 2.49; 95% CI, 1.15–5.40) and intracerebral hemorrhage (adjusted OR, 4.06; 95% CI, 1.01–16.32) were associated with an increased risk of more frequent CMBs at follow-up. Interestingly, higher low density lipoprotein cholesterol appeared to exert protective effects on CMB progression (adjusted OR, 0.30; 95% CI, 0.14–0.68).

Although the significance of these studies is not yet apparent, it seems clear that CMBs are a dynamically changing phenomenon rather than a static marker of small vessel damage. The rapid evolution in acute stroke suggests a widespread small vessel pathological process associated with acute ischemia; the relationship to temperature suggests a possible role for inflammation. Much more work is needed to establish the significance of these imaging changes for acute or long-term outcome. The clinical consequences of CMB evolution over longer periods of time also require further investigation (particularly regarding functional and cognitive outcomes) in larger prospective cohorts.

Prognostic value of cerebral microbleeds

With increasing evidence of CMBs reflecting hemorrhage-prone microangiopathy, it has been speculated that CMBs may be an important factor for hemorrhagic stroke risk stratification. Fan et al. followed 121 patients with acute ischemic stroke and reported that stroke survivors with CMBs on baseline MRI scans had higher risk of hemorrhagic stroke, but the number of outcome events was very small [10]. In a CAA cohort, Greenberg et al. also reported that the count of micro- or macrohemorrhages on baseline GRE MRI was proportional to the heightened risk of hemorrhagic stroke [31]. An elevated risk of hemorrhagic stroke by the presence of CMBs was also noted in a prospective study of 112 survivors of ICH [32]. The predictive value of CMBs for ICH in patients with advanced white matter lesions was also

documented [27]. Studies of the association between CMBs and larger ICH volume has shown conflicting results [64,65]. In addition to hemorrhagic stroke, patients with CMBs were reported to be 2.8 times more likely to have a subsequent disabling or fatal stroke [17].

It has been hypothesized that CMBs, as a marker of bleeding-prone microangiopathy, might predict the risk of hemorrhagic transformation in acute ischemic stroke. Kidwell et al. suggested in 2002 that hemorrhagic transformation after thrombolysis was associated with the presence of CMBs [66]. Nighoghossian et al. also found that CMBs were associated with early hemorrhagic transformation in 100 patients with acute ischemic stroke [54]. Moreover, case reports have been published that showed hemorrhagic transformation occurring after embolic stroke at the very site of previous CMBs [67,68].

However, in contrast to these positive associations, a retrospective study investigating 279 patients with acute ischemic stroke reported that CMB count and hemorrhagic transformation were not associated [69]. Moreover, CMBs were not associated with post-thrombolytic hemorrhagic transformation in an analysis of 70 patients with hyperacute stroke [70]. A pooled analysis of 570 patients with acute ischemic stroke recruited from 13 centers worldwide finally reported that CMBs were not associated with symptomatic hemorrhage after thrombolytic treatment [20]. A retrospective study based at a single hospital investigated findings in 1034 patients with acute stroke and came to similar conclusions [21]. (Ch. 19 has a detailed discussion of CMBs in the context of thrombolysis.)

Differential association of CMBs with development of primary ICH and hemorrhagic transformation may be explained by different pathogenic mechanisms for these two phenomena. Primary ICH is in essence rupture of fragile microvascular walls which have lipohyalinosis or microaneurysm under the chronic influence of hypertension. Therefore, as patients with CMBs have histologically been found to have a similar pattern of vasculopathy to those with ICH, CMBs may be interpreted as a primary ICH of very small scale. However, one recent study in CAA suggests that, in this disease, CMBs may be associated with increased vessel wall thickness [71]. By contrast with "spontaneous microbleeds," hemorrhagic transformation develops after acute lethal hypoxic injury to relatively healthy microvasculature; consequently

CMBs may only partially explain the development of hemorrhagic transformation.

As CMBs reflect the bleeding tendency of the brain through fragile microvascular walls, interest has increased in utilizing CMBs in risk stratification of hemorrhagic complications for patients with antithrombotic treatment. Wong et al. reported that CMBs were more frequent and extensive in patients with aspirin-associated ICH [72]. In a cross-sectional study, CMBs were more common in antithrombotic drug users, and aspirin was related to the lobar location of CMBs [53] Moreover, patients with complications of anticoagulation-associated hemorrhagic stroke were 3.6 times more likely to have CMBs compared with age- and sex-matched controls [73]. However, Orken et al. [74] reported that the frequency of CMBs was not associated with duration of warfarin treatment, which suggests that warfarin treatment may not contribute to cerebral microhemorrhage. The duration of anticoagulation itself may not be as important as a high prothrombin time (pre-existing CMBs) for warfarin-related ICH. Further high-quality prospective studies are needed to address the relevance of CMBs in risk prediction prior to oral anticoagulation treatment. The issue of antithrombotic management and CMBs is discussed in Ch. 19.

Conclusions

Cerebral microbleeds are frequently detected in patients with ischemic or hemorrhagic strokes, and our understanding of their clinical relevance is also rapidly developing. CMBs are, in essence, extravasation of blood components through fragile microvascular walls, thereby reflecting bleeding-prone vasculopathies. In this context, various clinical studies have reported that CMBs are associated with hemorrhagic stroke and hemorrhagic complications following antithrombotic medications. In the future, prospective studies are warranted to confirm the clinical implications of CMBs and set up predictive risk models for hemorrhagic stroke in various populations of patients with cerebrovascular diseases.

References

1. Koennecke HC. Cerebral microbleeds on MRI: prevalence, associations, and potential clinical implications. *Neurology* 2006;**66**:165–71.

2. Roob G, Schmidt R, Kapeller P et al. MRI evidence of past cerebral microbleeds in a healthy elderly population. *Neurology* 1999;**52**:991–4.

3. Kinoshita T, Okudera T, Tamura H, Ogawa T, Hatazawa J. Assessment of lacunar hemorrhage associated with hypertensive stroke by echo-planar gradient-echo T_2^*-weighted MRI. *Stroke* 2000;**31**:1646–50.

4. Horita Y, Imaizumi T, Niwa J et al.[Analysis of dot-like hemosiderin spots using brain dock system.] *No Shinkei Geka* 2003;**31**:263–7.

5. Jeerakathil T, Wolf PA, Beiser A et al. Cerebral microbleeds: prevalence and associations with cardiovascular risk factors in the Framingham study. *Stroke* 2004;**35**:1831–5.

6. Vernooij MW, van der Lugt A, Ikram MA et al. Prevalence and risk factors of cerebral microbleeds: the Rotterdam Scan Study. *Neurology* 2008;**70**: 1208–14.

7. Kato H, Izumiyama M, Izumiyama K, Takahashi A, Itoyama Y. Silent cerebral microbleeds on T_2^*-weighted MRI: correlation with stroke subtype, stroke recurrence, and leukoaraiosis. *Stroke* 2002;**33**:1536–40.

8. Tsushima Y, Aoki J, Endo K. Brain microhemorrhages detected on T_2^*-weighted gradient-echo MR images. *AJNR Am J Neuroradiol* 2003;**24**:88–96.

9. Hanyu H, Tanaka Y, Shimizu S et al. Cerebral microbleeds in Binswanger's disease: a gradient-echo T_2^*-weighted magnetic resonance imaging study. *Neurosci Lett* 2003;**340**:213–16.

10. Fan YH, Zhang L, Lam WW, Mok VC, Wong KS. Cerebral microbleeds as a risk factor for subsequent intracerebral hemorrhages among patients with acute ischemic stroke. *Stroke* 2003;**34**:2459–62.

11. Lee SH, Kwon SJ, Kim KS, Yoon BW, Roh JK. Cerebral microbleeds in patients with hypertensive stroke. Topographical distribution in the supratentorial area. *J Neurol* 2004;**251**:1183–9.

12. Lee SH, Bae HJ, Kwon SJ et al. Cerebral microbleeds are regionally associated with intracerebral hemorrhage. *Neurology* 2004;**62**:72–6.

13. Naka H, Nomura E, Wakabayashi S et al. Frequency of asymptomatic microbleeds on T_2^*-weighted MR images of patients with recurrent stroke: association with combination of stroke subtypes and leukoaraiosis. *AJNR Am J Neuroradiol* 2004;**25**:714–19.

14. Imaizumi T, Horita Y, Hashimoto Y, Niwa J. Dotlike hemosiderin spots on T_2^*-weighted magnetic resonance imaging as a predictor of stroke recurrence: a prospective study. *J Neurosurg* 2004;**101**:915–20.

15. Schonewille WJ, Singer MB, Atlas SW, Tuhrim S. The prevalence of microhemorrhage on gradient-echo magnetic resonance imaging in acute lacunar infarction. *J Stroke Cerebrovasc Dis* 2005;**14**: 141–4.

16. Werring DJ, Coward LJ, Losseff NA, Jager HR, Brown MM. Cerebral microbleeds are common in ischemic stroke but rare in TIA. *Neurology* 2005;**65**:1914–18.

17. Boulanger JM, Coutts SB, Eliasziw M *et al.* Cerebral microhemorrhages predict new disabling or fatal strokes in patients with acute ischemic stroke or transient ischemic attack. *Stroke* 2006;**37**:911–14.

18. Ovbiagele B, Saver JL, Sanossian N *et al.* Predictors of cerebral microbleeds in acute ischemic stroke and TIA patients. *Cerebrovasc Dis* 2006;**22**:378–83.

19. Wardlaw JM, Lewis SC, Keir SL, Dennis MS, Shenkin S. Cerebral microbleeds are associated with lacunar stroke defined clinically and radiologically, independently of white matter lesions. *Stroke* 2006;**37**:2633–6.

20. Fiehler J, Albers GW, Boulanger JM *et al.* Bleeding risk analysis in stroke imaging before thrombolysis (BRASIL): pooled analysis of T_2*-weighted magnetic resonance imaging data from 570 patients. *Stroke* 2007;**38**:2738–44.

21. Lee SH, Kang BS, Kim N, Roh JK. Does microbleed predict haemorrhagic transformation after acute atherothrombotic or cardioembolic stroke? *J Neurol Neurosurg Psychiatry* 2008;**79**:913–16.

22. Seo WK, Lee JM, Park MH, Park KW, Lee DH. Cerebral microbleeds are independently associated with arterial stiffness in stroke patients. *Cerebrovasc Dis* 2008;**26**:618–23.

23. Cho AH, Lee SB, Han SJ *et al.* Impaired kidney function and cerebral microbleeds in patients with acute ischemic stroke. *Neurology* 2009;**73**:1645–8.

24. Jeon SB, Kwon SU, Cho AH *et al.* Rapid appearance of new cerebral microbleeds after acute ischemic stroke. *Neurology* 2009;**73**:1638–44.

25. Roob G, Lechner A, Schmidt R *et al.* Frequency and location of microbleeds in patients with primary intracerebral hemorrhage. *Stroke* 2000;**31**:2665–9.

26. Jeong SW, Jung KH, Chu K *et al.* Clinical and radiologic differences between primary intracerebral hemorrhage with and without microbleeds on gradient-echo magnetic resonance images. *Arch Neurol* 2004;**61**:905–9.

27. Lee SH, Heo JH, Yoon BW. Effects of microbleeds on hemorrhage development in leukoaraiosis patients. *Hypertens Res* 2005;**28**:895–9.

28. Gorner A, Lemmens R, Schrooten M, Thijs V. Is leukoaraiosis on CT an accurate surrogate marker for the presence of microbleeds in acute stroke patients? *J Neurol* 2007;**254**:284–9.

29. Fazekas F, Kleinert R, Roob G *et al.* Histopathologic analysis of foci of signal loss on gradient-echo T_2*-weighted MR images in patients with spontaneous intracerebral hemorrhage: evidence of microangiopathy-related microbleeds. *AJNR Am J Neuroradiol* 1999;**20**:637–42.

30. Tanaka A, Ueno Y, Nakayama Y, Takano K, Takebayashi S. Small chronic hemorrhages and ischemic lesions in association with spontaneous intracerebral hematomas. *Stroke* 1999;**30**:1637–42.

31. Greenberg SM, Eng JA, Ning M, Smith EE, Rosand J. Hemorrhage burden predicts recurrent intracerebral hemorrhage after lobar hemorrhage. *Stroke* 2004;**35**:1415–20.

32. Jeon SB, Kang DW, Cho AH *et al.* Initial microbleeds at MR imaging can predict recurrent intracerebral hemorrhage. *J Neurol* 2007;**254**:508–12.

33. Kumar S, Goddeau RP, Jr., Selim MH *et al.* Atraumatic convexal subarachnoid hemorrhage: clinical presentation, imaging patterns, and etiologies. *Neurology* 2010;**74**:893–9.

34. Katoh M, Yoshino M, Asaoka K *et al.* A restricted subarachnoid hemorrhage in the cortical sulcus in cerebral amyloid angiopathy: could it be a warning sign? *Surg Neurol* 2007;**68**:457–60.

35. Lee SH, Kwon SJ, Kim KS, Yoon BW, Roh JK. Topographical distribution of pontocerebellar microbleeds. *AJNR Am J Neuroradiol* 2004;**25**:1337–41.

36. Jeong JH, Yoon SJ, Kang SJ, Choi KG, Na DL. Hypertensive pontine microhemorrhage. *Stroke* 2002;**33**:925–9.

37. Greenberg SM, Finklestein SP, Schaefer PW. Petechial hemorrhages accompanying lobar hemorrhage: detection by gradient-echo MRI. *Neurology* 1996;**46**:1751–4.

38. van den Boom R, Bornebroek M, Behloul F *et al.* Microbleeds in hereditary cerebral hemorrhage with amyloidosis-Dutch type. *Neurology* 2005;**64**:1288–9.

39. Kim M, Bae HJ, Lee J *et al.* ApoE epsilon2/epsilon4 polymorphism and cerebral microbleeds on gradient echo MRI. *Neurology* 2005;**65**:1474–5.

40. Lee SH, Kim SM, Kim N, Yoon BW, Roh JK. Cortico-subcortical distribution of microbleeds is different between hypertension and cerebral amyloid angiopathy. *J Neurol Sci.* 2007;**258**:111–14.

41. Rosand J, Muzikansky A, Kumar A *et al.* Spatial clustering of hemorrhages in probable cerebral amyloid angiopathy. *Ann Neurol* 2005;**58**:459–62.

42. Lee SH, Bae HJ, Ko SB *et al.* Comparative analysis of the spatial distribution and severity of cerebral microbleeds and old lacunes. *J Neurol Neurosurg Psychiatry* 2004;**75**:423–7.

43. Staals J, van Oostenbrugge RJ, Knottnerus IL *et al.* Brain microbleeds relate to higher ambulatory blood

pressure levels in first-ever lacunar stroke patients. *Stroke* 2009;**40**:3264–8.

44. Chen YF, Chang YY, Liu JS *et al.* Association between cerebral microbleeds and prior primary intracerebral hemorrhage in ischemic stroke patients. *Clin Neurol Neurosurg* 2008;**110**:988–91.

45. Lee SH, Park JM, Kwon SJ *et al.* Left ventricular hypertrophy is associated with cerebral microbleeds in hypertensive patients. *Neurology* 2004;**63**:16–21.

46. Viswanathan A, Chabriat H. Cerebral microhemorrhage. *Stroke* 2006;**37**:550–5.

47. Iso H, Jacobs DR, Jr., Wentworth D, Neaton JD, Cohen JD. Serum cholesterol levels and six-year mortality from stroke in 350 977 men screened for the Multiple Risk Factor Intervention Trial. *N Engl J Med* 1989;**320**:904–10.

48. Reed DM. The paradox of high risk of stroke in populations with low risk of coronary heart disease. *Am J Epidemiol* 1990;**131**:579–88.

49. Amarenco P, Bogousslavsky J, Callahan A, 3rd *et al.* High-dose atorvastatin after stroke or transient ischemic attack. *N Engl J Med* 2006;**355**:549–59.

50. Goldstein LB, Amarenco P, Szarek M *et al.* Hemorrhagic stroke in the Stroke Prevention by Aggressive Reduction in Cholesterol Levels study. *Neurology* 2008;**70**:2364–70.

51. Kim BJ, Lee S-H, Ryu W-S *et al.* Low level of low-density lipoprotein cholesterol increases hemorrhagic transformation in large artery atherothrombosis but not in cardioembolism. *Stroke* 2009;**40**:1627–32.

52. Lee SH, Bae HJ, Yoon BW *et al.* Low concentration of serum total cholesterol is associated with multifocal signal loss lesions on gradient-echo magnetic resonance imaging: analysis of risk factors for multifocal signal loss lesions. *Stroke* 2002;**33**: 2845–9.

53. Vernooij MW, Haag MD, van der Lugt A *et al.* Use of antithrombotic drugs and the presence of cerebral microbleeds: the Rotterdam Scan Study. *Arch Neurol* 2009;**66**:714–20.

54. Nighoghossian N, Hermier M, Adeleine P *et al.* Old microbleeds are a potential risk factor for cerebral bleeding after ischemic stroke: a gradient-echo T_2*-weighted brain MRI study. *Stroke* 2002;**33**:735–42.

55. Heo SH, Lee SH, Kim BJ, Kang BS, Yoon BW. Does glycated hemoglobin have clinical significance in ischemic stroke patients? *Clin Neurol Neurosurg* 2010;**112**:98–102.

56. Iseki K, Kinjo K, Kimura Y, Osawa A, Fukiyama K. Evidence for high risk of cerebral hemorrhage in chronic dialysis patients. *Kidney Int* 1993;**44**:1086–90.

57. O'Rourke MF, Safar ME. Relationship between aortic stiffening and microvascular disease in brain and kidney: cause and logic of therapy. *Hypertension* 2005;**46**:200–4.

58. Yokoyama S, Hirano H, Uomizu K *et al.* High incidence of microbleeds in hemodialysis patients detected by T_2*-weighted gradient-echo magnetic resonance imaging. *Neurol Med Chir (Tokyo)* 2005;**45**:556–60; discussion 560.

59. Watanabe A. Cerebral microbleeds and intracerebral hemorrhages in patients on maintenance hemodialysis. *J Stroke Cerebrovasc Dis* 2007;**16**: 30–3.

60. Shima H, Ishimura E, Naganuma T *et al.* Cerebral microbleeds in predialysis patients with chronic kidney disease. *Nephrol Dial Transplant* 2010;**25**:1554–9.

61. Ovbiagele B, Liebeskind DS, Pineda S, Saver JL. Strong independent correlation of proteinuria with cerebral microbleeds in patients with stroke and transient ischemic attack. *Arch Neurol* 2010;**67**: 45–50.

62. Gregoire SM, Brown MM, Kallis C *et al.* MRI detection of new microbleeds in patients with ischemic stroke: five-year cohort follow-up study. *Stroke* 2010;**41**:184–6.

63. Lee ST, Lee SH, Roh JK. Changes in cerebral microbleed numbers of stroke patients and their prognostic factors. *Proceedings of the International Stroke Conference of the American Stroke Association*, San Antonio, USA, 2010, p. 491.

64. Lee SH, Kim BJ, Roh JK. Silent microbleeds are associated with volume of primary intracerebral hemorrhage. *Neurology* 2006;**66**:430–2.

65. Imaizumi T, Honma T, Horita Y *et al.* Hematoma size in deep intracerebral hemorrhage and its correlation with dot-like hemosiderin spots on gradient echo T_2*-weighted MRI. *J Neuroimaging* 2006;**16**:236–42.

66. Kidwell CS, Saver JL, Villablanca JP *et al.* Magnetic resonance imaging detection of microbleeds before thrombolysis: an emerging application. *Stroke* 2002;**33**:95–8.

67. Kim BJ, Lee SH. Silent microbleeds and hemorrhagic conversion of an embolic infarction. *J Clin Neurol* 2007;**3**:147–9.

68. Vernooij MW, Heeringa J, de Jong GJ, van der Lugt A, Breteler MMB. Cerebral microbleed preceding symptomatic intracerebral hemorrhage in a stroke-free person. *Neurology* 2009;**72**:763–5.

69. Kim HS, Lee DH, Ryu CW *et al.* Multiple cerebral microbleeds in hyperacute ischemic stroke: impact on prevalence and severity of early hemorrhagic

transformation after thrombolytic treatment. *AJR Am J Roentgenol* 2006;**186**:1443–9.

70. Kakuda W, Thijs VN, Lansberg MG *et al.* Clinical importance of microbleeds in patients receiving iv thrombolysis. *Neurology* 2005;**65**:1175–8.

71. Atlas SW, Mark AS, Grossman RI, Gomori JM. Intracranial hemorrhage: gradient-echo MR imaging at 1.5 T. Comparison with spin-echo imaging and clinical applications. *Radiology* 1988;**168**:803–7.

72. Wong KS, Mok V, Lam WWM *et al.* Aspirin-associated intracerebral hemorrhage: clinical and radiologic features. *Neurology* 2000;**54**:2298–2301.

73. Lee SH, Ryu WS, Roh JK. Cerebral microbleeds are a risk factor for warfarin-related intracerebral hemorrhage. *Neurology* 2009;**72**:171–6.

74. Orken DN, Kenangil G, Uysal E, Forta H. Cerebral microbleeds in ischemic stroke patients on warfarin treatment. *Stroke* 2009;**40**:3638–40.

Cerebral microbleeds in relation to hypertensive arteriopathy

Eric E. Smith and Roland N. Auer

Introduction

Hypertension is an extremely common age-related condition with dramatic consequences for the cerebral vascular supply and the brain if not adequately treated. Over time, high blood pressure leads to thickening of the walls of small arteries (arteriosclerosis and arteriolosclerosis), loss of smooth muscle cells and decreased vascular integrity, with leaking of plasma and red blood cells into the arterial wall and the immediately adjacent neuropil. The cerebral consequences of hypertension include brain infarction from accelerated large artery atherosclerosis or small artery arteriosclerosis, white matter lesions and hemorrhaging. The clinical consequences of untreated hypertension are dire and include stroke and vascular cognitive impairment.

The pathological and clinical consequences of arteriosclerosis, predominantly caused by untreated hypertension, were beginning to be recognized in the late nineteenth century by neuropathologists such as Kraepelin, Binswanger and others, not long after the invention of sphygmomanometry. Alois Alzheimer described brain atrophy secondary to arteriosclerosis 13 years before the seminal report on the disease that now bears his name [1]. Prior to the Nobel-prize winning discovery of propanolol in the 1950s, the first effective oral antihypertensive, options to treat chronic hypertension were limited and mostly confined to dietary changes. Because there were no studies of the modern epidemiological type during this period, we can only speculate on the true impact of hypertensive disease. The development of pharmacological approaches to blood pressure lowering, and subsequent dramatic improvement in the population control of hypertension, must rank as one of the most important medical advances of the twentieth century.

Because of effective treatments, the cerebral consequences of hypertension have been muted and delayed, but not abolished. Hypertensive brain disease in treated hypertensives is still common but is predominantly a disease of the elderly. The advent of modern neuroimaging has provided a better understanding of the high prevalence of hypertensive cerebral changes in vivo. This chapter reviews the pathophsyiology and pathology of hypertensive arteriopathy of the brain and its relationship to neuroimaging findings, particularly cerebral microbleeds (CMBs).

Epidemiology of hypertension

The prevalence of hypertension is highly age dependent. National surveys with blood pressure measurement have provided estimates of rates in the community. The prevalence is approximately 30% in persons aged 40–59 years but is more than 60% in those ≥60 years, based on a study in the USA [2]. A similarly high prevalence of hypertension has been found in China, although recognition and control were worse [3]. Consequently, it appears that most elderly persons suffer from hypertension, although in up to 30% it is not recognized by the person themselves [2]. The prevalence of diastolic hypertension reaches a plateau by approximately 60 years of age while the prevalence of systolic hypertension increases throughout life; therefore, many elderly have isolated systolic hypertension.

There are many possible causes of hypertension. A comprehensive discussion of these causes is outside the scope of this chapter but has recently been

---

Cerebral Microbleeds, ed. David J. Werring. Published by Cambridge University Press. © Cambridge University Press 2011.

reviewed [4]. Most commonly, no secondary cause is identified, thus leaving a diagnosis of *essential hypertension* [5]. The events that lead to essential hypertension are unclear and controversial. There is wide acceptance, however, that abnormal renal sodium excretion plays a significant role [6]. Risk factors for the development of hypertension have been identified and include age, male sex, obesity and high dietary sodium. Common genetic variation may play a role in susceptibility to hypertension, but aside from rare monogenic conditions the genes involved in hypertension are not well known.

Hypertension is a risk factor for cardiac, renal and cerebral diseases, among others. Hypertension-related cerebral diseases include hypertensive encephalopathy, stroke and vascular cognitive impairment. Hypertension is the strongest modifiable risk factor for ischemic or hemorrhagic stroke [7]. Hypertensive small vessel disease may lead to lacunar stroke and is a major cause of primary intracerebral hemorrhage (ICH) [8]. Mid-life hypertension is now recognized as a risk factor for late-life cognitive impairment and dementia [9]. Hypertension may promote cognitive impairment by causing silent brain infarction and white matter lesions or overt stroke with post-stroke cognitive impairment, but it may also increase the risk of clinically diagnosed Alzheimer's disease [9]. It is not entirely clear whether this increased risk of Alzheimer's disease in hypertensive persons is caused by increased Alzheimer pathology or an increased prevalence of silent brain infarction and white matter lesions that decrease cognitive reserve.

Vascular dysfunction and vascular remodeling in hypertension

Chronic exposure to increased blood pressure leads to reactive changes in the vascular wall, termed remodeling. This remodeling is ultimately accompanied by endothelial dysfunction, changes in smooth muscle cell contractility and loss of vascular integrity.

Under conditions of chronic increased blood pressure, there is hypertrophy of vascular smooth muscle cells and an increase in arterial wall thickness with fibrosis [10]. The lumen of the arteriole narrows such that resistance is increased, which prevents potentially harmful hyperperfusion of the distal capillary bed. A narrowed arteriolar lumen diameter at maximal dilation shifts the limits of the autoregulatory curve to the right [11]. Smooth muscle cells become more react-

ive to contractile stimuli. The vascular wall becomes thicker, possibly to maintain normal wall shear stress and preserve vascular integrity, such that the wall-to-lumen ratio is increased. Distensibility of the larger cerebral arteries is decreased in hypertension; paradoxically, the distensibility of the cerebral arterioles in hypertension may be increased [12].

Most germane to the development of CMB are the effects of high blood pressure on vascular integrity. With more long-standing and severe hypertension, there is disruption of the blood–brain barrier with deposition of fibrin and other serum proteins in the vessel wall [13], which is described in further detail in the subsequent section. Wall necrosis and disruption of the blood–brain barrier lead to a loss of vascular integrity, with leakage of serum, serum proteins or red blood cells into the perivascular space. Increased expression of matrix metalloproteinases and elastase may promote helpful adaptive changes in early hypertension but could play a role in disruption of the basement membrane in more long-standing hypertension [14].

Neuropathology of hypertensive arteriopathy

Although the term arteriopathy includes both arteries and arterioles, this chapter focuses on the intrinsic vascular pathology of arterioles in hypertension. Arteries certainly undergo accelerated atherosclerosis when hypertension is present. There are many other risk factors for atherosclerosis beside hypertension, and the process of atherosclerosis is left to other reviews.

The two principal vascular lesions seen at the arteriolar level in hypertension are blockade and leaking. Both can occur in a graded matter. That is, arterioles can be variably stenotic and show variable leakage. Moreover, both leakage and occlusion can simultaneously occur. The functional consequences of the arterial disease in hypertension are, therefore, complicated, but encompass the two kinds of stroke – infarcts and hemorrhages – at a smaller level than that seen after major arterial occlusion. The structural alterations that occur in hypertension will now be considered at the arteriolar level.

The earliest changes shown by arterioles in hypertension are usually termed hyperplastic arteriolosclerosis. Arterioles normally have a high wall-to-lumen ratio, and this must be considered in assessing arterioles in tissue sections. One useful feature seen early in hypertension is the tortuosity that arterioles show when subjected to chronically increased pressure. The increased length of the vessel, rather than further increase in medial wall thickness, causes multiple profiles to appear in tissue sections. These glomeruloid formations offer a clue to early arteriolar insult (Fig. 11.1A).

Over time, smooth muscle cells in the tunica media undergo cell death. This leaves acellular walls in tissue sections. Often, ill-defined nuclear outlines are seen as basophilic spindle-shaped nuclear remnants in the tunica media (Fig. 11.1B), signifying cell death.

Although collagen replaces the smooth muscle parenchyma that is lost in hypertension, additional material of an ill-defined nature is deposited; this has been termed fibrinoid. There is a heated debate on the nature of fibrinoid changes, but this is outside the scope of this chapter [15]. It is likely that plasma components leaking into the wall of the vessels supplements local collagen deposition to give the histological appearance seen (Fig. 11.1C).

The classic appearance of Charcot–Bouchard aneurysms is the subject of some debate [16]. We consider these sacs of collagen to be dilatations along the length of the arterioles, rather than blind ending cul-de-sacs as seen in berry aneurysm pathology on a larger spatial scale. Rarely, these aneurysms can be seen in surgical hematoma resection material as remnants of collagenous sacs in large areas of otherwise unenlightening hemorrhage. The relationship between CMBs on MRI and these small aneurysmal or hemorrhagic lesions is considered in more detail in Ch. 1.

Disrupted vascular integrity and microbleeds/bleeding

The issue of vascular integrity and microbleeding within the brain is surprisingly vexatious. It is highly likely that CMBs occur within the brain physiologically, possibly during transient, normal increases in blood pressure occurring during various activities through force dilatation in normal vessels [17]. Microbleeds are seen in routine autopsy material, even in the absence of accompanying vascular changes suggesting hypertension or a clinical history of hypertension before death (Fig. 11.2A).

Perivascular iron in the Virchow–Robin space is more common in hypertension. Bleeding ranges from slight (Fig. 11.2B) to almost circumferential

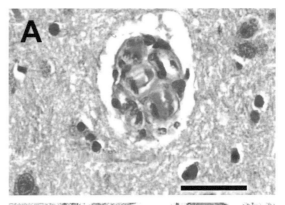

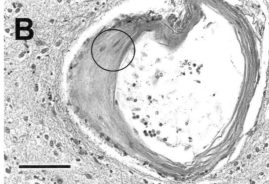

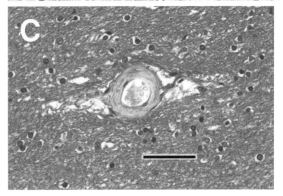

Fig. 11.1 Arteriolar changes caused by hypertension. (A) Tortuous hyperplastic arteriolar change, with six lumena visible in section. Abundant smooth muscle nuclei are seen, prior to the stage of medial cell death. Sections from a hypertensive male, aged 82, heart weight 660 g. Bar = 100 mm. (B) Loss of smooth muscle cells in tunica media, with only faint nuclear outlines seen (encircled). Bar = 100 mm. (C) Masson trichrome stain showing collagen (blue) to be a major part of the arteriolar change seen in hypertension. Although two endothelial cells are seen, the tunica media is acellular collagen. Bar = 100 mm. See the color plate section.

(Fig. 11.2C), so-called ball hemorrhages (also termed bleeding globes; see Ch. 1), which can presumably enlarge to fatal hemorrhages if fibrin polymerization does not occur (Fig. 11.2D).

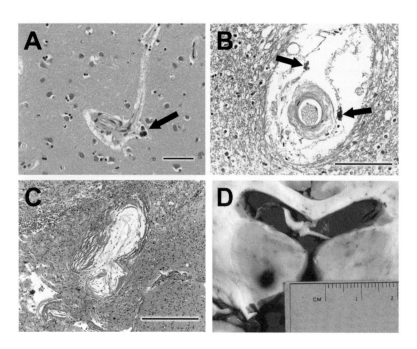

Fig. 11.2 Arteriolar bleeding. (A) Two brown macrophages containing iron (arrow) attest to microbleeding around a relatively normal arteriole (at a branch point). Such findings may relate to transient increases in blood pressure even in the absence of significant arteriolary pathology (see text). Bar = 150 mm. (B) Leakage of blood from acellular arterioles. The tunica media of a brain arteriole in hypertension (same patient as in Fig. 11.1) is acellular. Two brown-colored, iron-laden macrophages are seen (arrows), signifying previous microbleeding into the Virchow–Robin space. Bar = 200 mm. (C) Larger arteriole showing simultaneous leakage and dilatation. Leakage is seen as bright yellow-colored hematoidin (biliverdin) pigment, derived from blood. Hemorrhage approaches detectable size in current MR methodology (see text). Bar 500 mm. (D) Small ball hemorrhage in the thalamus in an asymptomatic patient, visible on gross pathology. See the color plate section.

Distribution in the brain

Within the brain, the gross general distribution of hypertensive arteriolar disease is an inverse negative of the distribution of arteriolar disease resulting from amyloid angiography (Ch. 12). Hypertension tends to affect arterioles close to the circle of Willis and vertebrobasilar circulation. This is in accord with the physiological function of arterioles in bringing down the blood pressure from arteriolar levels to capillary levels (Fig. 11.3). The centrencephalic arteries, arising directly from the low-resistance capacitance arteries at the base of the brain, are exposed to much larger pressure differential than the lobar arterial branches.

Neuroimaging findings of hypertensive arteriopathy

Current neuroimaging techniques do not have the spatial resolution to directly visualize the arterial wall abnormalities described in the preceding section. Hypertension-related arterial changes can be seen, however, in the larger vessels of the circle of Willis. These changes may include dolichoectasia of the larger arteries, particularly the basilar artery or the terminal portion of the intracranial internal carotid artery [18]. Intracranial atherosclerosis of large arteries is more common in hypertension [19]. The presence

of hypertensive arteriolosclerosis must be inferred indirectly, however. Characteristic parenchymal abnormalities in the setting of a history of hypertension, particularly when it has been poorly controlled over a long period, are suggestive of the presence of cerebral arteriosclerosis caused by hypertension. These parenchymal abnormalities include white matter lesions, lacunar lesions and microbleeds. Additionally there is some evidence that brain atrophy, more than expected for age, may be more common in hypertensives [20,21].

Cerebral microbleeds and hypertensive arteriopathy

Cerebral microbleeds are detected on MRI as small foci of signal loss (hypointensity) resulting from local dephasing of the MRI magnetic field caused by the presence of paramagnetic iron atoms. This paramagnetic iron derives from breakdown of the hemoglobin molecule after perivascular leakage of red blood cells [22]. Perivascular deposits of iron-containing proteins, predominantly hemosiderin, are frequently seen in autopsy specimens from individuals who had suffered from hypertension, arteriosclerosis and vascular remodeling, as discussed in the previous section. Therefore, it would be expected that some patients with hypertension would have CMBs. This section will

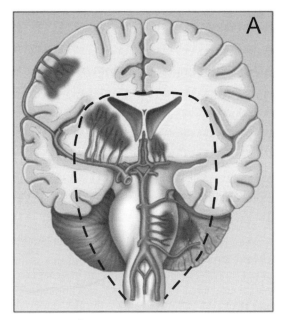

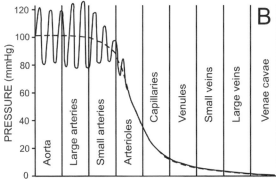

Fig. 11.3 Distribution of hypertensive microbleeds and macrobleeds to the centrencephalon (within dashed line in A). Hypertensive vascular changes are most severe in the centrencephalic arteries arising directly from the major branches of the Circle of Willis (A), where the pulse pressure and blood pressure in the vascular tree are highest (B). By contrast, the lobar arteries are exposed to lower pulse pressure and blood pressure and are less severely affected. See the color plate section.

review data on the relationship between hypertension and CMBs.

Because pathology studies show that hypertensive arteriopathy is more prominent in centrencephalic small arteries than in lobar small arteries, a similar relative distribution of CMBs in the two locations might be expected: that is, that CMBs caused by hypertensive arteriopathy are more likely to be located in the centrencephalic deep hemispheric structures (such

as the thalamus and basal ganglia) than in the cerebral cortex. By contrast cerebral amyloid angiopathy (CAA), probably the second most common small vessel arteriopathy associated with loss of vascular integrity, has almost an inverse pathological distribution, affecting the lobar small arteries with essentially no involvement of the centrencephalic small arteries [23]. Consistent with these varying distributions, neuroimaging studies of CMBs show that patients presenting with symptomatic deep hemispheric ICH, predominantly considered to be caused by hypertension, are more likely to have deep hemispheric CMBs, and patients presenting with symptomatic lobar ICH, frequently caused by CAA, are more likely to have lobar CMBs [24–26]. Research criteria for CAA take advantage of these distinct distributions by defining *probable* CAA based on the presence of multiple lobar CMBs without any deep hemispheric CMBs, in the absence of any other identified cause, and *possible* CAA based on the presence of a single lobar CMB without any other cause [27].

This section considers the risk factors and consequences of CMBs based on these patterns (deep hemispheric, lobar, or mixed lobar and deep hemispheric) when reported by studies.

Hypertension as a risk factor for cerebral microbleeds

Four population-based studies have suggested that high blood pressure is a risk factor for CMBs [28–31]. In the Austrian Stroke Prevention Study ($n = 280$; mean age 60 ± 6 years), CMBs were found in 14.1% of hypertensives but 2.6% of non-hypertensives [28]. Additionally systolic and diastolic blood pressures were significantly higher in those with CMBs. In the Framingham Study ($n = 472$; mean age 64 ± 12 years) the prevalence of CMBs was similar in hypertensives (5.1%) as in non-hypertensives (4.9%) [29]. Higher systolic blood pressure was associated with CMBs in univariate analysis but not after adjusting for age and sex. In the Age Gene/Environment Susceptibility (AGES)-Rekjavik study ($n = 1962$), CMBs were found in 11.9% of hypertensives and 8.2% of non-hypertensives; blood pressures were not reported [30]. The association of hypertension with CMBs was attenuated and of borderline significance after controlling for age and sex ($p = 0.07$). The Rotterdam Study ($n = 1062$; mean age 70 ± 7 years) used a substantially different MRI protocol that included a high-resolution three-dimensional T_2*-weighted gradient-recalled echo (GRE) sequence with a long echo time, which was shown to have approximately double the sensitivity for CMBs compared with conventional T_2*-weighted GRE sequences. In this study, there was no relationship between CMBs and either mild or severe hypertension, but there was an independent relationship between higher systolic (but not diastolic) blood pressure and the likelihood of CMBs (odds ratio 1.16 per standard deviation increase in systolic blood pressure) [31]. Across all studies, approximately 30–40% of CMBs were in deep hemispheric or posterior fossa locations. Only the Rotterdam Study systematically looked at risk factors separately in those with purely lobar CMBs, suggesting the presence of CAA, and those with non-lobar CMBs. The association between systolic blood pressure and CMBs was stronger after excluding patients with strictly lobar CMBs, and additionally a relationship with pulse pressure emerged [31].

Therefore, the aggregate evidence from population-based studies of healthy stroke-free persons demonstrates a relationship between CMBs, particularly non-lobar CMBs, and higher blood pressure. Relationships between CMBs and measured blood pressures seem to be stronger than for CMBs and history of hypertension. This suggests a graded relationship between blood pressure and the prevalence of CMBs, such that mild or treated hypertension may confer little increased risk. None of these population-based studies have included longitudinal measurements of CMBs; consequently, the incidence of new CMBs over a defined period of time in the general population is unknown.

Clinic-based cohort studies of neurologically healthy adults have also found a relationship between CMBs and hypertension [32,33]. An MRI substudy of the Prospective Study of Pravastatin in the Elderly at Risk (PROSPER) showed that hypertension was strongly associated with basal ganglia CMBs but not lobar CMBs [34]. Furthermore, studies in other small vessel arteriopathies such as CADASIL (cerebral autosomal dominant arteriopathy with subcortical infarcts and leukoencephalopathy) [35] and CAA [26] suggest that hypertension may have an added effect on the risk of CMBs in those conditions. A systematic review of all relevant studies confirmed an association between CMBs and hypertension [36].

Cerebral microbleeds in hypertension-related conditions including stroke

A relationship between CMBs and hypertensive arteriopathy is suggested by the high prevalence of CMBs in hypertension-related diseases such as stroke. A number of studies have identified CMBs in patients who have had a stroke; the prevalence of CMBs in ischemic stroke is approximately 20–30%, substantially higher than in the general population [24,37–50]. Additionally when CMBs are present in these patients, they are more likely to be multiple. Among patients with ischemic stroke, CMBs are more common in lacunar stroke (35–60%) [37,40,44,48,50] than in stroke caused by large artery atherosclerosis (12–26%) or cardioembolic stroke (4–30%) [44,50,51]. Studies undertaken after stroke have shown that CMBs are more frequent in patients who have a past history of lacunar stroke or ICH [38,40] and in those with neuroimaging evidence of past silent lacunar infarcts [46,50,52] than in the general population [28,31]. The prevalence of CMBs in patients with ICH is even higher, at 50–70% [24–26,38,43,45,50,53,54]. These data suggest that CMB are more frequent in small vessel stroke, which is more closely associated with hypertension than is large vessel stroke.

Cerebral microbleeds have been associated with chronic kidney disease, which may either result from hypertension or be a cause of hypertension. Two studies have reported a high prevalence of CMBs in patients with clinically diagnosed chronic kidney disease not on dialysis [55] or on dialysis [56]. Studies in patients after ischemic stroke have found associations between CMBs and lower estimated glomerular filtration rate [42] and the presence of proteinuria [57]. However, CMBs may also occur in hypertensives without other signs of end-organ damage such as kidney disease or cardiac disease [58].

Distribution of cerebral microbleeds in hypertension

Hypertensive arteriopathy may be seen pathologically in any of the brain vessels, but there is a predilection for the centrencephalic arteries supplying the deep

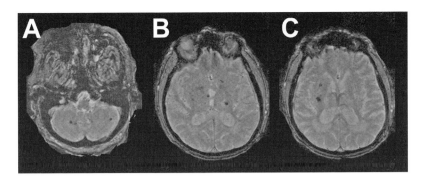

Fig. 11.4 Cerebral microbleeds in the cerebellum, thalami and basal ganglia in a 70-year-old patient with chronic hypertension, measured on MRI T_2^*-weighted gradient-recalled echo sequence. Microbleeds in these locations are typical for hypertensive arteriopathy.

hemispheric structures including the basal ganglia and thalamus. A population-based study has associated hypertension with an increased frequency of deep hemispheric CMBs [31]. Other studies have used MRI performed in hypertensive patients with stroke to map the distribution of CMBs according to brain region.

Overall, the distribution of CMBs in hypertension is similar to the distribution of hypertension-related symptomatic ICH (Fig. 11.4). In a study of 164 patients with 824 CMBs who presented with hypertension and stroke, supratentorial non-lobar CMBs were distributed as follows: caudate 5.0%, putamen 29.3%, internal capsule 6.9% and thalamus 58.8% [39]. Most CMBs were found in the gray matter structures, rather than the white matter of the diencephalon [39]. In the posterior fossa, CMBs were most frequently detected in the middle portion of the central pons and in the cerebellum in the region of the dentate nucleus [59].

Lobar CMBs may also occur as a result of hypertensive arteriopathy, although the pattern of purely lobar CMBs, with no deep hemispheric CMBs, appears to be quite specific for CAA [27]. A study of hypertensive patients with ischemic or hemorrhagic stroke showed a greater prevalence of CMBs in the cortico-subcortical regions of the temporal lobe (37.2% of all cortico-subcortical CMB) and occipital lobe (34.8%) than in the parietal lobe (15.1%) or the larger frontal lobe (10.5%) [39]. A limitation of this study is that some of the lobar CMBs could have been caused by CAA, because both hypertension arteriopathy and CAA are common pathologies of aging and must sometimes co-exist. Future studies incorporating in vivo amyloid imaging may in the future allow better sensitivity for exclusion of patients with CAA, and thus provide a clearer picture of the distribution of lobar CMBs in hypertension [60].

Risk factors for cerebral microbleeds among persons with hypertension

Relatively little work has been done to distinguish which patients with hypertension are likely to have CMBs. There does seem to be a correlation between hypertension severity, as inferred by blood pressure measured at a single study visit, and the presence of CMBs [31]. There are few data relating CMBs to the duration of hypertension, the combination of duration and severity of hypertension, or the timing and intensity of antihypertensive treatments. In one study, there was a correlation between higher left ventricular mass index, which is increased in proportion to the duration and severity of hypertension, and the presence of CMBs [61].

Twenty-four hour blood pressure recordings reveal that hypertensives with CMB have persistently higher blood pressure during the day than at night [48,62]. In one study, the association was attenuated and not significant when considering lobar CMBs alone [48]. An association with nocturnal dipping was not identified [62].

Studies relating measures of arterial stiffness to CMBs have produced somewhat conflicting results. Two studies, one in individuals with lacunar stroke and one in healthy volunteers, found an association between the presence of CMBs and higher brachial–ankle pulse wave velocity [63,64]. However, a study of stroke-free hypertensives found no association between CMBs and higher aortic pulse wave velocity [65]. Likewise, a study of patients with type 1 diabetes mellitus found no association with higher aortic pulse wave velocity [66].

Conclusions and future directions

Hypertension is a common age-related disease that is accompanied by loss of vascular integrity, with leakage of red blood cells and perivascular hemosiderin deposition. Larger deposits may be detectable as CMBs. Because the pathological prevalence of perivascular hemosiderin deposits appears to be much higher than the radiological prevalence of CMBs, it is likely that the measured prevalence and severity of CMBs will continue to increase as more sensitive MRI sequences, for example susceptibility-weighted imaging, are developed and used. Blood pressure recordings, and possibly measures of arterial stiffness and end-organ damage, are better predictors of CMBs than a clinical history of hypertension, possibly because a history of hypertension may reflect widely different severities of hypertension. Cerebral microbleeds caused by hypertensive arteriopathy may be seen in the deep hemispheric regions, brainstem, cerebellum and cerebral lobes; however, the pattern of purely lobar CMBs strongly suggests CAA rather than hypertensive arteriopathy.

There are many unanswered questions and avenues for future research. Cerebral microbleeds may be a marker of cerebral end-organ damage from hypertension and thus a useful surrogate marker for research studies. However, this requires more investigation and validation in longitudinal studies, because nearly all previous studies have been cross-sectional. It is tempting to hypothesize that CMBs are a radiological surrogate of disrupted vascular integrity in hypertensive arteriopathy and would predict future risk of hypertensive brain hemorrhage [67]. However, this hypothesis requires further testing in large studies. Preliminary evidence suggests that patients with CMBs are at risk for developing new CMBs, and that patients with high blood pressure are at the highest risk [68]. This suggests that patients with hypertension and CMBs may be a population in which more aggressive blood pressure lowering is warranted. However there is currently insufficient evidence to confidently recommend different blood pressure targets in patients with CMBs. There is a need for additional larger longitudinal studies to relate blood pressure, blood pressure treatment and changes in blood pressure over time with the incidence of CMBs and parenchymal hemorrhages.

References

1. Alzheimer A. On arteriosclerotic atrophy of the cortex. *Neurolog Zentralblat* 1894;**13**:765–8.

2. Hajjar I, Kotchen TA. Trends in prevalence, awareness, treatment, and control of hypertension in the United States, 1988–2000. *JAMA* 2003;**290**:199–206.

3. Gu D, Reynolds K, Wu X *et al.* Prevalence, awareness, treatment, and control of hypertension in China. *Hypertension* 2002;**40**:920–7.

4. Taler SJ. Secondary causes of hypertension. *Prim Care* 2008;**35**:489–500, vi.

5. Staessen JA, Wang J, Bianchi G *et al.* Essential hypertension. *Lancet* 2003;**361**:1629–41.

6. Strazzullo P, Galletti F, Barba G. Altered renal handling of sodium in human hypertension: short review of the evidence. *Hypertension* 2003;**41**:1000–5.

7. Goldstein LB, Adams R, Alberts MJ *et al.* Primary prevention of ischemic stroke: a guideline from the American Heart Association/American Stroke Association Stroke Council: cosponsored by the Atherosclerotic Peripheral Vascular Disease Interdisciplinary Working Group; Cardiovascular Nursing Council; Clinical Cardiology Council; Nutrition, Physical Activity, and Metabolism Council; and the Quality of Care and Outcomes Research Interdisciplinary Working Group: the American Academy of Neurology affirms the value of this guideline. *Stroke* 2006;**37**:1583–1633.

8. Fisher CM. Pathological observations in hypertensive cerebral hemorrhage. *J Neuropathol Exp Neurol* 1971;**30**:536–50.

9. Kivipelto M, Helkala EL, Laakso MP *et al.* Midlife vascular risk factors and Alzheimer's disease in later life: longitudinal, population based study. *BMJ* 2001;**322**:1447–51.

10. Bund SJ, Lee RM. Arterial structural changes in hypertension: a consideration of methodology, terminology and functional consequence. *J Vasc Res* 2003;**40**:547–57.

11. Strandgaard S, Olesen J, Skinhoj E *et al.* Autoregulation of brain circulation in severe arterial hypertension. *BMJ* 1973;**1**:507–10.

12. Baumbach GL, Heistad DD. Adaptive changes in cerebral blood vessels during chronic hypertension. *J Hypertens* 1991;**9**:987–91.

13. Sutherland GR, Auer RN. Primary intracerebral hemorrhage. *J Clin Neurosci* 2006;**13**:511–17.

14. Yasmin, McEniery CM, Wallace S *et al.* Matrix metalloproteinase-9 (MMP-9), MMP-2, and serum elastase activity are associated with systolic hypertension and arterial stiffness. *Arterioscler Thromb Vasc Biol* 2005;**25**:372.

15. Rosenblum WI. Fibrinoid necrosis of small brain arteries and arterioles and miliary aneurysms as causes of hypertensive hemorrhage: a critical reappraisal. *Acta Neuropathol* 2008;**116**:361–9.

16. Challa VR, Moody DM, Bell MA. The Charcot–Bouchard aneurysm controversy: impact of a new histologic technique. *J Neuropathol Exp Neurol* 1992;**51**:264–71.

17. Osol G, Brekke JF, McElroy-Yaggy K *et al.* Myogenic tone, reactivity, and forced dilatation: a three-phase model of in vitro arterial myogenic behavior. *Am J Physiol Heart Circ Physiol* 2002;**283**:H2260–7.

18. Pico F, Labreuche J, Touboul PJ *et al.* Intracranial arterial dolichoectasia and its relation with atherosclerosis and stroke subtype. *Neurology* 2003;**61**:1736–42.

19. Bae HJ, Lee J, Park JM *et al.* Risk factors of intracranial cerebral atherosclerosis among asymptomatics. *Cerebrovasc Dis* 2007;**24**: 355–60.

20. Goldstein IB, Bartzokis G, Guthrie D *et al.* Ambulatory blood pressure and the brain: a 5-year follow-up. *Neurology* 2005;**64**: 1846–52.

21. Heijer T, Skoog I, Oudkerk M *et al.* Association between blood pressure levels over time and brain atrophy in the elderly. *Neurobiol Aging* 2003;**24**:307–13.

22. Fazekas F, Kleinert R, Roob G *et al.* Histopathologic analysis of foci of signal loss on gradient-echo T_2*-weighted MR images in patients with spontaneous intracerebral hemorrhage: evidence of microangiopathy-related microbleeds. *AJNR Am J Neuroradiol.* 1999;**20**:637–42.

23. Auer RN, Sutherland GR. Primary intracerebral hemorrhage: pathophysiology. *Can J Neurol Sci* 2005;**32**(Suppl. 2):S3–12.

24. Lee SH, Bae HJ, Kwon SJ *et al.* Cerebral microbleeds are regionally associated with intracerebral hemorrhage. *Neurology* 2004;**62**:72–6.

25. Roob G, Lechner A, Schmidt R *et al.* Frequency and location of microbleeds in patients with primary intracerebral hemorrhage. *Stroke* 2000;**31**: 2665–9.

26. Smith EE, Nandigam KRN, Chen Y-W *et al.* MRI markers of small vessel disease in lobar and deep hemispheric intracerebral hemorrhage. *Stroke* 2010;**41**:1933–8.

27. Knudsen KA, Rosand J, Karluk D *et al.* Clinical diagnosis of cerebral amyloid angiopathy: validation of the Boston criteria. *Neurology* 2001;**56**:537–9.

28. Roob G, Schmidt R, Kapeller P *et al.* MRI evidence of past cerebral microbleeds in a healthy elderly population. *Neurology* 1999;**52**:991–4.

29. Jeerakathil T, Wolf PA, Beiser A *et al.* Cerebral microbleeds: prevalence and associations with cardiovascular risk factors in the Framingham Study. *Stroke* 2004;**35**:1831–5.

30. Sveinbjornsdottir S, Sigurdsson S, Aspelund T *et al.* Cerebral microbleeds in the population based AGES–Reykjavik study: prevalence and location. *J Neurol Neurosurg Psychiatry* 2008;**79**:1002–6.

31. Vernooij MW, van der Lugt A, Ikram MA *et al.* Prevalence and risk factors of cerebral microbleeds: the Rotterdam Scan Study. *Neurology* 2008;**70**: 1208–14.

32. Tsushima Y, Tanizaki Y, Aoki J *et al.* MR detection of microhemorrhages in neurologically healthy adults. *Neuroradiology* 2002;**44**:31–6.

33. Igase M, Tabara Y, Igase K *et al.* Asymptomatic cerebral microbleeds seen in healthy subjects have a strong association with asymptomatic lacunar infarction. *Circ J* 2009;**73**:530–3.

34. van Es AC, van der Grond J, de Craen AJ *et al.* Risk factors for cerebral microbleeds in the elderly. *Cerebrovasc Dis* 2008;**26**:397–403.

35. Viswanathan A, Guichard JP, Gschwendtner A *et al.* Blood pressure and haemoglobin A1c are associated with microhaemorrhage in CADASIL: a two-centre cohort study. *Brain* 2006;**129**:2375–83.

36. Cordonnier C, Al-Shahi Salman R, Wardlaw J. Spontaneous brain microbleeds: systematic review, subgroup analyses and standards for study design and reporting. *Brain* 2007;**130**:1988–2003.

37. Fan YH, Mok VC, Lam WW *et al.* Cerebral microbleeds and white matter changes in patients hospitalized with lacunar infarcts. *J Neurol* 2004;**251**:537–41.

38. Imaizumi T, Horita Y, Chiba M *et al.* Dot-like hemosiderin spots on gradient echo T_2*-weighted magnetic resonance imaging are associated with past history of small vessel disease in patients with intracerebral hemorrhage. *J Neuroimaging* 2004;**14**:251–7.

39. Lee SH, Kwon SJ, Kim KS *et al.* Cerebral microbleeds in patients with hypertensive stroke. Topographical distribution in the supratentorial area. *J Neurol* 2004;**251**:1183–9.

40. Imaizumi T, Honma T, Horita Y *et al.* Dotlike hemosiderin spots are associated with past

hemorrhagic strokes in patients with lacunar infarcts. *J Neuroimaging* 2005;**15**:157–63.

41. Werring DJ, Coward LJ, Losseff NA *et al.* Cerebral microbleeds are common in ischemic stroke but rare in TIA. *Neurology* 2005;**65**:1914–18.

42. Cho AH, Lee SB, Han SJ *et al.* Impaired kidney function and cerebral microbleeds in patients with acute ischemic stroke. *Neurology* 2009;**73**:1645–8.

43. Alemany M, Stenborg A, Terent A *et al.* Coexistence of microhemorrhages and acute spontaneous brain hemorrhage: correlation with signs of microangiopathy and clinical data. *Radiology* 2006;**238**:240–7.

44. Ovbiagele B, Saver JL, Sanossian N *et al.* Predictors of cerebral microbleeds in acute ischemic stroke and TIA patients. *Cerebrovasc Dis* 2006;**22**:378–83.

45. Jeon SB, Kang DW, Cho AH *et al.* Initial microbleeds at MR imaging can predict recurrent intracerebral hemorrhage. *J Neurol* 2007;**254**:508–12.

46. Han J, Gao P, Lin Y *et al.* Three-tesla magnetic resonance imaging study of cerebral microbleeds in patients with ischemic stroke. *Neurol Res* 2009;**31**:900–3.

47. Orken DN, Kenangil G, Uysal E *et al.* Cerebral microbleeds in ischemic stroke patients on warfarin treatment. *Stroke* 2009;**40**:3638–40.

48. Staals J, van Oostenbrugge RJ, Knottnerus IL *et al.* Brain microbleeds relate to higher ambulatory blood pressure levels in first-ever lacunar stroke patients. *Stroke* 2009;**40**:3264–8.

49. Sun J, Soo YO, Lam WW *et al.* Different distribution patterns of cerebral microbleeds in acute ischemic stroke patients with and without hypertension. *Eur Neurol* 2009;**62**:290–303.

50. Kato H, Izumiyama M, Izumiyama K *et al.* Silent cerebral microbleeds on T$_2$*-weighted MRI: correlation with stroke subtype, stroke recurrence, and leukoaraiosis. *Stroke* 2002;**33**:1536–40.

51. Gao T, Wang Y, Zhang Z. Silent cerebral microbleeds on susceptibility-weighted imaging of patients with ischemic stroke and leukoaraiosis. *Neurol Res* 2008;**30**:272–6.

52. Lee SH, Bae HJ, Ko SB *et al.* Comparative analysis of the spatial distribution and severity of cerebral microbleeds and old lacunes. *J Neurol Neurosurg Psychiatry* 2004;**75**:423–7.

53. Lim JB, Kim E. Silent microbleeds and old hematomas in spontaneous cerebral hemorrhages. *J Korean Neurosurg Soc* 2009;**46**:38–44.

54. Copenhaver BR, Hsia AW, Merino JG *et al.* Racial differences in microbleed prevalence in primary intracerebral hemorrhage. *Neurology* 2008;**71**:1176–82.

55. Shima H, Ishimura E, Naganuma T *et al.* Cerebral microbleeds in predialysis patients with chronic kidney disease. *Nephrol Dial Transplant* 2010;**25**:1554–9.

56. Yokoyama S, Hirano H, Uomizu K *et al.* High incidence of microbleeds in hemodialysis patients detected by T$_2$*-weighted gradient-echo magnetic resonance imaging. *Neurol Med-Chir* 2005;**45**:556–60; discussion 560.

57. Ovbiagele B, Liebeskind DS, Pineda S *et al.* Strong independent correlation of proteinuria with cerebral microbleeds in patients with stroke and transient ischemic attack. *Arch Neurol* 2010;**67**:45–50.

58. Henskens LH, van Oostenbrugge RJ, Kroon AA *et al.* Detection of silent cerebrovascular disease refines risk stratification of hypertensive patients. *J Hypertens* 2009;**27**:846–53.

59. Lee SH, Kwon SJ, Kim KS *et al.* Topographical distribution of pontocerebellar microbleeds. *AJNR Am J Neuroradiol.* 2004;**25**:1337–41.

60. Johnson KA, Gregas M, Becker JA *et al.* Imaging of amyloid burden and distribution in cerebral amyloid angiopathy. *Ann Neurol* 2007;**62**:229–34.

61. Lee SH, Park JM, Kwon SJ *et al.* Left ventricular hypertrophy is associated with cerebral microbleeds in hypertensive patients. *Neurology* 2004;**63**:16–21.

62. Henskens LH, van Oostenbrugge RJ, Kroon AA *et al.* Brain microbleeds are associated with ambulatory blood pressure levels in a hypertensive population. *Hypertension* 2008;**51**:62–8.

63. Seo WK, Lee JM, Park MH *et al.* Cerebral microbleeds are independently associated with arterial stiffness in stroke patients. *Cerebrovasc Dis* 2008;**26**:618–23.

64. Ochi N, Tabara Y, Igase M *et al.* Silent cerebral microbleeds associated with arterial stiffness in an apparently healthy subject. *Hypertens Res* 2009;**32**:255–60.

65. Henskens LH, Kroon AA, van Oostenbrugge RJ *et al.* Increased aortic pulse wave velocity is associated with silent cerebral small-vessel disease in hypertensive patients. *Hypertension* 2008;**52**:1120–6.

66. van Elderen SG, Brandts A, Westenberg JJ *et al.* Aortic stiffness is associated with cardiac function and cerebral small vessel disease in patients with type 1 diabetes mellitus: assessment by magnetic resonance imaging. *Eur Radiol* 2010;**20**:1132–8.

67. Soo YO, Yang SR, Lam WW *et al.* Risk vs benefit of anti-thrombotic therapy in ischaemic stroke patients with cerebral microbleeds. *J Neurol* 2008;**255**:1679–86.

68. Gregoire SM, Brown MM, Kallis C *et al.* MRI detection of new microbleeds in patients with ischemic stroke: five-year cohort follow-up study. *Stroke* 2010;**41**:184–6.

Chapter

12

Cerebral microbleeds in relation to cerebral amyloid angiopathy

M. Ayaz Khan, Anand Viswanathan and Steven M. Greenberg

Introduction

Cerebral amyloid angiopathy (CAA) is small vessel disease that occurs commonly in the elderly population. It results in thickening of the vessel wall, primarily in small arteries and arterioles of the leptomeninges and cerebral cortex [1]. It can also affect cerebellar vessels [2]. The primary constituent of the vascular amyloid deposits is the beta-amyloid peptide (Aβ), also the main component of the senile plaques observed in Alzheimer's disease (AD). The earliest detectable vascular Aβ deposits typically occur between the smooth muscle cells of the media and the connective tissue of the adventitia. As the disease progresses, amyloid replaces the media with loss of smooth muscle cells [1]. Autopsy studies indicate that CAA is a common pathology of older individuals, with 10–40% prevalence in the general population and at least 80% among individuals with AD [3].

Although the precise origin of the vascular amyloid has not been definitively established, the predominant source appears to be neuronal [4]. According to this model, Aβ derived from amyloid precursor protein can deposit in the brain parenchyma to form senile plaques or can be carried via the interstitial fluid into the perivascular space to become cerebrovascular deposits in CAA [5]. Deposition of Aβ causes injury to the vessel wall, which can give rise to small infarctions [6,7] or to rupture of the vessel wall, with leakage of blood, and formation of small cerebral microbleeds (CMB) or larger symptomatic intracerebral hemorrhage (ICH).

Cerebral amyloid angiopathy and intracerebral hemorrhage

Primary ICH in the elderly is the result of disease of the small cerebral vessels, in particular hypertensive vasculopathy or CAA. Mild CAA may cause no evident vessel damage, but moderate to severe disease results in breakdown of the vessel wall, including loss of smooth muscle cells, splitting of the vessel wall, microaneurysms, fibrinoid necrosis and leakage of blood products [8,9]. These changes give rise to large CAA-related hemorrhagic strokes, the most severe recognized clinical manifestation of CAA.

The CAA-related ICH occurs in cortical or cortico-subcortical (lobar) brain regions, reflecting the location of the underlying vascular amyloid deposits [10]. This location contrasts with the typical deep hemispheric or infratentorial locations of hypertensive ICH. Within lobar brain regions, CAA-related ICH tends to favor the occipital cortex; one study found 25% of symptomatic hemorrhages in this region [11] although this lobe only makes up 18.3% of cortical volume [12]. The occipital predilection again likely reflects increased occipital burden of the underlying vascular pathology [10].

Although lobar ICH is associated with CAA, the prevalence of CAA-related ICH is considerably lower than the overall prevalence of CAA. It is, therefore, only the most severely affected minority of patients with CAA who develop ICH.

Cerebral Microbleeds, ed. David J. Werring. Published by Cambridge University Press. © Cambridge University Press 2011.

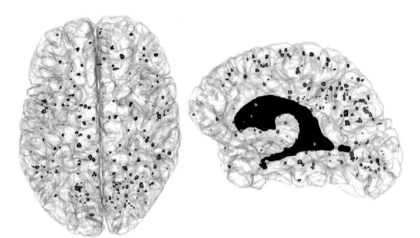

Fig. 12.1 Three-dimensional templates of hemorrhage distribution related to cerebral amyloid angiopathy. The axial (A) and sagittal (B) images display the composite locations of all identified hemorrhages in a subject imaged with T_2*-weighted MRI. Each dot represents a single bleed. Notice that most are located in the posterior part of the brain (occipital region). See the color plate section.

Cerebral amyloid angiopathy-related cerebral microbleeds

The introduction of T_2*-weighted MRI enabled the detection of CMBs as focal hypointensities generally not seen with conventional spin echo sequences [13]. Histopathological correlation has shown that these MRI lesions occur in association with small vessel diseases of the brain such as CAA [14]. Although these signal voids are generally considered clinically silent, a growing literature supports the idea that CMB are not only markers of cerebral microvasculopathy but may also contribute to neurological decline [11,15,16].

The CAA-related CMBs, like other types of microbleed, consist primarily of macrophages containing hemosiderin, a degraded form of ferritin. Based on counting CMBs in patients presenting with CAA-related ICH, there appear to be approximately 2.5 times as many CMBs as symptomatic "macrobleeds" [11]. This cross-sectional estimate is biased by the fact that all patients in the study were required to have at least one lobar ICH, thus undercounting CMB that occur without associated lobar ICH.

The distribution of CAA-related CMB appears similar to CAA-related symptomatic ICH. As noted for larger hemorrhages, CMB in CAA occur preferentially in posterior lobar regions (Fig. 12.1) [15,17]. There is also a tendency within individual subjects for hemorrhagic lesions (both micro- and macrobleeds) to cluster within the same lobe [17]. These findings suggest that differences in brain regions (arising either from general brain anatomy or specific changes in CAA) play an important role in promoting CAA-related ICH.

Incident CMBs or symptomatic ICH can be demonstrated in longitudinally followed individuals diagnosed with CAA [11,15,16]. Based on clinical follow-up (for ICH) and serial T_2*-weighted MRI (for CMB), the incidence of CAA-related CMB appears to be approximately 10-fold greater than for symptomatic hemorrhages [11]. Similar to the clustering of hemorrhagic lesions noted in cross-sectional studies, incident CMBs tend to occur in brain regions with prior hemorrhages (Fig. 12.2) [15,17].

The number of CAA-related CMBs at baseline is a strong predictor of incident CMBs on serial imaging [18] and of recurrent ICH on clinical follow-up (Fig. 12.3A) [11]. In a study of patients presenting with lobar ICH, the 2-year cumulative rate of recurrent ICH was 14% in those subjects with only one total (ICH plus

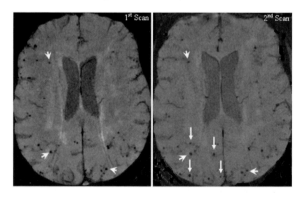

Fig. 12.2 New cerebral microbleed (CMB). Susceptibility-weighted images (4 mm slice thickness) from two different scans, performed 1 year apart, show development of incident CMB in lobar region (white arrows). Arrowheads in the first image show the CMBs observed in both scans. All CMB are located in lobar regions, consistent with the diagnosis of probable cerebral amyloid angiopathy.

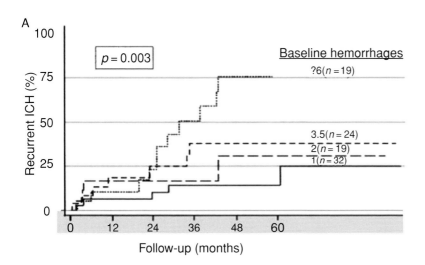

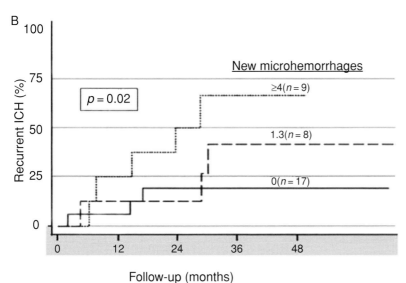

Fig. 12.3 Kaplan–Meier estimates of rate of recurrent lobar ICH. Data are stratified according to the number of hemorrhages detected on baseline MRI (A) or the number of new hemorrhages detected on follow-up MRI (B). Testing for significance is by Cox proportional-hazards regression model on the designated categories; the analysis in B also controls for the time interval between the two MRI scans. (Reproduced with permission from Greenberg *et al.* 2004 [11].)

CMBs) hemorrhagic lesion at baseline, 17% for subjects with two total baseline hemorrhages, 37% with three to five lesions and 51% for six or more lesions [11]. Appearance of new CMB also predicted subsequent recurrent ICH (Fig. 12.3B) [11], further underscoring the connection between these two types of hemorrhagic event.

Most studies of CAA-related CMB have relied on "conventional" T_2*-weighted MRI performed under standard clinical parameters. Newer T_2*-weighted techniques, however, appear to increase sensitivity for CMB detection [15,19,20], resulting in higher lesion counts. One such method, termed susceptibility-weighted imaging (SWI) [21], is a three-dimensional

T_2*-weighted technique with long echo time and incorporating both magnitude and phase information. Studies using SWI have detected CMBs as small as approximately 1 mm in diameter (Fig. 12.4) [15].

Role of cerebral microbleeds in the diagnosis of cerebral amyloid angiopathy: the Boston criteria

The most commonly employed criteria for diagnosis of CAA-related ICH, termed the Boston criteria (Box 12.1), are based on neuropathological examination or, more commonly, characteristic neuroimaging findings [22]. The diagnosis of "probable CAA"

Box 12.1 Boston criteria for diagnosis of cerebral amyloid angiopathy (CAA)-related intracranial hemorrhage

Definite cerebral amyloid angiopathy

Full autopsy examination demonstrating:

- lobar, cortical or cortico-subcortical hemorrhage
- severe CAA with vasculopathy
- absence of other diagnostic lesion.

Probable cerebral amyloid angiopathy with supporting pathology

Clinical data and pathological tissue (evacuated hematoma or cortical biopsy) showing:

- lobar, cortical or cortico-subcortical hemorrhage
- some degree of CAA in specimen
- absence of other cause of hemorrhage.[a]

Probable cerebral amyloid angiopathy

- Clinical data and MRI or CT demonstrating multiple hemorrhages restricted to lobar, cortical or cortico-subcortical regions (cerebellar hemorrhage allowed).
- Age ≥ 55 years.
- Absence of other cause of hemorrhage.[a]

Possible cerebral amyloid angiopathy

- Clinical data and MRI or CT demonstrating single lobar, cortical or cortico-subcortical hemorrhage.
- Age ≥ 55 years.
- Absence of other cause of hemorrhage.[a]

[a] Other causes of hemorrhage include antecedent head trauma or ischemic stroke, central nervous system tumor, warfarin therapy with international normalized ratio >3, vascular malformation or vasculitis.

in particular depends on identifying multiple (two or more) hemorrhagic lesions strictly localized to the lobar brain regions characteristic of this disorder. To meet these criteria, hemorrhages must entirely spare locations typical of hypertensive ICH such as basal ganglia, thalamus or pons; cerebellar hemorrhage is allowed. Diagnosis of probable CAA is also precluded by other definite causes of hemorrhage such as trauma, vasculitis or excessive anticoagulation.

The requirement for multiple strictly lobar hemorrhagic lesions to diagnose probable CAA pertains to CMB as well as ICH. The rationale for incorporating CMB into the diagnostic criteria is that lobar CMB and lobar ICH each represent independent vascular ruptures in brain regions characteristic of CAA-related hemorrhage and, therefore, offer equal evidence for the presence of CAA. Supporting this approach is the observation that CMBs and ICH tend to occur in the same brain compartment (i.e. both lobar in CAA, both deep hemispheric in hypertensive ICH) [23,24].

The *specificity* of the Boston criteria has been validated by correlation with neuropathology obtained at brain biopsy, hematoma evacuation or autopsy examination [22]. A more recent study using the genetic mutation associated with Dutch-type hereditary CAA as the basis for diagnosis found high *sensitivity* for the diagnosis of CAA in clinically symptomatic patients [25]. The sensitivity of the probable CAA diagnosis in this study was increased when CMBs as well as symptomatic ICH were included as hemorrhagic lesions. Of note, none of the patients demonstrated CMB in deep white matter, basal ganglia, thalamus or brainstem, again supporting the distinction drawn between lobar and non-lobar CMB in diagnosing underlying small vessel pathology.

Role of cerebral amyloid angiopathy-related microbleeds in neurological dysfunction

The neuroimaging and neuropathological evidence described above strongly implicate CMB as a marker of CAA (or other small vessel disease). It is less clear

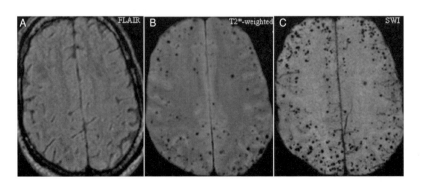

Fig. 12.4 Improved detection of cerebral microbleed (CMB) in "conventional" gradient-recalled echo (GRE) T_2*-weighted (B) and susceptibilty-weighted (SWI) (C) images relative to fluid attenuated inversion recovery (FLAIR) image (A). The CMB in both GRE and SWI images are located in a strictly lobar distribution.

whether, in addition to being a marker for CAA, CMBs also contribute directly to neurological dysfunction such as cognitive impairment. One study [11] found that higher numbers of baseline hemorrhagic lesions (ICH plus CMB) were associated with increased hazard for incident clinical decline (defined as incident dementia, functional dependence or death). This association remained detectable even when excluding patients with ICH during follow-up (Fig. 11.3A), indicating that it was not driven primarily by recurrent hemorrhagic stroke.

A direct contribution of CAA-related CMBs to cognitive impairment is consistent with other studies that suggest a deleterious effect for these lesions [15,26,27]. The interpretation of these findings is complicated, however, by the other manifestations of small vessel disease that typically accompany CMBs. In the case of CAA, it is difficult to tease apart the independent contribution of CMBs from the other types of CAA-related brain injury such as white matter hyperintensities [28,29], changes in diffusion tensor measurements [30] and microinfarcts [6,7]. If CMB indeed have an independent contribution to vascular cognitive impairment, it is most likely as part of a multifactorial process from multiple small vessel-related injuries together with other degenerative pathologies such as accompanying AD [31].

Relationship of cerebral amyloid angiopathy-related microbleeds and intracerebral hemorrhage: the effect of vascular structure

Despite the overall association noted above between CAA-related CMB and ICH, some individuals with CAA appear predisposed to large numbers of CMBs with few or no large hemorrhages, whereas others may have frequent recurrent macrobleeds without CMBs. This observation raises the general question as to exactly what determines whether a vessel rupture will result in a CMB or a larger macrobleed. One study of the volumes of CAA-related hemorrhagic lesions [32] found that the volumes fell into two distinct peaks of microbleeds and macrobleeds, rather than forming a single continuous distribution. The peaks were best separated by a cut-point diameter of 5.7 mm, a value similar to the conventionally chosen criteria for the upper size limit of a CMB [33]. These data suggest that microbleeding and macrobleeding, though shar-

ing common underlying etiologies (such as CAA), may represent distinct pathophysiological events.

Another finding from the same study [32] was that autopsied CAA subjects selected to represent extreme "microbleeders" (more than 50 CMBs) demonstrated significantly thicker vessel walls than those with macrobleeds and few CMB (fewer than three). Increased vessel thickness was observed only in amyloid-laden vessels and, therefore, did not appear to reflect a more general underlying vascular process. These results, yet to be confirmed in other series or other small vessel diseases, raise the possibility that particular properties of the diseased vessel wall may predispose to formation of microbleeds rather than macrobleeds or vice versa.

Detection of cerebral amyloid angiopathy-related microbleeds in the absence of intracerebral hemorrhage

Alzheimer's disease

Both CAA and AD are common pathologies of aging, with shared pathogenic features (such as deposition of $A\beta$), and thus demonstrate substantial overlap. In the CERAD study of 117 brains with confirmed AD for example, 97 (83%) demonstrated at least mild CAA, including 30 (26%) with moderate to severe CAA [34]. The increased overlap of AD with advanced CAA likely accounts for the high prevalence of CMB (approximately 20–25% by conventional T_2^*-weighted MRI) identified in studies of patients diagnosed with probable AD [35–37]. Like CAA-related CMBs, most AD-associated CMBs are lobar with predilection for posterior cortical lobes [37], further supporting the role of accompanying CAA in causing these lesions.

The question arises again whether AD-associated CMB, in addition to marking underlying vascular disease, are also contributors to cognitive impairment in AD. Some studies of CMB-positive patients with AD have suggested worse cognitive performance or shorter survival [38,39]. There is also clinical–pathological evidence that advanced CAA may be an independent contributor to cognitive impairment, in either the absence or the presence of AD pathology [40,41]. It remains to be determined, however, whether the CMBs per se are an important component of worsened neurological function in CMB-positive individuals with AD.

General aging population

The prevalence of CMBs in the general population increases with aging [42]. The highest estimates for CMB-positive individuals, obtained from optimized T_2^*-weighted MRI [19], range from 17.8% in those aged 60–69 years, to 31.3% for individuals aged 70–79 years and 38.3% for age $\geq$80 years [43]. Although CMBs in the healthy aging population most commonly arise from either hypertensive vasculopathy or advanced CAA, it is notable that the majority of these CMBs appear in a lobar distribution [43,44]. This observation raises the possibility that a substantial subset of apparently healthy elderly individuals have advanced (though clinically asymptomatic) CAA. Further support for this possibility comes from reported associations between strictly lobar CMBs and the *APOE ε*4 allele [43] or between any CMB and the *APOE ε*4/*ε*4 homozygous genotype [44]. These suggestive observations will require replication and corroboration from other methods to confirm the presence of advanced CAA.

Conclusions

Despite its high age-related prevalence, CAA has been difficult to detect non-invasively and is, therefore, likely to be underestimated in its effects on the aging process. The occurrence of CAA-related CMBs has emerged as the most useful diagnostic marker for CAA in clinical practice and investigation. Through sensitive MRI-based methods, these markers have served as the basis for reasonably specific and sensitive detection of CAA-related ICH. Further application of the same imaging methods to the general population has suggested that CAA of sufficient severity to cause CMBs may be common in apparently healthy elderly individuals.

The impact of CAA-related CMBs on neurological impairment and clinical decisions still remains to be defined. A key question in clinical practice is whether the increased risk for ICH associated with CAA-related CMBs is sufficient to tip treating clinicians away from prescribing antiplatelet or anticoagulant agents for patients with appropriate indications. Decision analysis of a hypothetical individual with non-valvular atrial fibrillation, typical stroke risk factors and CMBs suggests that anticoagulation remains the preferred strategy [45], but this important question requires further investigation. Detection of CAA via CMBs may also affect future use

of anti-Aβ immunotherapy for AD, as adverse effects in trials of these agents may have been driven by underlying CAA [46,47].

The study of CAA-related CMBs is likely to evolve rapidly with technical improvements not only in CMB imaging [15,20] but also in non-invasive detection of other aspects of CAA. Recent studies of the amyloid ligand Pittsburgh compound B, for example, have highlighted this agent's ability to detect CAA as well as plaque amyloid [48,49]. Multimodal imaging of the full spectrum of lesions associated with CAA offers the potential for establishing where CMBs fit in the pathogenesis of this increasingly recognized disorder.

References

1. Vinters HV. Cerebral amyloid angiopathy: a critical review. *Stroke* 1987;**18**:311–19.

2. Itoh Y, Yamada M, Hayakawa M, Otomo E, Miyatake T. Cerebral amyloid angiopathy: a significant cause of cerebellar as well as lobar cerebral hemorrhage in the elderly. *J Neurol Sci* 1993;**116**:135–41.

3. Jellinger KA. Alzheimer disease and cerebrovascular pathology: an update. *J Neural Transm* 2002;**109**: 813–36.

4. Smith EE, Greenberg SM. Beta-amyloid, blood vessels, and brain function. *Stroke* 2009;**40**:2601–6.

5. Weller RO, Massey A, Newman TA *et al.* Cerebral amyloid angiopathy: amyloid beta accumulates in putative interstitial fluid drainage pathways in Alzheimer's disease. *Am J Pathol* 1998;**153**:725–33.

6. Kimberly WT, Gilson A, Rost NS *et al.* Silent ischemic infarcts are associated with hemorrhage burden in cerebral amyloid angiopathy. *Neurology* 2009;**72**:1230–5.

7. Soontornniyomkij V, Lynch MD, Mermash S *et al.* Cerebral microinfarcts associated with severe cerebral beta-amyloid angiopathy. *Brain Pathol* 2010;**20**:459–67.

8. Mandybur TI. Cerebral amyloid angiopathy: the vascular pathology and complications. *J Neuropathol Exp Neurol* 1986;**45**:79–90.

9. Vonsattel JP, Myers RH, Hedley-Whyte ET *et al.* Cerebral amyloid angiopathy without and with cerebral hemorrhages: a comparative histological study. *Ann Neurol* 1991;**30**:637–9.

10. Vinters HV, Gilbert JJ. Cerebral amyloid angiopathy: incidence and complications in the aging brain. II. The distribution of amyloid vascular changes. *Stroke* 1983;**14**:924–8.

11. Greenberg SM, Eng JA, Ning M, Smith EE, Rosand J. Hemorrhage burden predicts recurrent intracerebral

hemorrhage after lobar hemorrhage. *Stroke* 2004;**35**:1415–20.

12. Kennedy DN, Lange N, Makris N *et al.* Gyri of the human neocortex: an MRI-based analysis of volume and variance. *Cereb Cortex* 1998;**8**:372–84.

13. Atlas SW, Mark AS, Grossman RI, Gomori JM. Intracranial hemorrhage: gradient-echo MR imaging at 1.5 T. Comparison with spin-echo imaging and clinical applications. *Radiology* 1988;**168**:803–7.

14. Fazekas F, Kleinert R, Roob G *et al.* Histopathologic analysis of foci of signal loss on gradient-echo T_2*-weighted MR images in patients with spontaneous intracerebral hemorrhage: evidence of microangiopathy-related microbleeds. *AJNR Am J Neuroradiol* 1999;**20**:637–42.

15. Ayaz M, Boikov AS, Haacke EM, Kido DK, Kirsch WM. Imaging cerebral microbleeds using susceptibility weighted imaging: one step toward detecting vascular dementia. *J Magn Reson Imaging* 2010;**31**:142–8.

16. Imaizumi T, Horita Y, Hshimoto Y, Niwa J. Dotlike hemosiderin spots on T_2*-weighted magnetic resonance imaging as a predictor of stroke recurrence: a prospective study. *J Neurosurg* 2004;**101**:915–20.

17. Rosand J, Muzikansky A, Kumar A *et al.* Spatial clustering of hemorrhages in probable cerebral amyloid angiopathy. *Ann Neurol* 2005;**58**:459–62.

18. Greenberg SM, O'Donnell HC, Schaefer PW, Kraft E. MRI detection of new hemorrhages: potential marker of progression in cerebral amyloid angiopathy. *Neurology* 1999;**53**:1135–38.

19. Vernooij MW, Ikram MA, Wielopolski PA *et al.* Cerebral microbleeds: accelerated 3D T_2*-weighted GRE MR imaging versus conventional 2D T_2*-weighted GRE MR imaging for detection. *Radiology* 2008;**248**:272–7.

20. Nandigam RN, Viswanathan A, Delgado P *et al.* MR imaging detection of cerebral microbleeds: effect of susceptibility-weighted imaging, section thickness, and field strength. *AJNR Am J Neuroradiol* 2009;**30**:338–43.

21. Haacke EM, Xu Y, Cheng YN, Reichenbach R. Susceptibility weighted imaging (SWI). *Magn Reson Med* 2004;**618**:612–18.

22. Knudsen KA, Rosand J, Karluk D, Greenberg SM. Clinical diagnosis of cerebral amyloid angiopathy: validation of the Boston Criteria. *Neurology* 2001;**56**:537–9.

23. Lee SH, Kim SM, Kim N, Yoon BW, Roh JK. Cortico-subcortical distribution of microbleeds is different between hypertension and cerebral amyloid angiopathy. *J Neurol Sci* 2007;**258**:111–14.

24. Smith EE, Nandigam KRN, Chen Y-W *et al.* MRI markers of small vessel disease in lobar and deep hemispheric intracerebral hemorrhage. *Stroke* 2010:**41**:1933–8.

25. van Rooden S, van der Grond J, van den Boom R *et al.* Descriptive analysis of the Boston criteria applied to a Dutch-type cerebral amyloid angiopathy population. *Stroke* 2009;**40**:3022–7.

26. Viswanathan A, Godin O, Jouvent E *et al.* Impact of MRI markers in subcortical vascular dementia: a multi-modal analysis in CADASIL. *Neurobiol Aging* 2010;**31**:1629–36.

27. Werring DJ, Frazer DW, Coward LJ *et al.* Cognitive dysfunction in patients with cerebral microbleeds on T_2*-weighted gradient-echo MRI. *Brain* 2004;**127**:2265–75.

28. Gurol ME, Irizarry MC, Smith EE *et al.* Plasma beta-amyloid and white matter lesions in AD, MCI, and cerebral amyloid angiopathy. *Neurology* 2006;**66**:23–9.

29. Haglund M, Englund E. Cerebral amyloid angiopathy, white matter lesions and Alzheimer encephalopathy: a histopathological assessment. *Dement Geriatr Cogn Disord* 2002;**14**:161–6.

30. Salat DH, Smith EE, Tuch DS *et al.* White matter alterations in cerebral amyloid angiopathy measured by diffusion tensor imaging. *Stroke* 2006;**37**:1759–64.

31. Schneider JA, Arvanitakis Z, Bang W, Bennett DA. Mixed brain pathologies account for most dementia cases in community-dwelling older persons. *Neurology* 2007;**69**:2197–2204.

32. Greenberg SM, Nandigam RN, Delgado P *et al.* Microbleeds versus macrobleeds: evidence for distinct entities. *Stroke* 2009;**40**:2382–6.

33. Cordonnier C, Al-Shahi Salman R, Wardlaw J. Spontaneous brain microbleeds: systematic review, subgroup analyses and standards for study design and reporting. *Brain* 2007;**130**:1988–2003.

34. Ellis RJ, Olichney JM, Thal LJ *et al.* Cerebral amyloid angiopathy in the brains of patients with Alzheimer's disease: the CERAD experience, Part XV. *Neurology* 1996;**46**:1592–6.

35. Cordonnier C, van der Flier WM, Sluimer JD *et al.* Prevalence and severity of microbleeds in a memory clinic setting. *Neurology* 2006;**66**:1356–60.

36. Atri A, Locascio JJ, Lin JM *et al.* Prevalence and effects of lobar microhemorrhages in early-stage dementia. *Neurodegener Dis* 2005;**2**:305–12.

37. Pettersen JA, Sathiyamoorthy G, Gao F-Q *et al.* Microbleed topography, leukoaraiosis, cognition in probable Alzheimer disease from the Sunnybrook Dementia Study. *Arch Neurol* 2008;**65**:790–5.

38. Goos JD, Kester MI, Barkhof F *et al.* Patients with Alzheimer disease with multiple microbleeds: relation with cerebrospinal fluid biomarkers and cognition. *Stroke* 2009;**40**:3455–60.

39. Henneman WJ, Sluimer JD, Cordonnier C *et al.* MRI biomarkers of vascular damage and atrophy predicting mortality in a memory clinic population. *Stroke* 2009;**40**:492–8.

40. Arvanitakis Z, Leurgans SE, Wang Z *et al.* Cerebral amyloid angiopathy pathology and cognitive domains in older persons. *Ann Neurol* 2010; epub ahead of print.

41. Pfeifer LA, White LR, Ross GW, Petrovitch H, Launer LJ. Cerebral amyloid angiopathy and cognitive function: the HAAS autopsy study. *Neurology* 2002;**58**:1629–34.

42. Greenberg SM, Vernooij MW, Cordonnier C *et al.* Cerebral microbleeds: a guide to detection and interpretation. *Lancet Neurol* 2009;**8**:165–74.

43. Vernooij MW, van der Lugt A, Ikram MA *et al.* Prevalence and risk factors of cerebral microbleeds: the Rotterdam Scan Study. *Neurology* 2008;**70**: 1208–14.

44. Sveinbjornsdottir S, Sigurdsson S, Aspelund T *et al.* Cerebral microbleeds in the population based AGES–Reykjavik study: prevalence and location. *J Neurol Neurosurg Psychiatry* 2008;**79**:1002–6.

45. Eckman MH, Wong LK, Soo YO *et al.* Patient-specific decision-making for warfarin therapy in nonvalvular atrial fibrillation: how will screening with genetics and imaging help? *Stroke* 2008;**39**:3308–15.

46. Nicoll JA, Wilkinson D, Holmes C *et al.* Neuropathology of human Alzheimer disease after immunization with amyloid-beta peptide: a case report. *Nat Med* 2003;**9**:448–52.

47. Salloway S, Sperling R, Gilman S *et al.* A phase 2 multiple ascending dose trial of bapineuzumab in mild to moderate Alzheimer disease. *Neurology* 2009;**73**:2061–70.

48. Johnson KA Amyloid imaging of Alzheimer's disease using Pittsburgh Compound B. *Curr Neurol Neurosci Rep* 2006;**6**:496–503.

49. Ly JV, Donnan GA, Villemagne VL *et al.* ^{11}C-PIB binding is increased in patients with cerebral amyloid angiopathy-related hemorrhage. *Neurology* 2010;**74**:487–93.

Chapter

13

Cerebral microbleeds and Alzheimer's disease

Charlotte Cordonnier and Wiesje M. van der Flier

Introduction

In Alzheimer's disease (AD), cerebral microbleeds (CMBs) are of special interest as they may have a crucial role in the pathophysiology of the disorder. Moreover, they may affect the clinical course of the disease and may have therapeutic consequences. This chapter will review the available data that help in considering the meaning of CMBs in clinical terms and the underlying pathology in the context of AD.

Prevalence of cerebral microbleeds in Alzheimer's disease

Five studies have reported the prevalence of CMBs in patients with AD (Table 13.1) [1–5]. One study reported the prevalence of lobar CMBs in 61 demented patients, half having AD [6]. Unfortunately, data from the AD subgroup could not be extracted. In total, we have extracted data from 450 patients with AD and the prevalence of CMBs was 22% (95% confidence interval (CI), 18–26) (Table 13.1). Figure 13.1 shows the prevalence of CMBs in different disease settings compared with that in AD. Even when CMBs are quite prevalent in a disorder, the majority of patients with CMBs only show one CMB. It is possible that CMBs exert their effect in a dose-dependent manner, so a high number of CMBs would predispose to a more aggressive disease course. Whether or not one or only a few CMBs should be regarded as silent lesions without clinical implications, remains to be demonstrated in large studies of sufficient power.

Table 13.1 Publications reporting prevalence of cerebral microbleeds in Alzheimer's disease populations

Source	No. patients	No. patients with CMB	Prevalence of CMBs (% [95% CI])
Nakata et al. 2002 [5]	38	7	18 (9–33)
Hanyu et al. 2003 [4]	59	19	32 (22–45)
Cordonnier et al. 2006 [3]	223	41	18 (14–24)
Nakata-Kudo et al. 2006 [2]	50	8	16 (8–29)
Pettersen et al. 2008 [1]	80	23	29 (20–39)
Overall	**450**	**98**	**22 (18–26)**

CMB, cerebral microbleeds; CI, confidence interval.

Significance of cerebral microbleeds in Alzheimer's disease

Cerebral microbleeds are a radiological construct that is considered to represent perivascular collections of hemosiderin deposits. These microscopic hemorrhages are observed on MRI as rounded signals of hypointensity on gradient-recalled echo $T_2{}^*$-weighted sequence, but what is their relevance in AD? This question can be approached from two angles: what do they represent and what are their clinical consequences?

What do cerebral microbleeds represent?

Evidence on the underlying pathology of CMBs can be sought from neuropathology studies, anatomical distribution in AD and clinical studies on related factors.

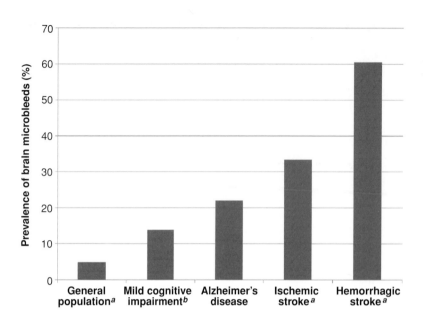

Fig. 13.1 Prevalences of brain microbleeds in different disease settings. (Data were extracted from [a]Cordonnier *et al.* 2007 [17] and [b]Staekenborg *et al.* 2009 [34].)

Neuropathology

To demonstrate the neuropathological correlates of the radiological construct, autopsy imaging studies combined with histology are required. However, at present there are only a limited number of pathological studies regarding CMBs: three studies gathering 3 controls, 11 with intracerebral hemorrhages (ICH) and 8 with AD have been published [9–11]. Fazekas *et al.* were the first to demonstrate (in a sample of patients who died from ICH) that, histologically, CMBs represent focal leakage of hemosiderin from abnormal small blood vessels [11]. Because of the nature of the sample (mostly hypertensive patients who died from ICH), CMBs in this study were strongly associated with hypertensive vasculopathy. This association was also reported in a single case report of an elderly hypertensive woman [10]. In AD, only eight brains have been reported to date [9]. The majority of the lesions appeared in a cortico-subcortical location and beta-amyloid deposition was present in the vessel walls adjacent to the bleeds, suggesting that cortico-subcortical CMBs are a consequence of underlying cerebral amyloid angiopathy (CAA). Some argue that *all* amyloid plaques arise from bleeds, based on the co-location of CMBs and amyloid deposition in the brain, but this finding remains to be replicated [12,13]. Available data suggest that different mechanisms can lead to CMBs. Typically, deep and infratentorial CMBs are presumed to result from hypertensive

vasculopathy, while cortico-subcortical CMBs seem to be closely related to cerebral amyloid angiopathy. This dichotomy is particularly relevant in AD for two reasons:

- patients with AD often have a past history of arterial hypertension even if at the time of diagnosis they are no longer hypertensive [14]
- CAA occurs in 78–98% of patients with AD, is frequently considered to be a major pathological feature of AD [15] and is also considered to contribute to the cognitive decline in AD [16].

Specifically in AD, it is conceivable that CMBs can develop through both pathways, as neurodegenerative (including CAA) and cerebrovascular pathology both play a role in the pathophysiology of the disease (see the discussion of the hypotheses of neuropathogenesis in AD below).

Anatomical distribution of cerebral microbleeds in Alzheimer's disease

Most studies on CMBs in AD demonstrated a cortico-subcortical predominance (Figs. 13.2 and 13.3), but with some patients exhibiting CMBs both in deep and cortico-subcortical locations. One study specifically focused on the anatomical distribution of CMBs and revealed that the topography of CMBs had cortico-subcortical predominance in 92% of patients with AD,

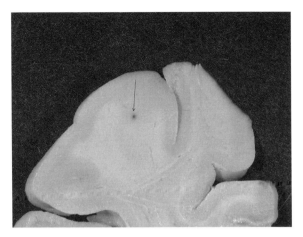

Fig. 13.2 Coronal section through a cerebral hemisphere showing a cortical brain microbleed (arrow) in a patient with Alzheimer's disease and cerebral amyloid angiopathy. (Courtesy of Pr Jacques De Reuck, Lille.)

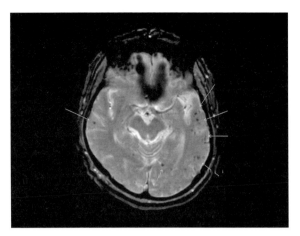

Fig. 13.3 Gradient echo T_2*-weighted image of a 68-year-old man suffering from Alzheimer's disease. Axial slice showing multiple cortico-subcortical brain microbleeds (arrows).

with occipital lobes accounting for 57% of these CMBs [1]. Interestingly, the cortico-subcortical pattern of distribution was similar to the CAA-related ICH distribution, indirectly suggesting that CMBs in AD in cortico-subcortical locations are linked to CAA [17]. Notably, in a study focusing on patients with AD and multiple CMBs, in the patients severely affected by AD, the CMBs were found almost invariably in the cortico-subcortical regions of the brain [18].

Factors associated with cerebral microbleeds

Arterial hypertension

Cerebral microbleeds are strongly linked to hypertensive vasculopathy; CMBs occur more frequently in hypertensive people, both in general (odds ratio [OR], 3.9; 95% CI, 2.4–6.4) and in cerebrovascular (OR, 2.3; 95% CI, 1.7–3.0) populations [7]. In AD, data on arterial hypertension in relation to CMBs are available from two studies ($n = 88$)[2,5]. The OR associated with hypertension was 1.24 (95% CI, 0.41–3.78), which suggests that the association between hypertension and CMBs is weaker among those with AD than among those with cerebrovascular disease or the healthy general population. Possible explanations are that hypertension was underdiagnosed since the patients with AD were not hypertensive at the time of the study but had been in the past [14] and that CMBs in AD are more likely to be associated with CAA than with hypertensive vasculopathy.

Imaging measures of small vessel disease

Vascular pathology is important in AD [19,20]. Associations between CMBs and white matter hyperintensities have often been found [1,3,18,21]. Likewise, CMBs have been shown to be associated with lacunes [22–24]. This provides evidence for microangiopathy as an underlying mechanism for CMBs. Three studies in AD reported a correlation between the severity of white matter hyperintensities and the existence of CMBs [1,2,4]. Unfortunately, they all used different scales, thus precluding any meta-analysis. These associations suggest that CMBs can be interpreted as a third expression of small vessel disease on MRI, next to white matter hyperintensities and lacunes.

APOE genotype

In an analysis of *APOE* genotype in healthy elderly subjects subdivided according to CMB distribution, the Rotterdam Scan Study found an association with the *APOE* ε4 allele pertaining only to the subgroup with isolated cortico-subcortical CMBs and not the subgroup with deep hemispheric or infratentorial CMBs [21]. Given the relationship between *APOE* ε4 and CAA [25], these results provide further evidence that isolated cortico-subcortical CMBs often reflect the presence of advanced CAA. No association with *APOE* genotype was found in two studies in AD ($n = 139$) [1,4]. Sample sizes were not designed to disclose any significant results. In a study comparing patients with AD and many CMBs and those without any CMBs, the patients with many CMBs were more likely to be homozygous for *APOE* ε4 [18].

Beta-amyloid as a cerebrospinal fluid biomarker

Cerebrospinal fluid (CSF) is in direct contact with the brain, and as such it provides a window to the processes occurring in the brain. The concentration of amyloid $A\beta_{1-42}$ are reduced in patients with AD, probably reflecting the presence of senile plaques, one of the neuropathological hallmarks of AD [26–28]. In a preliminary study, patients with AD and multiple CMBs were shown to have even more severely reduced levels of $A\beta_{1-42}$ in CSF than patients with AD but no CMBs [18]. Congruent with this finding, it was recently shown that patients with CAA have more strongly reduced levels of CSF $A\beta_{1-42}$ than patients with AD [29]. In the latter study, $A\beta_{1-40}$ was also found to be reduced in patients with CAA, while such an effect was not found in patients with AD. The described associations with this CSF biomarker provide support for the notion that CMBs are in some way directly linked to (vascular) amyloid, one of the major pathological hallmarks of AD.

Clinical significance of cerebral microbleeds

Studies on the clinical significance of CMBs are slowly emerging, but mostly in populations other than those with AD.

Cognitive dysfunction

In patients with stroke and non-demented patients, CMBs have been associated with cognitive decline [30–32]. As a first step towards elucidating the meaning of CMBs in dementia, a study demonstrated that CMBs are an important factor causing cognitive decline in subcortical vascular dementia [33]. There is only one study investigating relationships between CMBs and neuropsychological performance in a relatively large number of patients with AD ($n = 80$) [1]. The authors were not able to find any association with neuropsychological performance. Previous studies, focusing only on the Mini-Mental State Examination (MMSE) score, failed to demonstrate the impact of CMBs on cognition[1,2,5]. Potentially, those studies were hampered by their relatively small sample size (overall number of patients, 168), low number of CMBs and the crude nature of the MMSE.

To overcome the problem of low numbers of CMBs, a proof of principle approach was taken in a study comparing patients with AD and multiple CMBs with those with AD but no CMBs [18]. Patients with multiple CMBs had more severe cognitive impairment, which could not be explained by disease duration, degree of atrophy or white matter hyperintensities.

Predicting dementia in mild cognitive impairment

Mild cognitive impairment (MCI) is characterized by isolated memory impairment, not sufficient for a diagnosis of dementia [34]. Patients with MCI are at an increased risk to develop dementia, mostly AD, with a rate of 12–15% per year (compared with 1–2% in the normal population). A study on the predictive value of CMBs in patients with MCI showed that the observation of at least one CMB on MRI yielded a more than twofold increased, although non-significant, risk of non-Alzheimer dementia [8]. Another study showed that occurrence of CMBs on susceptibility-weighted MRI in patients with MCI predicted subsequent cognitive decline [35].

Mortality

One study investigated the association of CMBs with subsequent mortality in a memory clinic [36]. Finding CMBs in the presenting MRI was associated with a more than twofold increased risk of mortality, which could not be explained by other expressions of small vessel disease on MRI (i.e. white matter hyperintensities) or vascular comorbidity. There was a clear dose-effect relationship, with a higher number of CMBs being related with an increased risk, while one or a few CMBs had little impact. It is tempting to assume that the increased risk of mortality reflects increased occurrence of hemorrhage, but at present, this remains speculative.

Cerebral microbleeds and treatment decisions in Alzheimer's disease

To date, there are no evidence-based data to guide the clinician for treatment decisions in a patient with CMBs [37] and there are no specific data available for AD. In a population-based setting, CMBs were more prevalent among users of antiplatelet agents (OR, 1.7; 95% CI, 1.2–2.4) while anticoagulants failed to show a significant effect (OR, 1.5; 95% CI, 0.8–2.7) [38].

Because of the cross-sectional design of this study, the causal relationship remains unclear: antithrombotic drug use may give rise to the development of CMBs, or patients with vascular disease requiring antithrombotic treatment may have more CMBs to start with because of their vascular disease. Given the current lack of evidence, at present the benefits of antithrombotic agents seem to outweigh the potential risks in secondary prevention of vascular diseases.

Do cerebral microbleeds signify an increased risk of intracerebral hemorrhage?

There are no data on the natural history of ICH in AD, nor are there any data on CMBs in relation to ICH in AD. However, in some interventional trials with low dose of acetylsalicylic acid in AD, the occurrence of ICH was described. Among 156 patients receiving acetylsalicylic acid, four suffered from an ICH compared with none among the 154 receiving placebos [39]. The same tendency was found in a recent trial where 3 of 65 patients with AD receiving acetylsalicylic acid suffered from an ICH whereas none did so in the cohort of 58 patients with AD receiving placebos [40]. Although the small numbers of patients preclude a definitive conclusion, the finding might suggest that a subgroup of patients with AD who use acetylsalicylic acid might be at greater risk of ICH. Even so, these studies did not take into account the presence of CMBs.

Use of cerebral microbleeds in clinical trials

With studies on the relevance of CMBs in AD emerging, CMBs have become a factor of interest in the design of clinical trials, particularly with regard to the new generation of immunization therapies, which have been linked to the development of new CMBs. However, there are few published data on which any recommendations could be made regarding how to handle CMBs in the context of clinical trials.

Pathophysiology of Alzheimer's disease

Cerebral microbleeds may form the missing link between the two most important theories on the neuropathogenesis of AD: the amyloid cascade hypothesis and the vascular hypothesis.

Amyloid cascade hypothesis

The most widely accepted theory regarding the pathogenesis of AD is the amyloid cascade hypothesis [41]. In short, this hypothesis states that the development of AD is initiated by abnormal cleavage of the amyloid precursor protein (APP), resulting in an imbalance of production and clearance of beta-amyloid. As a consequence, beta-amyloid accumulates in the brain in the form of senile plaques. Despite extensive research, the amyloid hypothesis has not provided definitive answers. There are a number of problems with the hypothesis: first, amyloid deposition does not correlate with dementia severity or extent of neurodegeneration; second, there are many cognitively intact elderly with abundant beta-amyloid plaques in their brains, while conversely, many demented elderly do not have a sufficient number of plaques for an AD diagnosis [42].

Vascular hypothesis

The alternative hypothesis, the vascular hypothesis, has been developed from the late 1990s, and states that vascular pathology plays an important role in the pathogenesis of AD [43–45]. On MRI, expressions of cerebrovascular disease, such as white matter hyperintensities and lacunes, are more often observed in patients with AD than in controls [19,20]. However, despite much research, the vascular hypothesis has also not led to a breakthrough, as correlations of cerebrovascular disease with cognitive impairment are only modest [46–48]. Based on pathological and epidemiological evidence, both amyloid and cerebrovascular pathology are implicated in AD, but until now it has been unclear how the two could interact [43,49]. Amyloid deposition may be a necessary prerequisite for the development of AD, but there seems to be a missing link or additional factor that determines whether the disease develops or not.

Are cerebral microbleeds the missing link between the hypotheses?

We propose that CMBs are an important factor in the pathogenesis of AD. Moreover, they may be an important candidate to bridge the amyloid and vascular hypotheses, as illustrated in Fig. 13.4 [50]. However, CMBs are strongly related to hypertensive vasculopathy [11,51]; on the other hand, they are seemingly a marker of CAA [9,12,51]. The specific underlying pathology of CMBs may differ by brain

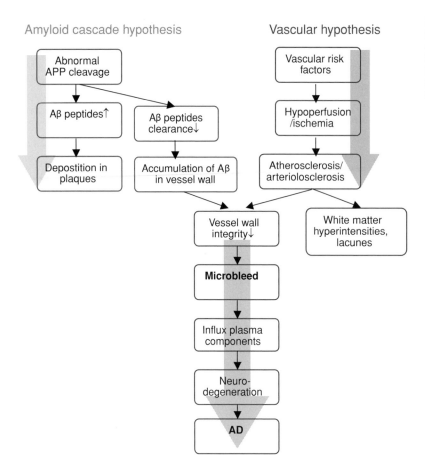

Fig. 13.4 Proposed representation of the pathophysiological pathway of Alzheimer's disease with a prominent role for brain microbleeds, suggesting that they act as a major link between the two pathways. Aβ, beta-amyloid; APP, amyloid precursor protein.

location. In the deep gray matter and infratentorial regions, CMBs may be the result of microangiopathy, including ischemia and arteriosclerosis (vascular route). In contrast, in cortico-subcortical regions, CMBs may result from deposition of amyloid in the vessels (amyloid route). Hence, CMBs could be the common downstream product of two separate pathways that each acts as a catalyst towards subsequent degeneration.

Conclusions and future directions

Certain conclusions can be drawn from the studies on CMBs and on CMBs in AD:

- one in five patients with AD has at least one CMB, which is more than in the general population
- CMBs may be a common downstream product of the two prevailing pathways suggested for the pathophysiology of AD – the amyloid cascade and vascular pathology – and acting, in turn, as a catalyst for further neurodegeneration

- CMBs in AD are mainly cortico-subcortical
- while CMBs have long been considered as "silent lesions," evidence is now emerging suggesting that the presence of CMBs in AD is related to a more aggressive disease course, with more severe cognitive decline and a higher risk of death.

Research should now focus on numbers (and location) of lesions rather than just on prevalence. Whether or not one or only a few CMBs should be regarded as silent lesions without clinical implications remains unsettled.

To date, there are no evidence-based data to guide the clinician for treatment decision in a patient with AD and CMBs. Given the current lack of evidence, the benefits of antithrombotic drugs seem to outweigh the potential risks in secondary prevention of vascular diseases. Monitoring CMBs in clinical trials dedicated to patients with AD should provide more data on which to base treatment decisions when patients have both CMBs and AD.

References

1. Pettersen JA, Sathiyamoorthy G, Gao FQ *et al.* Microbleed topography, leukoaraiosis, and cognition in probable Alzheimer disease from the Sunnybrook Dementia Study. *Arch Neurol* 2008;**65**:790–5.

2. Nakata-Kudo Y, Mizuno T, Yamada K *et al.* Microbleeds in Alzheimer disease are more related to cerebral amyloid angiopathy than cerebrovascular disease. *Dement Geriatr Cogn Disord* 2006;**22**:8–14.

3. Cordonnier C, van der Flier WM, Sluimer JD *et al.* Prevalence and severity of microbleeds in a memory clinic setting. *Neurology* 2006;**66**:1356–60.

4. Hanyu H, Tanaka Y, Shimizu S, Takasaki M, Abe K. Cerebral microbleeds in Alzheimer's disease. *J Neurol* 2003;**250**:1496–7.

5. Nakata Y, Shiga K, Yoshikawa K *et al.* Subclinical brain hemorrhages in Alzheimer's disease: evaluation by magnetic resonance T_2^*-weighted images. *Ann NY Acad Sci* 2002;**977**:169–72.

6. Atri A, Locascio JJ, Lin JM *et al.* Prevalence and effects of lobar microhemorrhages in early-stage dementia. *Neurodegener Dis* 2005;**2**:305–12.

7. Cordonnier C, Al-Shahi Salman R, Wardlaw J. Spontaneous brain microbleeds: systematic review, subgroup analyses and standards for study design and reporting. *Brain* 2007;**130**:1988–2003.

8. Staekenborg SS, Koedam EL, Henneman WJ *et al.* Progression of mild cognitive impairment to dementia: contribution of cerebrovascular disease compared with medial temporal lobe atrophy. *Stroke* 2009;**40**:1269–74.

9. Schrag M, McAuley G, Pomakian J *et al.* Correlation of hypointensities in susceptibility-weighted images to tissue histology in dementia patients with cerebral amyloid angiopathy: a postmortem MRI study. *Acta Neuropathol* 2010;**119**:291–302.

10. Tatsumi S, Shinohara M, Yamamoto T. Direct comparison of histology of microbleeds with postmortem MR images: a case report. *Cerebrovasc Dis* 2008;**26**:142–6.

11. Fazekas F, Kleinert R, Roob G *et al.* Histopathologic analysis of foci of signal loss on gradient-echo T_2^*-weighted MR images in patients with spontaneous intracerebral hemorrhage: evidence of microangiopathy-related microbleeds. *AJNR Am J Neuroradiol* 1999;**20**:637–42.

12. Cullen KM, Kocsi Z, Stone J. Microvascular pathology in the aging human brain: evidence that senile plaques are sites of microhaemorrhages. *Neurobiol Aging* 2006;**27**:1786–96.

13. Stone J. What initiates the formation of senile plaques? The origin of Alzheimer-like dementias in capillary haemorrhages. *Med Hypotheses* 2008;**71**:347–59.

14. Skoog I, Lernfelt B, Landahl S *et al.* 15-year longitudinal study of blood pressure and dementia. *Lancet* 1996;**347**:1141–5.

15. Kalaria RN, Ballard C. Overlap between pathology of Alzheimer disease and vascular dementia. *Alzheimer Dis Assoc Disord* 1999;**13**(Suppl. 3):S115–23.

16. Pfeifer LA, White LR, Ross GW, Petrovitch H, Launer LJ. Cerebral amyloid angiopathy and cognitive function: the HAAS autopsy study. *Neurology* 2002;**58**:1629–34.

17. Rosand J, Muzikansky A, Kumar A *et al.* Spatial clustering of hemorrhages in probable cerebral amyloid angiopathy. *Ann Neurol* 2005;**58**:459–62.

18. Goos JD, Kester MI, Barkhof F *et al.* Patients with Alzheimer disease with multiple microbleeds: relation with cerebrospinal fluid biomarkers and cognition. *Stroke* 2009;**40**:3455–60.

19. Schneider JA, Wilson RS, Bienias JL, Evans DA, Bennett DA. Cerebral infarctions and the likelihood of dementia from Alzheimer disease pathology. *Neurology* 2004;**62**:1148–55.

20. DeCarli CS. When two are worse than one: stroke and Alzheimer disease. *Neurology* 2006;**67**:1326–7.

21. Vernooij MW, van der Lugt A, Ikram MA *et al.* Prevalence and risk factors of cerebral microbleeds: the Rotterdam Scan Study. *Neurology* 2008;**70**:1208–14.

22. Roob G, Schmidt R, Kapeller P *et al.* MRI evidence of past cerebral microbleeds in a healthy elderly population. *Neurology* 1999;**52**:991–4.

23. Horita Y, Imaizumi T, Niwa J *et al.* [Analysis of dot-like hemosiderin spots using brain dock system.] *No Shinkei Geka* 2003;**31**:263–7.

24. Wardlaw JM, Lewis SC, Keir SL, Dennis MS, Shenkin S. Cerebral microbleeds are associated with lacunar stroke defined clinically and radiologically, independently of white matter lesions. *Stroke* 2006;**37**:2633–6.

25. Greenberg SM, Rebeck GW, Vonsattel JP, Gomez-Isla T, Hyman BT. Apolipoprotein E epsilon 4 and cerebral hemorrhage associated with amyloid angiopathy. *Ann Neurol* 1995;**38**:254–9.

26. Blennow K, Hampel H. CSF markers for incipient Alzheimer's disease. *Lancet Neurol* 2003;**2**:605–13.

27. Mulder C, Verwey NA, van der Flier WM *et al.* Amyloid-beta(1–42), total tau, and phosphorylated tau as cerebrospinal fluid biomarkers for the diagnosis of Alzheimer disease. *Clin Chem* 2010;**56**:248–53.

28. Mattsson N, Zetterberg H, Hansson O *et al.* CSF biomarkers and incipient Alzheimer disease in patients with mild cognitive impairment. *JAMA* 2009;**302**:385–93.

29. Verbeek MM, Kremer BP, Rikkert MO *et al.* Cerebrospinal fluid amyloid beta(40) is decreased in cerebral amyloid angiopathy. *Ann Neurol* 2009;**66**: 245–9.

30. Greenberg SM, Eng JA, Ning M, Smith EE, Rosand J. Hemorrhage burden predicts recurrent intracerebral hemorrhage after lobar hemorrhage. *Stroke* 2004;**35**: 1415–20.

31. Werring DJ, Frazer DW, Coward LJ *et al.* Cognitive dysfunction in patients with cerebral microbleeds on T_2^*-weighted gradient-echo MRI. *Brain* 2004;**127**: 2265–75.

32. Yakushiji Y, Nishiyama M, Yakushiji S *et al.* Brain microbleeds and global cognitive function in adults without neurological disorder. *Stroke* 2008;**39**:3323–8.

33. Won Seo S, Hwa Lee B, Kim EJ *et al.* Clinical significance of microbleeds in subcortical vascular dementia. *Stroke* 2007;**38**:1949–51.

34. Petersen RC, Doody R, Kurz A *et al.* Current concepts in mild cognitive impairment. *Arch Neurol* 2001;**58**: 1985–92.

35. Kirsch W, McAuley G, Holshouser B *et al.* Serial susceptibility weighted MRI measures brain iron and microbleeds in dementia. *J Alzheimers Dis* 2009;**17**: 599–609.

36. Henneman WJ, Sluimer JD, Cordonnier C *et al.* MRI biomarkers of vascular damage and atrophy predicting mortality in a memory clinic population. *Stroke* 2009; **40**:492–8.

37. Cordonnier C. Brain microbleeds. *Pract Neurol* 2010; **10**:94–100.

38. Vernooij MW, Haag MD, van der Lugt A *et al.* Use of antithrombotic drugs and the presence of cerebral microbleeds: the Rotterdam Scan Study. *Arch Neurol* 2009;**66**:714–20.

39. Bentham P, Gray R, Sellwood E *et al.* Aspirin in Alzheimer's disease (AD2000): a randomised open-label trial. *Lancet Neurol* 2008;**7**:41–9.

40. Richard E, Kuiper R, Dijkgraaf MG, van Gool WA. Vascular care in patients with Alzheimer's disease with cerebrovascular lesions-a randomized clinical trial. *J Am Geriatr Soc* 2009;**57**:797–805.

41. Hardy J, Selkoe DJ. The amyloid hypothesis of Alzheimer's disease: progress and problems on the road to therapeutics. *Science* 2002;**297**:353–6.

42. Neuropathology Group of the Medical Research Council. Pathological correlates of late-onset dementia in a multicentre, community-based population in England and Wales. Medical Research Council Cognitive Function and Ageing Study (MRC CFAS). *Lancet* 2001;**357**:169–75.

43. Breteler MM. Vascular risk factors for Alzheimer's disease: an epidemiologic perspective. *Neurobiol Aging* 2000;**21**:153–60.

44. Snowdon DA, Greiner LH, Mortimer JA *et al.* Brain infarction and the clinical expression of Alzheimer disease. The Nun Study. *JAMA* 1997;**277**: 813–17.

45. de la Torre JC. Is Alzheimer's disease a neurodegenerative or a vascular disorder? Data, dogma, and dialectics. *Lancet Neurol* 2004;**3**: 184–90.

46. van der Flier WM, van Straaten EC, Barkhof F *et al.* Small vessel disease and general cognitive function in non-disabled elderly: the LADIS study. *Stroke* 2005; **36**:2116–20.

47. Prins ND, van Dijk EJ, den Heijer T *et al.* Cerebral small-vessel disease and decline in information processing speed, executive function and memory. *Brain* 2005;**128**:2034–41.

48. Schmidt R, Ropele S, Enzinger C *et al.* White matter lesion progression, brain atrophy, and cognitive decline: the Austrian Stroke Prevention Study. *Ann Neurol* 2005;**58**:610–16.

49. Casserly I, Topol E. Convergence of atherosclerosis and Alzheimer's disease: inflammation, cholesterol, and misfolded proteins. *Lancet* 2004;**363**: 1139–46.

50. Cordonnier C, van der Flier W. Brain microbleeds and Alzheimer's disease: innocent observation or key player? *Brain* 2001;**134**: in press.

51. Greenberg SM, Vernooij MW, Cordonnier C *et al.* Cerebral microbleeds: a guide to detection and interpretation. *Lancet Neurol* 2009;**8**:165–74.

Cerebral microbleeds in relation to brain trauma

Rainer Scheid

Introduction

Traumatic brain injury (TBI) is arguably the most common neurological disorder. Including mild TBI, which is its most frequent variant, incidence rates may be >650/100 000 per year – more than triple the incidence rate of stroke [1,2]. The injury is caused by the effects of direct and indirect mechanical forces to the brain. There is no universally accepted classification scheme of TBI. With respect to severity, it is commonly classified as mild, moderate or severe according to the Glasgow Coma Scale [3]. A general dichotomy is the distinction of primary and secondary injuries. Primary injuries are directly caused by the mechanical forces themselves and develop at the moment of the trauma. Parenchymal damage through depressed skull fractures, cortical contusions, rupture and dissection of intracranial blood vessels, and also the complex of diffuse or traumatic axonal injury (DAI/TAI), belong in this category [4].

Formation of a TBI is a dynamic process. All of the above-mentioned primary injuries can lead to or can be complicated by secondary injuries or secondary damage to the brain. Edema, ischemia and secondary hematoma formation are the best-known examples. However, in recent years, it has become more and more clear that TBIs are accompanied by a cascade of biochemical, cellular and molecular processes, with potentially deleterious effects on the brain and its functions. Impact depolarization, excitotoxicity and cellular apoptosis are keywords for these three processes, respectively [5–8].

Another important and often used distinction is the differentiation of focal and diffuse injuries [9,10]. There is no clear-cut dividing line between the two.

Cortical contusions are focal injuries, but can also be multifocal. Occurrence of DAI/TAI is usually regarded as a diffuse injury, but this view has also been questioned [4,11–13].

An additional model for classification, which is often used in the radiological literature, is the distinction between intra- and extra-axial injuries. All intra-parenchymal traumatic pathologies are subsumed under the former. The latter denotes pathological findings beyond the parenchyma itself, like epidural and subdural hematomas, but also intraventricular bleedings [14].

Imaging of traumatic brain injury

Several excellent reviews on imaging of TBI have been published recently [15–17]. There is no doubt that MRI is the method of choice for demonstrating structural damage after brain trauma [18]. Nevertheless, cranial CT still has its merits in the acute setting and is particularly useful for the rapid identification of patients who will need invasive treatment (neurosurgery).

Most of the pathologies mentioned in the introduction can reliably be depicted by neuroimaging. However, DAI/TAI, which in the true sense is a microscopic if not a molecular biological diagnosis, is an important exception [4,19]. Particularly in the context of DAI/TAI, increased attention has been given to the neuroradiological finding of microbleeds in patients with TBI. These are referred to as traumatic microbleeds (TMBs) or traumatic microhemorrhages (Fig. 14.1) and will now be considered.

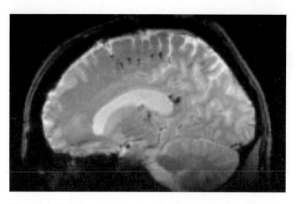

Fig. 14.1 Multiple traumatic microbleeds mainly at the gray matter–white matter interface of the frontal lobe shown in a $T_2{}^*$-weighted gradient-recalled echo image at 3 T (sagittal slice). Two somewhat larger hemorrhages (see also text) are depicted in the splenium of the corpus callosum. On the whole, such a finding is a strong argument for a diagnosis of diffuse axonal injury/traumatic axonal injury.

Traumatic microbleeds

History

What we now call TMBs were already known in patients with TBI in the pre-MRI era when CT was the sole available modality; they were then called petechial white matter hemorrhages. Together with isolated intraventricular or subarachnoid hemorrhage, diffuse swelling or even a normal CT, they constituted the radiological definition of DAI/TAI [20–22]. Early MRI studies after TBI then reported diffuse, often multiple, small focal abnormalities limited to white matter tracts, which were also used as a defining criterion for DAI/TAI [23]. However, in the majority, these abnormalities were first reported to be non-hemorrhagic, which may be because of the MRI sequences used (T_1- and T_2-weighted and fluid attenuated inversion recovery [FLAIR] images) [23,24]. With the advent of $T_2{}^*$-weighted gradient-recalled echo (GRE) MRI, more and more hemorrhagic lesions were reported, which were first referred to as "hemorrhagic shearing injuries" and gave rise to the distinction of hemorrhagic and non-hemorrhagic DAI [25–27].

The first systematic studies on TMBs date from the early 2000s and were unequivocal in showing that these can often be found in the acute as well as in the chronic stages of TBI, and that, at longer time intervals from the actual injury, hypointense lesions on $T_2{}^*$-weighted GRE images (i.e. hemorrhagic) appear to be much more frequent than hyperintense lesions

on T_2-weighted MRI (i.e. non-hemorrhagic lesions) [28,29].

Etiology, neuropathology and differential diagnosis

It is assumed that the radiological finding of microbleeds on MRI after head injury or trauma to the head is diagnostic of TBI [15,17]. However, in its original sense, this assumption has never been proven, since – for obvious reasons – there is generally no such thing as before and after imaging. This consideration is not trivial, because "spontaneous" microbleeds, which might be indistinguishable from TMBs, have been reported to be present in 5–6% of healthy adults (see Ch. 10), and their prevalence has particularly been correlated with advanced age and endemic diseases such as hypertension and diabetes mellitus [30,31].

However, for the interpretation of TMBs, these associations seem to be no major limitation, because in most of the studies, patients with hypertension, diabetes and cerebrovascular disorders, for example, have been excluded [28,29,32]. In this context, it should also be particularly noted that TBI study populations are usually characterized by a lower age than stroke cohorts, and that several studies on this subject were performed in otherwise healthy children, where incidental microbleeds are even less likely [33–35]. Moreover, in addition to patient history, concomitant radiological findings of TBI, such as contusion(s) or extra-axial hemorrhages, support the interpretation of microbleeds as traumatic. Nevertheless, TMBs as the sole radiological finding after TBI have been convincingly demonstrated [18,29,32,34,36,37]. In such a setting, the clinically most relevant problem concerning interpretation (artefactual versus incidental versus traumatic) may arise if there are only one or two TMBs detected [36,38].

In addition to the above-mentioned criteria, the regional distribution of TMBs can also be used for differentiation from microbleeds of other etiologies. The TMBs are typically localized in the white matter of the frontal lobes, particularly of superior frontal gyrus and corpus callosum, and at the gray matter–white matter interface of the frontal and temporal lobes (Fig. 14.2) [29,34]. These sites are clearly different from the areas where microbleeds can be seen in hypertensive vasculopathy or cerebral microangiopathy, in which the basal ganglia, thalamus, brainstem and cerebellum are often affected [30,39,40]. However, with the exception

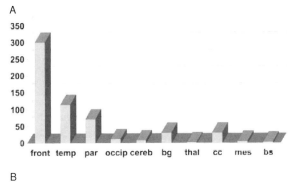

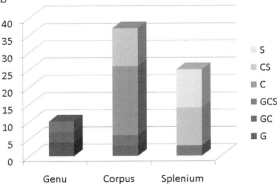

Fig. 14.2 Occurrence of traumatic microbleeds (TMBs). (A) Frequency and site of TMBs according to 10 brain areas ($n = 66$). The total number of TMBs in each brain area is shown. (front, frontal lobe; temp, temporal lobe; par, parietal lobe; occip, occipital lobe; cereb, cerebellum; bg, basal ganglia; thal, thalamus; cc, corpus callosum; mes, mesencephalon; bs, brainstem). (B) Absolute and relative frequencies of singular and multiple traumatic microbleeds in the corpus callosum ($n = 148$). (S, splenium; CS, corpus + splenium; C, corpus; GCS, genu + corpus + splenium; GC, genu + corpus; G, genu). (Reproduced with permission from Scheid *et al.* 2003 [29].)

of the corpus callosum, the sites of TMBs may resemble those of cerebral amyloid angiopathy (CAA), where microbleeds are usually present in cortico-subcortical areas [30,39,40]. With respect to CAA, the patient's age may be an important criterion for differentiation, as bleeds in CAA are more common in older people. Furthermore, it should be noted that microbleeds in CAA tend to favor the occipital lobe, which is clearly different from the TMBs associated with brain trauma [29,40].

It is obvious that TMBs, like microbleeds from other etiologies, must also be differentiated from artefacts. There is a complete chapter in this book dedicated to this issue (see Ch. 5.).

The neuropathology of microbleeds has been studied in cerebrovascular disorders by several investigators [41–44], although I am not aware of direct comparative radiology–neuropathology studies in TBI. The extent to which radiology–neuropathology correlations of non-traumatic microbleeds can be adapted to TMBs requires further study or modification.

Based on the classical neuropathology descriptions of DAI/TAI, TMBs are most likely the radiological substrates of the "tissue tear hemorrhages" that typically accompany this disorder [10,12,19,45–47]. In "macroscopic" DAI/TAI, these lesions are most often 3–5 mm in size, but they may extend over an anterior–posterior distance of several centimeters [10,12,19,45]. Since the preferential sites of neuropathologically proved DAI/TAI also closely match those of the radiological descriptions of microbleeds after TBI, TMBs can most likely be regarded as radiological markers or biomarkers of DAI/TAI [15,17,29,32,34]. However, based on present knowledge, it cannot be emphasized strongly enough that TMBs and DAI/TAI are not synonymous. The TMBs are merely an accompaniment of the latter, and the sensitivity of TMB as a marker of DAI/TAI remains to be investigated. With the exception of the sparse neuropathological literature on microbleeds that indicate some kind of surrounding tissue damage [41–44], there is no information about the structural and functional integrity of nerve fibers within or in close proximity to a TMB, nor about the grade of disruption of functional circuits that a TMB might generate [32]. However, since it seems that most of the pathobiological processes of DAI/TAI take place on a biochemical, cellular and molecular level that is, for the time being, not readily visualized by neuroradiology, current neuroimaging most likely only depicts the tip of the iceberg of the problem [4,7,13,48,49]. Consequently, pending further studies, TMBs may best be viewed as a relatively inexact, but clinically useful, diagnostic marker for DAI/TAI.

Imaging

The imaging modality of choice for the diagnosis of microbleeds in relation to brain trauma is MRI [15,17,29,34,35]. The most suitable MRI methods are T_2*-weighted GRE and, particularly, susceptibility-weighted imaging (SWI). In comparison with T_2*-weighted GRE, SWI has been reported to depict approximately sixfold more lesions in TBI (in children) and is also able to depict smaller lesions [33,34]. Lesions of 1–15 mm have been used to classify TMBs [28,29,33]. Based on the neuropathological literature,

3–5 mm would be expected to be particularly typical [10,19,45]; however, in T_2*-weighted GRE and SWI (and in comparisons of these) "blooming," which leads to an overestimation of the original size of the lesion, can be expected [40,50].

An upper cut-off point of 15 mm had been chosen in some studies [29,32] because classic radiological reports defined the neuroradiological correlates of DAI as diffuse, small (5–15 mm) focal lesions, limited to white matter tracts [23,24]. The choice of such a size may also be supported by the extrapolation of the "lacune hypothesis," denoting the parenchymal damage resulting from the obliteration of a single small penetrating vessel [51]. Several studies lack clear size definition information [18,26,37,52–54]. However, this proviso should be qualified by noting that the choice of precise size parameters has not seemed to have had a major effect on the classification of microbleeds, as pointed out by Greenberg et al. in a recent review [40]. (Semi)automated volumetric analyses of imaging data have also been performed [27,35,55,56] but may carry the risk of misinterpretation through insufficient differentiation of lesions from artefacts; this is a particular challenge for detecting microbleeds as there are many mimics (see Ch. 5.).

For medical and logistic reasons, MRI may not be performed in the acute stage of TBI. However, in the subacute and chronic stages of TBI, MRI can be applied to most patients if it is deemed necessary [49]. Although vanishing of TMBs has been reported anecdotally [57,58], the majority of TMBs, if present, seem to last for months or years after the injury [36]. Therefore, the possible delay in imaging in individual patients most likely does not have any significance in terms of the diagnosis made. The general considerations concerning detection and interpretation of microbleeds, which are reviewed in detail in Section I of this book, also apply to TMBs and will, therefore, not be repeated here. Table 14.1 gives an overview of several important studies in the particular field of microbleeds in relation to brain trauma.

Clinical significance

Although as discussed above, the strict proof of principle is awaited, there is reasonable evidence for the use of TMBs as a surrogate marker of DAI/TAI. Not less important, however, and independent from the specific pathobiological interpretations, the presence

of TMBs in the vast majority of patients with TBI at least signifies the occurrence of a structural alteration in the brain. This may be of special importance in the context of mild TBI and concussion, where the results of "conventional" neuroimaging have often been reported as unremarkable, or, as in the case of concussion, traditionally even been required to be negative [15,17,59,60]. Meanwhile, the radiological presence of TMBs as the only imaging abnormality in mild TBI has been well documented [18,36,37,54,61]. It is of particular interest that, in a comparative study of MRI and CT in mild TBI, most of the lesions missed by CT were indeed TMBs [18].

The fact that TMBs can also be caused by mild or minor TBI could also be of some importance for the interpretation of the results from larger epidemiological studies and studies on microbleeds in association with specific non-traumatic disorders (cerebrovascular, neurodegenerative, etc.) [40,62–65]. These studies are usually performed in adults, many of whom are of advanced age. Since, on the one hand, the risk of mild TBI is high during an individual lifespan, and, on the other hand, it may often go undetected and/or unremembered, it may well be a specific but so far under-recognized confounder in such studies. For the time being, this subject has not been adequately discussed in the major reviews on microbleeds in general [30,31,40,66,67].

Conflicting results have been reported about the impact of TMBs on cognition and outcome. In particular, several SWI studies in children and adolescents have reported significant correlations between SWI hemorrhagic lesion number and lesion volume with cognitive measures and outcome (Pediatric Cerebral Performance Category Scale, Glasgow Outcome Scale) at 6 months to 4 years after injury [34,35,55,68]. However, it is very interesting that in the most recent study by the same group of researchers, which was performed in 38 adults with TBI, SWI was clearly the MRI method that depicted the largest number of lesions (compared with CT, T_2-weighted and FLAIR-weighted MRI; see also Table 14.1), but it was nevertheless not able to discriminate between good and poor outcomes [56].

There are also studies (T_2*-weighted GRE and SWI) with adults that have reported significant correlations between the number and site of TMBs and outcomes, as measured by the Glasgow Outcome Scale and "post-traumatic neurological deficits"

Table 14.1 Important studies of microbleeds in brain trauma

Study	No. patients (age [years] (mean or range)	GCS score (mean or range)	Mean time since injury	Methodology	Important results	Comments
Yanagawa et al. 2000 [28]	34 (27)	9.3	2.4 weeks	MRI (1.5 T), T_2-FSE, T_2*-GRE	More lesions detected by T_2*-GRE than by T_2-FSE[a] Correlation between LOC/GOS and number of lesions detected by T_2*-GRE[a]	No differentiation between micro- and macrobleeds (>2 mm) Poor description of the clinical manifestations that were "strongly and positively correlated" with the traumatic lesions detected on the T_2*-GRE images
Scheid et al. 2003 [29]	66 (33)	6	23.5 months	MRI (3 T), T_1-MDEFT, T_2-FSE, T_2*-GRE	More lesions detected by T_2*-GRE than by T_1-FSE and T_2-FSE[a] TMBs present in ~70% of patients; T_2-hyperintense foci present in ~23% of patients Correlation between GCS and number of lesions detected by T_2*-GRE;[a] no correlation with GOSE	Upper cut-off for TMBs possibly too large (1–15 mm)
Tong et al. 2003 [33]	7 (14)	7	5 days	MRI (1.5 T), T_1-SE, FLAIR, T_2*-GRE, SWI	Number and volume of lesions detected by SWI greater than by T_2*-GRE[a]	Poor definition of "DAI-lesion"
Tong et al. 2004 [34]	40 (12)	3–15	7 days	MRI (1.5 T), T_1-SE, FLAIR, T_2*-GRE, SWI, DWI	Majority of lesions hemorrhagic Correlation between GCS/LOC/GOS and number/volume of lesions detected by SWI[a]	Poor definition of "DAI-lesion" Semiautomatic volumetry
Scheid et al. 2006 [32]	18 (22.5)	5	9 months	MRI (3 T), T_1-MDEFT, T_2-FSE, T_2*-GRE	No correlation between TMB number and specific or global cognitive performance measured by detailed neuropsychological assessment	Patient population with "pure DAI" Upper cut-off for TMBs possibly too large (1–15 mm) No serial neuropsychological testing
Scheid et al. 2007 [36]	14 (28)	3.5	61 months	MRI (1.5/3 T), T_2*-GRE	More lesions detected by T_2*-GRE at 3 T than by T_2*-GRE at 1.5 T[a] Negative correlation between TMB number and the time interval between injury and imaging, particularly for imaging at 1.5 T	Upper cut-off for TMBs possibly too large (1–15 mm) Longitudinal data only from a subgroup of 9 patients
Lee et al. 2008 [18]	36 (30)	13–15	≤24 h, ≤2 weeks	CT MRI (3 T), T_1-FSPGR, FLAIR, T_2*-GRE	Intraparenchymal lesions on MRI in 75% of patients; TMBs most often missed by CT No significant correlation between imaging findings (particularly number of lesions detected by T_2*-GRE) and cognitive impairment	Exclusively mild TBI

(cont.)

Table 14.1 (cont.)

Study	No. patients (age [years] (mean or range)	GCS score (mean or range)	Mean time since injury	Methodology	Important results	Comments
Chastein et al. 2009 [56]	38 (18–66)	3–15	5.6 days	MRI (1.5 T), T_1-SE, T_2-SE, FLAIR, T_2*-GRE, SWI	Lesions of smallest volume and greatest number of lesions detected by SWI No significant correlations between lesion number/volume detected by SWI and outcome (GOS) Correlation between greater superficial injury and poor outcome (GOS)[a]	Semiautomatic volumetry Poor differentiation DAI/TAI versus other types of injury

DAI: diffuse axonal injury; GCS: Glasgow Coma Scale; GOS: Glasgow Outcome Scale; GOSE: extended Glasgow Outcome Scale; LOC: loss of consciousness; TAI: traumatic axonal injury; TMB, traumatic microbleed.
MRI: DWI, diffusion-weighted imaging; FLAIR, fluid attenuated inversion recovery; FSE, fast spin echo; FSPGR, fast spoiled gradient-recalled echo; GRE, gradient recalled echo; MDEFT, modified driven equilibrium Fourier transform; SE, spin echo; SWI, susceptibility-weighted imaging.
[a] Statistically significant result.

or the "clinical symptoms of head injury" [28,37]. However, in these studies, there is no clear differentiation between TMBs and traumatic lesion belonging to different etiological categories. Moreover, the majority of the clinical neurological abnormalities are only poorly and insufficiently described in these reports (e.g. "abnormal behavior," "frontal lobe signs" or even "Parkinson's syndrome"); consequently, a definite causal relation between TMBs and neurological abnormalities remains questionable.

There are, however, several reports in which no significant correlations have been demonstrated between the number and, in part, site (e.g. corpus callosum) of TMBs and cognition or outcome (psychometric assessment, extended Glasgow Outcome Scale) between 1 year and several years after TBI [18,29,32,49]. The results of these studies fit with the recent study by Chastein et al. [56], mentioned above, and also with considerations concerning non-traumatic microbleeds, where the prognostic utility of the microbleeds remains to be proven [31,40]. Currently, results favor the interpretation that TMBs, despite their usefulness as a diagnostic and categorical marker (see above), are by no means a sufficient parameter for the assessment of DAI/TAI severity or outcome. Since most of the pathology, and possibly also the most relevant pathology, of DAI/TAI takes place at a microstructural level, other imaging modalities (diffusion tensor imaging, MR spectroscopy, functional MRI or magnetoencephalography) may be

better suited to this purpose [60,69–71]. In addition, but clearly closely related to this issue, the overall significance of the distribution of TMBs is unclear at present.

Unresolved problems

Several issues of open debate have already been mentioned in the previous paragraph. The inconsistencies and uncertainties about the prognostic value of TMBs are probably clinically most important. A new and potentially clinically useful observation is the possible lower risk for post-traumatic epilepsy in patients with isolated TMBs compared with patients with other and/or additional traumatic cerebral abnormalities on MRI, which has recently been reported in a retrospective analysis [49].

At present, it is not clear whether TMBs (and microbleeds in general) directly disrupt brain function [40]. A case–control study in a cohort of patients with stroke and transient ischemic attack found an association of microbleeds with frontal-executive dysfunction [62], but despite careful matching this association could have been confounded by other types of cerebrovascular disease accompanying microbleeds. Since the co-existence of other vascular disease may be less likely in TBI, the issue of cognitive function and microbleeds in TBI warrants further study. It is intriguing to speculate about additional potential long-term toxic effects of associated iron accumulation in the brain [72,73]. The quantification of punctate brain iron sources could also turn out to be a valuable and objective surrogate marker of iron-mediated tissue damage in TBI [74].

As in other disorders accompanied by cerebral microbleeds, and with regard to the associated functional effects, the role of the location of TMBs in TBI still needs to be clarified. As has been suggested, detailed anatomical mapping of TMBs could be a promising approach [40]. However, it is difficult to say how many TMBs should constitute the lower cut-off, or whether the reliable and reproducible depiction of one TMB should be sufficient for a diagnosis.

Since there is no generally accepted standard for the MRI in TMBs, a first step for a meaningful comparison of the results of different studies also should be strict specification of imaging parameters. The definition of a standard sequence would be welcome for future studies. Nevertheless, before this can be done, more research is necessary to evaluate the clinical advantages of SWI over T_2*-weighted GRE, and imaging at higher field strengths [36,38,56]. A second area where standardization would assist is in the description and documentation of the images that show TMBs. Here a standardized tool, such as the Microbleed Anatomical Rating Scale, would be very welcome in both a research and clinical setting [75]. A further topic that needs to be pursued is the temporal characteristics of TMBs [36,57,58].

Conclusions

With the increasing availability of appropriate MRI sequences and methods, increased attention has been given to the radiological finding of microbleeds in relation to brain trauma in recent years. Although there are a number of unresolved questions, as outlined above, there is at least reasonable evidence for the following three statements:

- when a definite trauma to the head has occurred, MRI proof of TMBs indicates a structural alteration in the brain and, therefore, a TBI; the spatial distribution of these TMBs may be used to differentiate them from microbleeds of other origins
- after TBI, particularly mild TBI, TMBs can be found as the sole radiological abnormality

- identification of TMBs seem to be a useful clinical marker of DAI/TAI.

Therefore, the finding of TMBs may have diagnostic, prognostic and medicolegal implications. However, as long as the qualitative and quantitative relationships of TMBs with the accompanying axonal and neuronal damage remain unclear, drawing of oversimplistic structure–function correlations should be avoided. Caution is also needed in the design of functional outcome studies. The ultimate test of the value of TMB detection will be whether finding them has clinical relevance for physicians' decision making and on the development, selection (or monitoring) of therapeutic strategies.

References

1. Ryu WH, Feinstein A, Colantonio A, Streiner DL, Dawson DR. Early identification and incidence of mild TBI in Ontario. *Can J Neurol Sci* 2009;**36**:429–35.

2. Feigin VL, Lawes CM, Bennett DA, Barker-Collo SL, Parag V. Worldwide stroke incidence and early case fatality reported in 56 population-based studies: a systematic review. *Lancet Neurol* 2009;**8**:355–69.

3. Teasdale G, Jennett B. Assessment of coma and impaired consciousness. A practical scale. *Lancet* 1974;**ii**:81–84.

4. Povlishock JT, Katz DI. Update on neuropathology and neurological recovery after traumatic brain injury. *J Head Trauma Rehabil* 2005;**20**:76–94.

5. Bullock R, Zauner A, Woodward JJ *et al.* Factors affecting excitatory amino acid release following severe human head injury. *J Neurosurg* 1998;**89**:507–18.

6. Zhang X, Chen Y, Jenkins LW, Kochanek PM, Clark RS. Bench-to-bedside review: apoptosis/programmed cell death triggered by traumatic brain injury. *Crit Care* 2005;**9**:66–75.

7. Kochanek PM, Clark RSB, Jenkins LW. Pathobiology. In Zasler ND, Katz DI, Zafonte RD (eds.) *Brain Injury Medicine: Principles and Practice.* New York: Demos Medical, 2007, pp. 81–96.

8. Miñambres E, Ballesteros MA, Mayorga M *et al.* Cerebral apoptosis in severe traumatic brain injury patients: an in vitro, in vivo, and postmortem study. *J Neurotrauma* 2008;**25**:581–91.

9. Gennarelli TA, Spielman GM, Langfitt TW *et al.* Influence of the type of intracranial lesion on outcome from severe head injury. *J Neurosurg* 1982;**56**:26–32.

10. Graham DI, Gennarelli TA, McIntosh TA. Trauma. In Graham DI, Lantos PI (eds.) *Greenfield's Neuropathology,* 7th edn. London: Arnold, 2002, pp. 823–98.

11. Adams JH, Graham DI, Gennarelli TA, Maxwell WL. Diffuse axonal injury in non-missile head injury. *J Neurol Neurosurg Psychiatry* 1991;**54**: 481–83.

12. Graham DI, Gennarelli TA. Pathology of brain damage after head injury. In Cooper PR, Golfinos JG (eds.) *Head Injury*, 4th edn. New York: McGraw-Hill, 2000, pp. 133–53.

13. Büki A, Povlishock JT. All roads lead to disconnection? Traumatic axonal injury revisited. *Acta Neurochir (Wien)* 2006;**148**:181–94.

14. Barkley JM, Morales D, Hayman LA, Diaz-Marchan PJ. Static neuroimaging in the evaluation of TBI. In Zasler ND, Katz DI, Zafonte RD (eds.) *Brain Injury Medicine: Principles and Practice*. New York: Demos Medical, 2007, pp. 129–48.

15. Metting Z, Rödiger LA, de Keyser J, Van Der Naalt J. Structural and functional neuroimaging in mild-to-moderate head injury. *Lancet Neurol* 2007;**6**:699–710.

16. Maas AI, Stocchetti N, Bullock R. Moderate and severe traumatic brain injury in adults. *Lancet Neurol* 2008;**7**:728–41.

17. Provenzale JM. Imaging of traumatic brain injury: a review of the recent medical literature. *AJR Am J Roentgenol* 2010;**194**:16–19.

18. Lee H, Wintermark M, Gean AD *et al.* Focal lesions in acute mild traumatic brain injury and neurocognitive outcome: CT versus 3 T MRI. *J Neurotrauma* 2008;**25**:1049–56.

19. Adams JH, Doyle D, Ford I *et al.* Diffuse axonal injury in head injury: definition, diagnosis and grading. *Histopathology* 1989;**15**:49–59.

20. Cordobés F, Lobato RD, Rivas JJ *et al.* Post traumatic diffuse axonal brain injury. Analysis of 78 patients studied with computed tomography. *Acta Neurochir (Wien)* 1986;**81**:27–35.

21. Marshall LF, Marshall SB, Klauber MR *et al.* A new classification of head injury based on computerized tomography. *J Neurosurg* 1991;**75**:S14–20.

22. Katz DI, Alexander MP. Traumatic brain injury. Predicting course of recovery and outcome for patients admitted to rehabilitation. *Arch Neurol* 1994;**51**:661–70.

23. Gentry LR, Godersky JC, Thompson B. MR imaging of head trauma: review of the distribution and radiopathologic features of traumatic lesions. *AJR Am J Roentgenol* 1988;**150**:663–72.

24. Gentry LR. Imaging of closed head injury. *Radiology* 1994;**191**:1–17.

25. Atlas SW, Mark AS, Grossman RI, Gomori JM. Intracranial haemorrhage: gradient-echo MR imaging at 1.5 T. Comparison with spin echo imaging and clinical applications. *Radiology* 1988;**168**:803–7.

26. Mittl RL, Grossman RI, Hiehle JF *et al.* Prevalence of MR evidence of diffuse axonal injury in patients with mild head injury and normal head CT findings. *AJNR Am J Neuroradiol* 1994;**15**:1583–9.

27. Pierallini A, Pantano P, Fantozzi LM *et al.* Correlation between MRI findings and long-term outcome in patients with severe brain trauma. *Neuroradiology* 2000;**42**:860–7.

28. Yanagawa Y, Tsushima Y, Tokumaru A *et al.* A quantitative analysis of head injury using T_2*-weighted gradient-echo imaging. *J Trauma* 2000;**49**:272–7.

29. Scheid R, Preul C, Gruber O *et al.* Diffuse axonal injury associated with chronic traumatic brain injury: evidence from T_2*-weighted gradient-echo imaging at 3 T. *AJNR Am J Neuroradiol* 2003;**24**:1049–56.

30. Koennecke HC. Cerebral microbleeds on MRI: prevalence, associations, and potential clinical implications. *Neurology* 2006;**66**:165–71.

31. Cordonnier C, Al-Shahi Salman R, Wardlaw J. Spontaneous brain microbleeds: systematic review, subgroup analyses and standards for study design and reporting. *Brain* 2007;**130**:1988–2003.

32. Scheid R, Walther K, Guthke T, Preul C, von Cramon DY. Cognitive sequelae of diffuse axonal injury. *Arch Neurol* 2006;**63**:418–24.

33. Tong KA, Ashwal S, Holshouser BA *et al.* Hemorrhagic shearing lesions in children and adolescents with posttraumatic diffuse axonal injury: improved detection and initial results. *Radiology* 2003;**227**: 332–9.

34. Tong KA, Ashwal S, Holshouser BA *et al.* Diffuse axonal injury in children: clinical correlation with hemorrhagic lesions. *Ann Neurol* 2004;**56**:36–50.

35. Sigmund GA, Tong KA, Nickerson JP *et al.* Multimodality comparison of neuroimaging in pediatric traumatic brain injury. *Pediatr Neurol* 2007;**36**:217–26.

36. Scheid R, Ott DV, Roth H, Schroeter ML, von Cramon DY. Comparative magnetic resonance imaging at 1.5 and 3 Tesla for the evaluation of traumatic microbleeds. *J Neurotrauma* 2007;**24**:1811–16.

37. Park JH, Park SW, Kang SH *et al.* Detection of traumatic cerebral microbleeds by susceptibility-weighted image of MRI. *J Korean Neurosurg Soc* 2009;**46**:365–9.

38. Stehling C, Wersching H, Kloska SP *et al.* Detection of asymptomatic cerebral microbleeds: a comparative study at 1.5 and 3.0 T. *Acad Radiol* 2008;**15**:895–900.

39. Blitstein MK, Tung GA. MRI of cerebral microhemorrhages. *AJR Am J Roentgenol* 2007;**189**:720–5.

40. Greenberg SM, Vernooij MW, Cordonnier C for the Microbleed Study Group. Cerebral microbleeds: a guide to detection and interpretation. *Lancet Neurol* 2009;**8**:165–74.

41. Fazekas F, Kleinert R, Roob G *et al.* Histopathologic analysis of foci of signal loss on gradient-echo T_2*-weighted MR images in patients with spontaneous intracerebral hemorrhage: evidence of microangiopathy-related microbleeds. *AJNR Am J Neuroradiol* 1999;**20**:637–42.

42. Roob G, Kleinert R, Seifert T *et al.* MRI evidence of cerebral microbleeds. Comparative histopathologic data and possible clinical implications. *Nervenarzt* 1999;**70**:1082–7.

43. Tanaka A, Ueno Y, Nakayama Y, Takano K, Takebayashi S. Small chronic hemorrhages and ischemic lesions in association with spontaneous intracerebral hematomas. *Stroke* 1999;**30**:1637–42.

44. Tatsumi S, Shinohara M, Yamamoto T. Direct comparison of histology of microbleeds with postmortem MR images: a case report. *Cerebrovasc Dis* 2008;**26**:142–6.

45. Gennarelli TA, Thibault LE, Adams JH *et al.* Diffuse axonal injury and traumatic coma in the primate. *Ann Neurol* 1982;**12**:564–74.

46. Povlishock JT. Traumatically induced axonal injury: pathogenesis and pathobiological implications. *Brain Pathol* 1992;**2**:1–12.

47. Meythaler JM, Peduzzi JD, Eleftheriou E, Novack TA. Current concepts: diffuse axonal injury-associated traumatic brain injury. *Arch Phys Med Rehabil* 2001;**82**:1461–71.

48. Smith DH, Meaney DF, Shull WH. Diffuse axonal injury in head trauma. *J Head Trauma Rehabil* 2003;**18**:307–16.

49. Scheid R, von Cramon DY. Clinical findings in the chronic phase of traumatic brain injury: data from 12 years' experience in the Cognitive Neurology Outpatient Clinic at the University of Leipzig. *Dtsch Arztebl Int* 2010;**107**:199–205.

50. Nandigam RN, Viswanathan A, Delgado P *et al.* MR imaging detection of cerebral microbleeds: effect of susceptibility-weighted imaging, section thickness, and field strength. *AJNR Am J Neuroradiol* 2009;**30**:338–43.

51. Fisher CM. Lacunar infarcts: a review. *Cerebrovas Dis* 1991;**1**:311–20.

52. Giugni E, Sabatini U, Hagberg GE, Formisano R, Castriota-Scanderbeg A. Fast detection of diffuse axonal damage in severe traumatic brain injury: comparison of gradient-recalled echo and turbo proton echo-planar spectroscopic imaging MRI sequences. *AJNR Am J Neuroradiol* 2005;**26**:1140–8.

53. Hähnel S, Stippich C, Weber I *et al.* Prevalence of cerebral microhemorrhages in amateur boxers as detected by 3 T MR imaging. *AJNR Am J Neuroradiol* 2008;**29**:388–91.

54. Topal NB, Hakyemez B, Erdogan C *et al.* MR imaging in the detection of diffuse axonal injury with mild traumatic brain injury. *Neurol Res* 2008;**30**:974–8.

55. Babikian T, Freier MC, Tong KA *et al.* Susceptibility weighted imaging: neuropsychologic outcome and pediatric head injury. *Pediatr Neurol* 2005;**33**:184–94.

56. Chastain CA, Oyoyo U, Zipperman M *et al.* Predicting outcomes of traumatic brain injury by imaging modality and injury distribution. *J Neurotrauma* 2009;**26**:1183–96.

57. Messori A, Polonara G, Mabiglia C, Salvolini U. Is haemosiderin visible indefinitely on gradient-echo MRI following traumatic intracerebral haemorrhage? *Neuroradiology* 2003;**45**:881–6.

58. Ezaki Y, Tsutsumi K, Morikawa M, Nagata I. Lesions identified on T_2*-weighted gradient echo images in two patients with suspected diffuse axonal injury that resolved in less than ten days. *Acta Neurochir* (*Wien*) 2006;**148**:547–50.

59. Ropper AH, Gorson KC. Concussion. *N Engl J Med* 2007;**356**:166–72.

60. Bigler ED. Neuroimaging in mild traumatic brain injury. *Psychol Inj Law* 2010;**3**:36–9.

61. Tong KA, Ashwal S, Obenaus A *et al.* Susceptibility-weighted MR imaging: a review of clinical applications in children. *AJNR Am J Neuroradiol* 2008;**29**:9–17.

62. Werring DJ, Frazer DW, Coward LJ *et al.* Cognitive dysfunction in patients with cerebral microbleeds on T_2*-weighted gradient-echo MRI. *Brain* 2004;**127**:2265–75.

63. Cordonnier C, van der Flier WM, Sluimer JD *et al.* Prevalence and severity of microbleeds in a memory clinic setting. *Neurology* 2006;**66**:1356–60.

64. Vernooij MW, van der Lugt A, Ikram MA *et al.* Prevalence and risk factors of cerebral microbleeds: the Rotterdam Scan Study. *Neurology* 2008;**70**:1208–14.

65. Sveinbjornsdottir S, Sigurdsson S, Aspelund T *et al.* Cerebral microbleeds in the population-based AGES–Reykjavik study: prevalence and location. *J Neurol Neurosurg Psychiatry* 2008;**79**:1002–6.

66. Fiehler J. Cerebral microbleeds: old leaks and new haemorrhages. *Int J Stroke* 2006;**1**:122–30.

67. Werring DJ. Cerebral microbleeds: clinical and pathophysiological significance. *J Neuroimaging* 2007;**17**:193–203.

68. Ashwal S, Babikian T, Gardner-Nichols J *et al.* Susceptibility-weighted imaging and proton magnetic resonance spectroscopy in assessment of outcome after pediatric traumatic brain injury. *Arch Phys Med Rehabil* 2006;**87**(Suppl. 2):S50–8.

69. Levine B, Fujiwara E, O'Connor C *et al.* In vivo characterization of traumatic brain injury neuropathology with structural and functional neuroimaging. *J Neurotrauma* 2006;**23**: 1396–1411.

70. Gasparovic C, Yeo R, Mannell M *et al.* Neurometabolite concentrations in gray and white matter in mild traumatic brain injury: an 1H-magnetic resonance spectroscopy study. *J Neurotrauma* 2009;**26**:1635–43.

71. Mayer AR, Ling J, Mannell MV *et al.* A prospective diffusion tensor imaging study in mild traumatic brain injury. *Neurology* 2010;**74**:643–50.

72. Koeppen AH. A brief history of brain iron research. *J Neurol Sci* 2003;**207**:95–7.

73. Sadrzadeh SM, Saffari Y. Iron and brain disorders. *Am J Clin Pathol* 2004;**121**(Suppl.): S64–70.

74. McAuley G, Schrag M, Sipos P *et al.* Quantification of punctate iron sources using magnetic resonance phase. *Magn Reson Med* 2010;**63**:106–15.

75. Gregoire SM, Chaudhary UJ, Brown MM *et al.* The Microbleed Anatomical Rating Scale (MARS): reliability of a tool to map brain microbleeds. *Neurology* 2009;**73**:1759–66.

Chapter

15

Cerebral microbleeds in CADASIL

Anand Viswanathan, Hugues Chabriat and Martin Dichgans

Introduction

Cerebral autosomal dominant arteriopathy with sub-cortical infarcts and leukoencephalopathy (CADASIL) is an arteriopathy caused by mutations of the gene *NOTCH3* [1,2]. The main clinical manifestations of the disease include attacks of migraine with aura, mood disturbances, recurrent ischemic strokes and progressive cognitive decline [3,4].

On MRI, there is evidence of widespread white matter hyperintensities (WMH) on T_2-weighted images [5–7], lacunar infarctions on T_1-weighted images [2,4,5,8,9] and evidence of cerebral microbleeds (CMB) on T_2^*-weighted or gradient-recalled echo (GRE) images [9–12]. These MRI lesions represent different consequences of the underlying angiopathy in the disease.

Epidemiology

It has been reported that CMB occur in 25–69% of patients affected with CADASIL (Fig. 15.1) [9–12]. A study of 15 Dutch families with CADASIL showed that CMB occurred in 10 of 40 carriers of the *NOTCH3* mutation [10]. In a small cohort of German CADASIL patients, 11 of 16 subjects harbored CMB and each individual commonly had multiple lesions [11]. Finally, in a Chinese study of 21 patients with CADASIL, evidence of small intracerebral hemorrhages (ICH; 8 cm in diameter) was found in six patients [1–3]. It is unclear whether these ICHs are a consequence of the Notch-3 changes or of other causes such as hypertension as five of these six subjects had elevated blood pressure [13]. This study did not assess CMB as GRE sequences were not taken.

Pathologically, there was autopsy evidence of hemosiderin-laden macrophages in six of seven subjects with CADASIL [11]. In all cases, these macrophages were found in the vicinity of small blood vessels (diameter: 100–300 mm) where the vessel walls showed characteristic degenerative changes. There was no evidence of amyloid deposition or vascular malformations, which strongly supports the involvement of CADASIL-related ultrastructural modifications of the vessel wall in these lesions.

Recent data from a large two-center cohort study of patients with CADASIL defined risk factors for CMB [14], which were detected in 35% (52/147) of patients. In those patients with CMB, lesions were most commonly multiple (median 3; mean 10.9 ± 24.8). In univariate analysis, the presence of CMB was strongly correlated with age ($p = 0.0002$), the diagnosis of hypertension ($p = 0.001$), decreased high density lipoprotein (HDL) cholesterol ($p = 0.02$), elevated hemoglobin A1c (HbA1c; $p = 0.04$) and anticoagulant treatment ($p = 0.008$), but not with antiplatelet use ($p = 0.28$). Additionally, individuals with CMB had, on average, higher systolic and diastolic blood pressure ($p = 0.001$ and $p = 0.008$, respectively).

The presence of CMB was also strongly associated with other MRI markers in the CADASIL cohort (Table 15.1). In univariate analysis, those patients with CMB had a larger total normalized lacunar infarct volume (nLV; $p = 0.0001$) and greater normalized WMH lesion volume (nWMH; $p = 0.0002$). Furthermore, regression models (Table 15.2) demonstrated that the number of CMB was independently associated with systolic blood pressure ($p = 0.005$; odds ratio [OR, risk per 10 mmHg increase], 1.42; 95% confidence

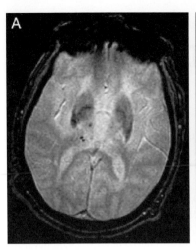
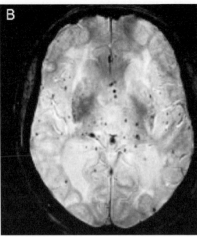

Fig. 15.1 Examples of cerebral microbleeds in CADASIL. (A) Gradient echo MRI sequences demonstrate several microbleeds in the thalamus. (B) Numerous microbleeds are seen in the thalamus and cortico-subcortical junction.

interval [CI], 1.11–1.81), the diagnosis of hypertension ($p = 0.0004$; OR, 5.19; 95% CI, 2.08–12.95), nWMH ($p = 0.0005$; OR, 1.16 [risk per percent increase in nWMH]; 95% CI, 1.07–1.26) and nLV ($p = 0.004$; OR, 1.96; 95% CI, 1.24–3.09).

In the final maximally adjusted multivariable logistic regression model, HbA1c ($p = 0.004$), systolic blood pressure ($p = 0.014$), nLV ($p = 0.010$) and nWMH ($p = 0.046$) were independently associated with the presence of CMB. The effect of systolic blood pressure remained significant ($p = 0.004$) when only individuals with normal blood pressure (systolic blood pressure <140 mmHg) were analyzed. These results are shown in Table 15.2. Finally, the independent risk factors predisposing subjects to CMB (hypertension, systolic blood pressure, HbA1c) were not found to be associated with white matter lesions or lacunar infarctions after performing similar univariate and multivariate analyses.

Interestingly, in this study, the average blood pressure in subjects with CMB and in those without were found to be in the normal range (<140/90 mmHg) (Table 15.1). In addition, when hypertensive patients were removed from the analysis, the association remained highly significant (Table 15.2). These results suggest that small increases in systolic blood pressure may contribute to CMB through an additive effect on the ultrastructural vessel wall modifications caused by *NOTCH3* mutations [15]. It remains to be elucidated which factors (pulsatility, cerebrovascular resistance or vessel wall stiffness) most strongly influence the rupture of the cerebral microvessel wall in the setting of moderate elevations of blood pressure. Importantly, these results emphasize that acceptable blood pres-

sure values in the setting of an existing cerebral microangiopathy may well differ from the established normal range.

The correlation between serum HbA1c and presence of CMB in multivariable modeling suggests that long-term serum glucose levels may also play a role in CADASIL vessel dysfunction. Although a specific association between Hb1Ac and CMB has not been previously reported in other cerebral disease pathologies, there is evidence to suggest that increased serum glucose increases the risk associated with ICH. Hyperglycemia and diabetes have been identified as independent risk factors for fatal outcome [16–19], and other observations suggest that hyperglycemia predisposes to increased bleeding [20–26]. There is some evidence in experimental models to suggest that increased HbA1c may alter erythrocyte deformability and increase shear stress on the microvessel wall [27]. Additionally, in the setting of ischemia, hyperglycemia leads to increased blood–brain barrier breakdown [28]. The observations of CMB in individuals with higher serum HbA1c (even in non-diabetic patients) may imply that chronically increased serum glucose levels in the setting of this genetic arteriopathy may lead to vessel fragility and microhemorrhage.

Vascular wall abnormalities in CADASIL may affect the vulnerability of certain blood vessels, resulting in rupture and microhemorrhage [11]. Certain vascular risk factors such as elevated blood pressure and HbA1c may favor the rupture of the vascular wall, and the cerebral angioarchitecture may promote the occurrence of CMB in locations different from those of ischemic lesions. Further studies are required to elucidate this potential mechanism.

Table 15.1 Characteristics of CADASIL cohort with and without cerebral microbleeds

Characteristic	Without CMB	With ≥1 CMB	*p* value
Male (No. [%])	39 (41)	24 (46)	0.55
Age (years [±SD])	49.4 ± 11.1	56.3 ± 10.0	0.0002
History of hypertension (No. [%])	10 (10.6)	17 (32.7)	0.001
Dementia (No. [%])	9 (9.8)	14 (26.9)	0.007
Past or current smoker (No. [%])	49 (51.6)	23 (44.2)	0.39
Diabetes mellitus (No. [%])	1 (1)	3 (5.8)	0.13
History of hypercholesterolemia (No. [%])	45 (48)	28 (54)	0.49
Anticoagulant use (No. [%])	1 (1)	6 (11.5)	0.008
Antithrombotic use (No. [%])	65 (68.4)	40 (76.9)	0.28
Any alcohol consumption (No. [%])	51 (58)	27 (57.5)	0.95
Systolic blood pressure (mmHg [±SD])	125 ± 15	135 ± 18	0.001
Diastolic blood pressure (mmHg [±SD])	74 ± 10	79 ± 10	0.008
Mini-Mental State Examination (score [±SD])	26.8 ± 4.2	24.6 ± 5.8	0.01
Total cholesterol (mmol/l [±SD])	5.42 ± 1.1	5.62 ± 1.1	0.30
LDL (mmol/l [±SD])	3.38 ± 0.90	3.61 ± 0.94	0.16
LDL ≥3.1mmol/l (No. [%])	59 (62.8)	38 (76)	0.11
HDL (mmol/l [±SD])	1.52 ± 0.45	1.37 ± 0.33	0.02
HbA1c (±SD)	5.4 ± 0.39	5.6 ± 0.48	0.04
HbA1c ≥5.6 (No. [%])	25 (26.9)	30 (58.8)	0.0002
Blood glucose (mmol/l [±SD])	5.24 ± 0.71	5.43 ± 0.71	0.18
nWMH (±SD)	6.7 ± 4.7	9.5 ± 4.8	0.0002
nLV (±SD)	0.7 ± 1.7	1.1 ± 0.9	0.0001

CADASIL, cerebral autosomal dominant arteriopathy with subcortical infarcts and leukoencephalopathy; CMB, cerebral microbleed; HbA1c, hemoglobin A1c; HDL, high density lipoprotein; LDL, low density lipoprotein; nLV, normalized lacunar infarct volume; nWMH, normalized white matter hyperintensity volume. *Source*: adapted from Viswanathan *et al.*, 2006 [14].

Location of cerebral microbleeds in CADASIL

The most common areas for CMBs in CADASIL are the thalamus (61.5% of patients with CMB), brain-

Table 15.2 Multivariable model of predictors of cerebral microbleeds in CADASIL

Predictor	Odds ratio	95% confidence interval	*p* value
Model 1, adjusted to include history of hypertension			
Hypertension	4.90	1.63–14.71	0.005
HbA1c ≥5.6	3.25	1.38–7.62	0.007
LDL ≥3.1 mmol/l	2.95	1.08–8.00	0.034
nWMH	1.09[a]	1.00–1.19	0.041
nLV	2.15[b]	1.47–4.22	0.001
Model 2, substituting hypertension history with measured blood pressure			
Systolic blood pressure (mmHg)	1.42[c]	1.07–1.88	0.014
HbA1c ≥5.6	3.49	1.49–8.13	0.004
nWMH	1.10[a]	1.00–1.12	0.046
nLV	1.99[b]	1.18–3.37	0.010
Model 3, effect of blood pressure in normotensive CADASIL (*n* = 125)			
Systolic blood pressure <140 mmHg	2.15[c]	1.27–3.65	0.004
HbA1c ≥5.6	3.68	1.40–9.68	0.008
nLV	2.23[b]	1.14–4.36	0.019
Age	1.06[d]	1.00–1.12	0.024

CADASIL, cerebral autosomal dominant arteriopathy with subcortical infarcts and leukoencephalopathy; HbA1c, hemoglobin A1c; LDL, low density lipoprotein; nLV, normalized lacunar infarct volume; nWMH, normalized white matter hyperintensity volume.
[a] Expressed as risk per percentage increase in nWMH.
[b] Expressed as risk per 0.1% increase in nLV.
[c] Expressed as risk per 10\mmHg increase in systolic blood pressure.
[d] Expressed as risk per year increase in age.
Source: adapted from Viswanathan *et al.* 2006 [14].

stem (38.5%), basal ganglia (38.5%) and cortex or cortico-subcortical junction in the temporal (36.5%) and occipital (26.9%) areas. Cerebral microbleeds are detected in the cerebellum in 25% of cases where lacunar infarcts or WMH are typically absent. This distribution differs from that observed for lacunar infarctions and WMH in CADASIL (Fig. 15.2).

Relationship between cerebral microbleeds and other imaging markers of small vessel disease in CADASIL

As one of the key imaging markers in cerebral small vessel disease [12], CMB are strongly correlated with WMHs and lacunar lesions in CADASIL. There was a

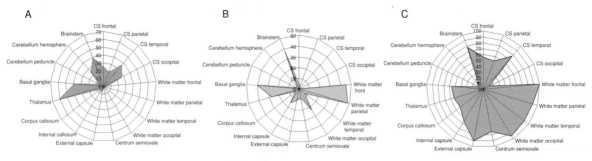

Fig. 15.2 Distribution of MRI lesions in 147 patients with CADASIL (cerebral autosomal dominant arteriopathy with subcortical infarcts and leukoencephalopathy). Radar plots show the frequency at each location of (A) cerebral microhemorrhages, (B) lacunar infarctions and (C) white matter hyperintensities. In each category, frequency is expressed as a percentage of the number of patients harboring a lesion at a given location divided by the total number of patients with that specific lesion. CS, cortical sulci. See the color plate section. (Adapted from Viswanathan *et al.* 2006 [14].)

strong positive correlation between WMHs and lacunar volumes and number of CMBs in 147 patients with CADASIL (Table 15.1). In univariate analysis, patients with CMB had larger nLV ($p = 0.0001$) and greater nWMH ($p = 0.0002$) [14].

As described above, in the two-center cohort study of CADASIL patients, the other MRI markers of CADASIL (lacunar infarctions and WMH) were not associated with the vascular risk factors for CMB. Additionally, there was a minimal overlap between regions of CMB and regions of lacunar infarction or prominent WMH (Fig. 15.2) [11,14]. The differences in risk factors and the location of CMB and the other MRI lesions in the disease suggest the presence of distinct pathophysiological pathways that lead to ischemic or hemorrhagic lesions in CADASIL.

The exact relationship between vessel pathology in CADASIL and each of these MRI markers of small vessel disease remains to be further elucidated and may require detailed neuroimaging–pathology studies.

Genetic determinants of cerebral microbleeds in CADASIL

The gene *NOTCH3* encodes a single-pass transmembrane protein. It is an evolutionarily conserved protein. The Notch signaling pathway plays a central role in the development and maturation of most vertebrate organs [29]. *NOTCH3* is predominantly expressed in vascular smooth muscle cells and its protein product, Notch-3, is critical for the structural and functional integrity of small arteries. Notch-3 is thought to control arterial differentiation and maturation of smooth muscle cells [30,31]. At the cell surface, the Notch-3

receptor is a heterodimer composed of a large extracellular domain, containing 34 epidermal growth factor-like (EGF-1) repeats (EGFRs), non-covalently attached to the membrane-tethered intracellular domain [30]. Ligand binding initiates a series of proteolytic cleavages that releases the Notch-3 intracellular domain for subsequent translocation to the nucleus. In the nucleus, the Notch-3 intracellular domain interacts with transcription factors to activate the transcription of target genes [32].

Although *NOTCH3* has 33 exons, CADASIL mutations occur in exons 2–24, which encode the EGFR domains. The mutations lead to an odd number of cysteine residues within one of the domains [33–36]. Recent studies suggest that disease may not be caused by compromised Notch-3 function in the majority of cases. Instead, it is thought that most mutations convey a non-physiological and deleterious activity to the Notch-3 receptor [36–41].

However, by contrast, certain naturally occurring mutations are predicted to result in loss of function in the Notch-3 receptor. These particular mutations affect repeats 10 and 11 of the EGF-1 region of the protein [36,38]. A recent study examining mutations affecting this region showed that these patients had increased volume of WMHs compared with patients with mutations altering repeats 2–5. Patients with mutations altering EGFR 10 and 11 seemed to have fewer CMB than patients with mutations affecting EGFR 2–5 (0.11 ± 0.33 versus 2.6 ± 5.8), although this was not statistically significant ($p = 0.21$) [42]. This does raise the possibility that specific *NOTCH3* mutations may influence the overall burden of CMB in patients with CADASIL. Further studies to investigate this possibility are required.

To date, no other convincing evidence has emerged to suggest that CMB burden or location varies by *NOTCH3* mutation in CADASIL. Neither have other genetic modifiers been found that may predispose CADASIL patients to microbleeds.

Cerebral microbleeds and brain function

Cerebral microbleeds have also been associated with clinical disability in CADASIL [14,43]. In a two-center cohort study of 147 patients with CADASIL, the number of CMBs was independently associated with functional dependence (defined as modified Rankin score ≥ 3) with an OR per additional microbleed of 1.16 (95% CI, 1.01–1.34; $p = 0.034$) after adjustment for other confounding variables [14]. Multivariable analysis to define correlates of cognition did not, however, find a similar independent association with CMB.

If CMBs indeed have direct effects on brain function (rather than simply marking the presence of other cerebrovascular pathologies), one would expect CMB location to play a role. In analyses of the two-center CADASIL cohort, CMB in the caudate were independently associated with lower global cognitive scores (based on the Mattis Dementia Rating Scale; $p = 0.027$) and CMB in the frontal lobes showed a trend toward lower global cognitive scores ($p = 0.056$) [14].

Recently, a small study has been performed that examined the change in number of cerebral microbleeds over time [44]. Twenty-five *NOTCH3* mutation carriers underwent baseline and follow-up neuropsychological testing and neuroimaging. Both global and domain-specific cognitive function was assessed using the cognitive section of the Cambridge Mental Disorders of the Elderly Examination (CAMCOG). The average follow-up time was 7.1 years (range, 6.4–7.6). Microbleeds were assessed on GRE sequences. The authors found that the average number of CMB increased from 1.6 to 3.5 ($p < 0.05$). Furthermore, in univariate analysis, the increase in the number of CMB was correlated with global cognitive function (change in CAMCOG total score; $p = 0.005$) and executive function (change in Trails B score; $p = 0.007$). In multivariate analysis, accounting for other MRI markers, increase in CMBs was independently associated with worsening executive dysfunction as measured by the Trails B score.

Conclusions

The recent data described above, together with previous cross-sectional studies [43], suggest that CMB have an independent impact on cognition in CADASIL. Their impact likely stems from total CMB burden and microbleed localization [43]. In the future, larger cohort studies with detailed neuroimaging should be performed to further define risk factors for CMB formation as well as the location of newly formed CMB. As it is established that CMBs have an impact on cognition and disability, the results from these studies may eventually be used to design therapeutic trials to prevent the formation of CMBs in patients with CADASIL.

References

1. Tournier-Lasserve E, Joutel A, Melki J *et al.* Cerebral autosomal dominant arteriopathy with subcortical infarcts and leukoencephalopathy maps to chromosome 19q12. *Nat Genet* 1993;3:256–9.

2. Joutel A, Corpechot C, Ducros A *et al.* Notch3 mutations in CADASIL, a hereditary adult-onset condition causing stroke and dementia. *Nature* 1996; **383**:707–10.

3. Dichgans M, Mayer M, Uttner I *et al.* The phenotypic spectrum of CADASIL: clinical findings in 102 cases. *Ann Neurol* 1998;**44**:731–9.

4. Chabriat H, Vahedi K, Iba-Zizen MT *et al.* Clinical spectrum of CADASIL: a study of 7 families. Cerebral autosomal dominant arteriopathy with subcortical infarcts and leukoencephalopathy. *Lancet* 1995;**346**: 934–9.

5. Chabriat H, Levy C, Taillia H *et al.* Patterns of MRI lesions in CADASIL. *Neurology* 1998;**51**:452–7.

6. Tournier-Lasserve E, Iba-Zizen MT, Romero N, Bousser MG. Autosomal dominant syndrome with strokelike episodes and leukoencephalopathy. *Stroke* 1991;**22**:1297–1302.

7. Auer DP, Putz B, Gossl C *et al.* Differential lesion patterns in CADASIL and sporadic subcortical arteriosclerotic encephalopathy: MR imaging study with statistical parametric group comparison. *Radiology* 2001;**218**:443–51.

8. O'Sullivan M, Rich PM, Barrick TR, Clark CA, Markus HS. Frequency of subclinical lacunar infarcts in ischemic leukoaraiosis and cerebral autosomal dominant arteriopathy with subcortical infarcts and leukoencephalopathy. *AJNR Am J Neuroradiol* 2003; **24**:1348–54.

9. van den Boom R, Lesnik Oberstein SA, Ferrari MD, Haan J, van Buchem MA. Cerebral autosomal

dominant arteriopathy with subcortical infarcts and leukoencephalopathy: MR imaging findings at different ages: 3rd–6th decades. *Radiology* 2003;**229**: 683–90.

10. Lesnik Oberstein SA, van den Boom R, van Buchem MA *et al.* Cerebral microbleeds in CADASIL. *Neurology* 2001;**57**:1066–70.

11. Dichgans M, Holtmannspotter M, Herzog J *et al.* Cerebral microbleeds in CADASIL: a gradient-echo magnetic resonance imaging and autopsy study. *Stroke* 2002;**33**:67–71.

12. Viswanathan A, Chabriat H. Cerebral microhemorrhage. *Stroke* 2006;**37**:550–5.

13. Lee YC, Liu CS, Chang MH *et al.* Population-specific spectrum of NOTCH3 mutations, MRI features and founder effect of CADASIL in Chinese. *J Neurol* 2009;**256**:249–55.

14. Viswanathan A, Guichard JP, Gschwendtner A *et al.* Blood pressure and haemoglobin A1c are associated with microhaemorrhage in CADASIL: a two-centre cohort study. *Brain* 2006;**129**:2375–83.

15. Ruchoux MM, Maurage CA. CADASIL: cerebral autosomal dominant arteriopathy with subcortical infarcts and leukoencephalopathy. *J Neuropathol Exp Neurol* 1997;**56**:947–64.

16. Wong KS. Risk factors for early death in acute ischemic stroke and intracerebral hemorrhage: a prospective hospital-based study in Asia. Asian Acute Stroke Advisory Panel. *Stroke* 1999;**30**:2326–30.

17. Arboix A, Massons J, Garcia-Eroles L, Oliveres M, Targa C. Diabetes is an independent risk factor for in-hospital mortality from acute spontaneous intracerebral hemorrhage. *Diabetes Care* 2000;**23**: 1527–32.

18. Passero S, Ciacci G, Ulivelli M. The influence of diabetes and hyperglycemia on clinical course after intracerebral hemorrhage. *Neurology* 2003;**61**:1351–6.

19. Rosand J, Eckman MH, Knudsen KA, Singer DE, Greenberg SM. The effect of warfarin and intensity of anticoagulation on outcome of intracerebral hemorrhage. *Arch Intern Med* 2004;**164**:880–4.

20. de Courten-Myers GM, Kleinholz M, Holm P *et al.* Hemorrhagic infarct conversion in experimental stroke. *Ann Emerg Med* 1992;**21**:120–6.

21. Williams SB, Goldfine AB, Timimi FK *et al.* Acute hyperglycemia attenuates endothelium-dependent vasodilation in humans in vivo. *Circulation* 1998; **97**:1695–1701.

22. Kase CS, Furlan AJ, Wechsler LR *et al.* Cerebral hemorrhage after intra-arterial thrombolysis for ischemic stroke: the PROACT II trial. *Neurology* 2001;**57**:1603–10.

23. Meigs JB, Mittleman MA, Nathan DM *et al.* Hyperinsulinemia, hyperglycemia, and impaired hemostasis: the Framingham Offspring Study. *JAMA* 2000;**283**:221–8.

24. Demchuk AM, Morgenstern LB, Krieger DW *et al.* Serum glucose level and diabetes predict tissue plasminogen activator-related intracerebral hemorrhage in acute ischemic stroke. *Stroke* 1999;**30**: 34–9.

25. Bruno A, Levine SR, Frankel MR *et al.* Admission glucose level and clinical outcomes in the NINDS rt-PA Stroke Trial. *Neurology* 2002;**59**:669–74.

26. Song EC, Chu K, Jeong SW *et al.* Hyperglycemia exacerbates brain edema and perihematomal cell death after intracerebral hemorrhage. *Stroke* 2003;**34**: 2215–20.

27. Tsukada K, Sekizuka E, Oshio C, Minamitani H. Direct measurement of erythrocyte deformability in diabetes mellitus with a transparent microchannel capillary model and high-speed video camera system. *Microvasc Res* 2001;**61**:231–9.

28. Dietrich WD, Alonso O, Busto R. Moderate hyperglycemia worsens acute blood–brain barrier injury after forebrain ischemia in rats. *Stroke* 1993;**24**: 111–16.

29. Gridley T. Notch signaling in vascular development and physiology. *Development* 2007;**134**:2709–18.

30. Joutel A, Andreux F, Gaulis S *et al.* The ectodomain of the Notch3 receptor accumulates within the cerebrovasculature of CADASIL patients. *J Clin Invest* 2000;**105**:597–605.

31. Domenga V, Fardoux P, Lacombe P *et al.* Notch3 is required for arterial identity and maturation of vascular smooth muscle cells. *Genes Dev* 2004;**18**: 2730–5.

32. Schweisguth F. Regulation of notch signaling activity. *Curr Biol* 2004;**14**:R129–38.

33. Oberstein SA, Ferrari MD, Bakker E *et al.* Diagnostic Notch3 sequence analysis in CADASIL: three new mutations in Dutch patients. Dutch CADASIL Research Group. *Neurology* 1999;**52**:1913–15.

34. Joutel A, Vahedi K, Corpechot C *et al.* Strong clustering and stereotyped nature of Notch3 mutations in CADASIL patients. *Lancet* 1997;**350**:1511–15.

35. Singhal S, Bevan S, Barrick T, Rich P, Markus HS. The influence of genetic and cardiovascular risk factors on the CADASIL phenotype. *Brain* 2004;**127**:2031–8.

36. Peters N, Opherk C, Zacherle S *et al.* CADASIL-associated Notch3 mutations have differential effects both on ligand binding and ligand-induced Notch3 receptor signaling through RBP-Jk. *Exp Cell Res* 2004;**299**:454–64.

37. Haritunians T, Chow T, de Lange RP *et al.* Functional analysis of a recurrent missense mutation in Notch3 in CADASIL. *J Neurol Neurosurg Psychiatry* 2005;**76**: 1242–8.

38. Joutel A, Monet M, Domenga V, Riant F, Tournier-Lasserve E. Pathogenic mutations associated with cerebral autosomal dominant arteriopathy with subcortical infarcts and leukoencephalopathy differently affect Jagged1 binding and Notch3 activity via the RBP/JK signaling pathway. *Am J Hum Genet* 2004;**74**:338–47.

39. Karlstrom H, Beatus P, Dannaeus K *et al.* A CADASIL-mutated Notch 3 receptor exhibits impaired intracellular trafficking and maturation but normal ligand-induced signaling. *Proc Natl Acad Sci USA* 2002;**99**:17119–24.

40. Low WC, Santa Y, Takahashi K, Tabira T, Kalaria RN. CADASIL-causing mutations do not alter Notch3 receptor processing and activation. *Neuroreport* 2006;**17**:945–9.

41. Opherk C, Duering M, Peters N *et al.* CADASIL mutations enhance spontaneous multimerization of NOTCH3. *Hum Mol Genet* 2009;**18**:2761–7.

42. Monet-Lepretre M, Bardot B, Lemaire B *et al.* Distinct phenotypic and functional features of CADASIL mutations in the Notch3 ligand binding domain. *Brain* 2009;**132**:1601–12.

43. Viswanathan A, Godin O, Jouvent E *et al.* Impact of MRI markers in subcortical vascular dementia: a multi-modal analysis in CADASIL. *Neurobiol Aging* 2010;**31**:1629–36.

44. Liem MK, Lesnik Oberstein SA, Haan J *et al.* MRI correlates of cognitive decline in CADASIL: a 7-year follow-up study. *Neurology* 2009;**72**: 143–8.

Miscellaneous conditions associated with cerebral microbleeds

David J. Werring and Hans Rolf Jäger

Introduction

Cerebral microbleeds (CMBs) have mainly generated interest in the context of common acquired cerebrovascular and neurodegenerative diseases – including ischemic stroke of various causes, spontaneous intracerebral hemorrhage (ICH) and Alzheimer's disease. However, since MRI sequences sensitive to CMBs are now established as a routine component of neuroradiological investigation in many different clinical settings, CMBs have been detected in a number of less common disorders in many different fields of medicine. This chapter provides an overview of CMBs in rarer conditions or clinical cohorts not covered elsewhere in the book. Where possible, the potential relevance for understanding pathophysiology or clinical impact of CMBs is discussed. Although the conditions considered in this chapter form a rather disparate grouping, they have been divided into the following categories: rare inherited cerebral microangiopathies (amyloid and non-amyloid related), cardiac conditions, hematological conditions, large vessel angiopathies (moyamoya syndrome), miscellaneous encephalopathies and renal disease. Although in the genetic disorders, the molecular pathology of the disorders clearly points to the mechanism by which CMBs may develop, in many of the other disorders the mechanism of association of CMBs with the condition under study can only be inferred. In some of the conditions, the patients have other risk factors for CMBs that may confound the interpretation of CMB prevalence data. Other associations consist of single case reports. The limitations and limited generalizability of some of these studies is recognized and acknowledged, but in the interests of

a comprehensive account, the available studies at the time of writing are discussed, if only briefly.

Cerebral microbleeds and rarer cerebral small vessel diseases

As we have seen in Chs. 10–12, the commonest cerebral microangiopathies are age-related processes associated first with hypertension and other conventional vascular risk factors and, second, with amyloid deposition (cerebral amyloid angiopathy [CAA]). However, there are other rarer small vessel disorders, including hereditary amyloid angiopathies and non-amyloid microangiopathies, in which CMBs have been described in recent years.

Familial cerebral amyloid angiopathies

Cerebral amyloid angiopathy covers a number of highly diverse sporadic and genetic disorders that, nevertheless, all share the same pathological hallmark: fibrils of amyloid, a highly insoluble protein, are deposited in the walls of small leptomeningeal and cortical vessels (mainly arterioles, but less commonly capillaries or venules). Although the end result is the same in all types of CAA, the amyloid fibrils may be formed from a range of different proteins. Beta-amyloid is the commonest protein found in amyloid angiopathies in vivo (including sporadic Alzheimer's disease or CAA, discussed in Chs. 13 and 12), but other types of amyloid may form in some rare hereditary amyloid disorders depending on the underlying molecular pathology. These proteins include ABri, ADan, cystatin C, transthyretins, prion proteins and

---

Table 16.1 Some familial amyloid angiopathies and their MRI findings

Disorder name	Abnormal amyloid protein	Clinical features	MRI findings
Hereditary cerebral hemorrhage with amyloidosis-Dutch type (HCHWA-D)	Beta-amyloid	Cerebral hemorrhage, dementia	Leukoaraisosis, CMBs
Familial British dementia (FBD)	ABri	Dementia	Leukoaraiosis; CMBs not studied
Familial Danish dementia (FDD)	ADan		Not available
Hereditary cerebral hemorrhage with amyloidosis Icelandic type (HCHWA-I)	Cystatin C	Early-onset severe cerebral hemorrhage, dementia	Not available
Oculoleptomeningeal amyloidisis	Transthyretins	Multiorgan involvement	CMBs
Finnish amyloidosis	Gelsolin	Multiorgan involvement	Not available
Hereditary dementia with intracerebral hemorrhage (single Finnish family)	Beta-amyloid	Dementia, cerebral hemorrhage	Leukoaraiosis, CMBs

CMB, cerebral microbleeds.

gelsolin. A range of different phenotypes – often named by the geographical locations where the disorders were first identified – have been described. Of these disorders, some have been studied using MRI and have radiological features of diffuse small vessel disease including CMBs. Some of the key familial amyloid angiopathies are summarized in Table 16.1.

Hereditary cerebral hemorrhage with amyloidosis-Dutch type (HCHWA-D) is a rare, autosomal dominant condition caused by a mutation on chromosome 21 at codon 693 of the gene for amyloid precursor protein [1–3]. Pathologically, as in sporadic CAA, the hallmark is the deposition of beta-amyloid in small leptomeningeal arterioles, making them fragile and prone to bleeding and also leading to ischemia in the territories supplied by the diseased vessels. The clinical phenotype is of cognitive impairment and recurrent lobar ICH. One study used $T_2{}^*$-weighted imaging in a cohort of 27 patients with confirmed HCHWA-D, 15 of whom were symptomatic [1]. Cerebral microbleeds were detected in 69% of all mutation carriers, including all of those who had clinical symptoms. The bleeds were located exclusively in the cerebral lobes (at the cortico-subcortical junction) or cerebellum; none was present in deep structures (basal ganglia, brainstem). Those patients with hypertension were more likely to have CMBs in the cerebellum, but not in other brain regions. In this study, CMBs had a predilection for the occipital and temporal lobes, a distribution similar to that reported in sporadic CAA. HCHWA-D may be a useful model to investigate how CMBs are related to amyloid deposition, and the findings of this small study are consistent with the hypothesis that exclu-

sively cortico-subcortical lobar CMBs may indeed be a marker for amyloid angiopathy. The Boston criteria for sporadic CAA (Ch. 6) have been applied to a cohort of patients with HCHWA-D, with and without the use of CMBs for the classification; in this cohort, using lobar CMBs increased the sensitivity of the criteria [2]. However, whether these findings can be extrapolated to sporadic CAA will require further studies, ideally including pathological confirmation of underlying small vessel damage. Figure 16.1 shows CMBs, ICH and siderosis in HCHWA-D.

Hereditary dementia with intracerebral hemorrhages and cerebral amyloid angiopathy

A distinct multisystem amyloidosis, termed the Finnish type, has been described where neurological, dermatological and ophthalmological manifestations result from mutations in the gene encoding gelsolin [4]. However, no neuroimaging studies of this disorder are available. A Finnish family with beta-amyloid deposition in cerebral vessels and brain parenchyma has been described, with cognitive decline and sometimes ICH [5]; neuroimaging disclosed confluent white matter abnormalities (leukoaraiosis) and CMBs in a striking occipito-parietal distribution. No molecular genetic basis could be identified.

Transthyretin amyloidosis

Amyloidosis may result from mutations in the gene encoding transthyretin, with a phenotype originally

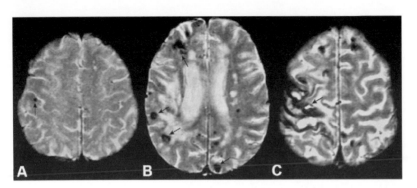

Fig. 16.1 Microbleeds in hereditary cerebral hemorrhage with amyloidosis-Dutch type (HCHWA-D). (A) Axial gradient-recalled echo (GRE) T_2*-weighted image shows a cerebral microbleed (CMB) in the cortical/cortico-subcortical brain region (arrow). (B) Several intracerebral hemorrhages in the cortical/cortico-subcortical brain region (arrows). (C) Superficial siderosis (arrow). (Reproduced with permission from van Rooden *et al.* 2009 [2].)

termed "oculoleptomeningeal amyloidosis" [6], which includes dementia, ICH, ataxia and seizures [7]. A case report recently described a patient who presented with a deep ICH in the context of hypertension and dementia [8]. The patient had a mutation in codon 122 of the gene for transthyretin, and imaging showed extensive CMBs in a mixed lobar and deep distribution. Although CMBs may have been directly related to amyloid deposition in relation to the transthyretin mutant, the co-existence of hypertensive arteriopathy or age-related sporadic CAA cannot be discounted as contributors.

Non-amyloid cerebral microangiopathies

COL4A1 mutations

Collagen type IV α1 (COL4A1) is an essential component for maintaining the integrity of the vascular basement membrane; disruption of the integrity of this structure may, therefore, be expected to lead to blood vessel leakage. A study in mice showed that mutations in *COL4A1* were associated with an increased risk of perinatal ICH [9], particularly during the increased stress associated with parturition. A Dutch family with a clinical syndrome of porencephaly (the presence of a fluid-filled cerebral cavity in communication with the lateral ventricle) related to a defect in *COL4A1* (heterozygous G3706A mutation) have been studied [10]; all patients had white matter changes on brain MRI (leukoencephalopathy) and CMBs were also noted in one of the three patients. Another study of a family with a heterozygous mutation in *COL41A* had a clinical phenotype of recurrent stroke and cataracts, but no porencephaly [11]. All patients showed leukoencephalopathy and CMBs, suggesting a diffuse small vessel angiopathy [12]. A single individual with recurrent spontaneous deep ICHs was

found to have a new *COL4A1* mutation (G805R) and on MRI had leukoencephalopathy and newly appearing deep CMBs [12]. Another clinical and genetic study, with 7 years of follow-up of a family with a different (G562E) *COL4A1* mutation [13], found that three of four patients had leukoencephalopathy and CMBs, but all patients remained clinically and radiologically stable over the 7 years; this was in marked contrast to two clinically affected family members, who died of traumatic or anticoagulant-related hemorrhage [9,14].

These studies confirm that *COL4A1* mutations are associated with imaging and clinical findings suggestive of a diffuse cerebral microangiopathy. However, there is a broad phenotype for at least some *COL4A1* mutations, and to what extent genetic and environmental factors account for this phenotypic variation requires further study in larger cohorts. A recent systematic review describes the phenotype spectrum associated with reported *COL41A* mutations, confirming an association with ischemic stroke, ICH and neuroimaging abnormalities [15].

CADASIL

Cerebral autosomal dominant arteriopathy with subcortical infarcts and leukoencephalopathy (CADASIL) is an important single gene disorder causing a "pure" cerebral small vessel disease. It is caused by a mutation in *NOTCH3*, encoding part of the cell signaling system, and has a characteristic phenotype including complex migraine, cognitive decline and recurrent ischemic stroke. CADASIL is considered in detail in Ch. 15.

Other angiopathies of retina and brain

A number of other hereditary disorders affecting blood vessels of the brain and retina have been

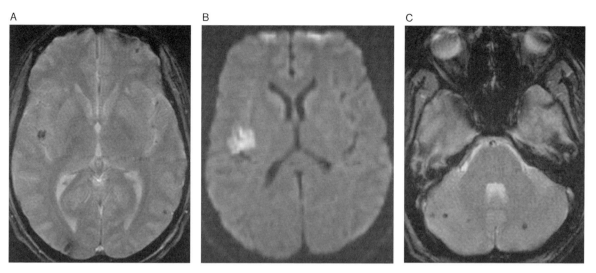

Fig. 16.2 Cerebral microbleeds in infective endocarditis. (A) Several peripheral microhemorrhages are shown on this gradient-recalled echo T_2^*-weighted image. The larger hypointense lesion in the right Sylvian fissure proved to be the site of a mycotic aneurysm on catheter and CT angiography. (B) The diffusion-weighted imaging demonstrates an infarct in the right insula, presumably resulting from vasospasm. (C) In the same patient there are also microbleeds in the cerebellum.

identified in recent years, including three autosomal dominant adult-onset conditions: cerebroretinal vasculopathy; hereditary endotheliopathy with retinopathy; and hereditary endotheliopathy with retinopathy, nephropathy and stroke (HERNS) [16]. All of these entities have been linked to a locus on chromosome 3p21 and show cerebral and retinal small vessel arteriopathy, but CMBs have not been systematically evaluated in these disorders. Imaging for CMB may be a useful addition to the investigation protocol for these and other cerebral and retinal small vessel diseases.

Cerebral microbleeds associated with cardiac disorders

Infective endocarditis

Two case reports have noted apparently asymptomatic CMBs in patients with clinical diagnosis of infective endocarditis [17,18]. We have also found small hemorrhagic lesions, including CMBs, in patients with endocarditis complicated by ICH (see example, Fig. 16.2). An association of CMBs with endocarditis has been confirmed by a recent case–control study from a single center that compared 60 patients with community-acquired infective endocarditis with 120 control subjects matched for age and sex, retrospec-

tively selected from a local radiology database. Systematic gradient-recalled echo (GRE) T_2^*-weighted imaging was undertaken on all cases within a week of admission [19]. The authors found CMBs in 57% of the endocarditis case group, compared with 15% of control subjects, with some morphological differences in CMB lesions between the groups. The association became stronger as the number of CMBs increased; moreover, CMBs located in cortical sulci were only found in patients with endocarditis and not in any controls. It remains unclear whether the lesions seen in these studies are histologically similar to those seen in CAA or hypertensive arteriopathy; it is possible that at least some of the lesions were, in fact, small mycotic aneurysms. Alternatively, microbleeding could occur as a result of hemorrhage into small emboli. Notwithstanding potential selection bias and confounding from case and control selection, these data suggest that CMBs may be a helpful diagnostic adjunct or marker of cerebral involvement in endocarditis, particularly in patients without other risk factors for CMBs; however, further studies in larger cohorts are required to assess their value in diagnosis or prognosis in this condition.

Atrial myxoma

Although CMBs are generally attributed to small previous leaks from cerebral small vessels, another potential mechanism is from hemorrhage into small emboli. One case report described a patient who presented with an acute stroke syndrome (hemiparesis) attributed to an atrial myxoma [20]. The patient was treated with intravenous thrombolysis after no evidence of ICH was found on CT. Subsequent MRI studies revealed multiple hyperintense areas on diffusion-weighted images, compatible with small areas of ischemia resulting from a proximal source embolism. Use of GRE T_2*-weighted imaging showed multiple CMBs in a similar distribution. Trans-oesophageal echocardiography revealed a left atrial myxoma. The authors undertook a positron emission tomography study using Pittsburgh B compound, an in vivo marker for amyloid deposition, and found no evidence of increased amyloid protein. They concluded that the CMBs were the result of hemorrhagic transformation of cardiac emboli from the atrial myxoma, possibly related to thrombolysis, although microaneurysms in the brain and retina have also been described in relation to atrial myxoma [21].

After cardiac surgery

A recent prospective study undertook pre- and post-operative MRI studies in 19 consecutive patients having cardiac valve surgery. Twelve patients developed 26 new lesions compatible with CMBs, most of which were asymptomatic. Further studies are needed to investigate the precise nature and clinical implications of new GRE-detectable lesions [22].

Cerebral microbleeds associated with hematological disorders

Many hematological disorders are associated with vascular damage or coagulopathies, which can increase the risk of ischemic stroke, ICH or cerebral venous thrombosis. Such processes could also theoretically lead to CMBs in the brain, but this possibility remains largely unexplored.

Paroxysmal cold hemaglobinuria

One case report describes a patient who presented with dizziness, confusion, drowsiness and right hemiparesis in the context of a hemolytic anemia, with diagnostic confirmation of paroxysmal cold hemoglobinuria [23]. Fibrinogen and D-dimers were elevated, and the international normalized ratio was prolonged. Diffusion-weighted MRI showed multiple areas of infarction, and

GRE T_2*-weighted imaging showed multiple CMBs in a cortico-subcortical distribution, which increased in number over a 1 week period. It was hypothesized that coagulopathy and a microangiopathy related to the hematological disorder could have contributed to the multiple evolving CMBs in this patient, but the mechanism remains speculative.

Idiopathic thrombocytopenic purpura

Idiopathic thrombocytopenic purpura (ITP) is an autoantibody-mediated thrombocytopenic disorder in which there is accelerated destruction of platelets. It is characterized by an increased risk of bruising or bleeding. Intracranial hemorrhage is the most feared complication of ITP [24]. Traditional treatments to reduce platelet destruction include steroids, immunoglobulin therapy and splenectomy. A combination of low platelets and vascular fragility could theoretically predispose to CMBs in the brain (Figs. 16.3 and 16.4). In ITP, ICH is a rare event that is difficult to predict; CMBs may have a role in helping to identify those patients at greatest risk, but further studies are needed.

Sneddon's syndrome

Sneddon's syndrome is a non-inflammatory arteriopathy of small to medium-sized vessels, characterized by young-onset stroke and a characteristic violaceous, mesh-like skin rash (livedo reticularis). Antiphospholipid antibodies may be detected. A case of familial Sneddon's syndrome has been reported in which the patient had multiple CMBs in both cerebral hemispheres; the distribution was not described in detail [25]. Since anticoagulation is often considered for patients with antiphospholipid antibodies and a history of thrombosis or stroke, CMBs may contribute to risk stratification for this treatment. (See Ch. 19. for a detailed discussion of CMBs in relation to anticoagulation treatment decisions.)

Systemic lupus erythematosus

Systemic lupus erythematosus may cause neurological dysfunction, including neuropsychiatric disturbances and stroke. A cerebral vasculitis has been suggested as a possible mechanism. We have found CMBs in some patients with systemic lupus erythematosus (Fig. 16.5), but the prevalence, underlying mechanisms and clinical significance of CMBs in this disorder have not yet been systematically investigated.

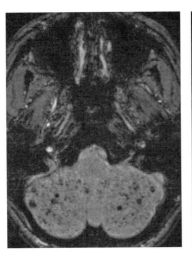
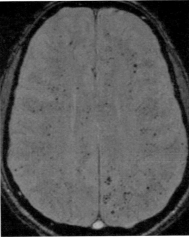
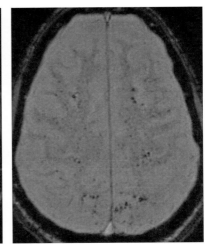

Fig. 16.3 Susceptibility-weighted imaging in a patient with idiopathic thrombocytopenic purpura showing a myriad of cerebral microbleeds (CMB) in the posterior fossa. The larger lesions were a result of an acute bleeding episode. Multiple CMBs are also seen in the cerebral hemispheres, mostly close to the gray–white matter junction.

Microbleeds associated with large vessel vasculopathy

Moyamoya syndrome

Moyamoya syndrome is a chronic cerebrovascular disorder resulting from progressive stenosis of the intracranial internal carotid arteries and their proximal branches. The name comes from the Japanese word for "puff of smoke," which refers to the characteristic appearance of fine tortuous collateral vessels in compensation for the compromise in carotid flow. Although first considered to be a disease of Asian populations, moyamoya is now recognized to occur throughout the world. Ischemic stroke and ICH are both recognized complications of the syndrome. Because moyamoya collateral vessels are pathological and potentially fragile, there has been interest in detecting CMBs in this condition, which might help to guide therapeutic decisions, particularly in relation to antithrombotic treatments. Several studies, all in Asian populations, have noted CMBs in patients with moyamoya disease [26–28], with a prevalence of up to 44% depending on the type of MRI sequence used: higher field strengths and susceptibility-weighted sequences detected CMBs in a higher proportion of patients. No systematic studies of CMBs in non-Asian cohorts have been reported, but experience at our own institution suggests that in European cohorts they may be

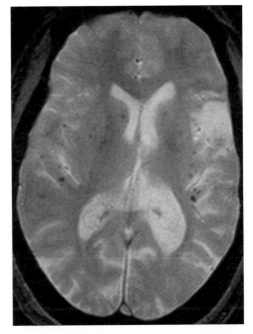

Fig. 16.4 A patient with idiopathic thrombocytopenic purpura shows a mature cortical infarct in the left insula in addition to several microbleeds in the basal ganglia and insula bilaterally.

less common (Martin Brown, personal communication). One study investigated the presence of CMBs as a predictor of future ICH risk [29] and found evidence that CMBs were indeed related to an increased

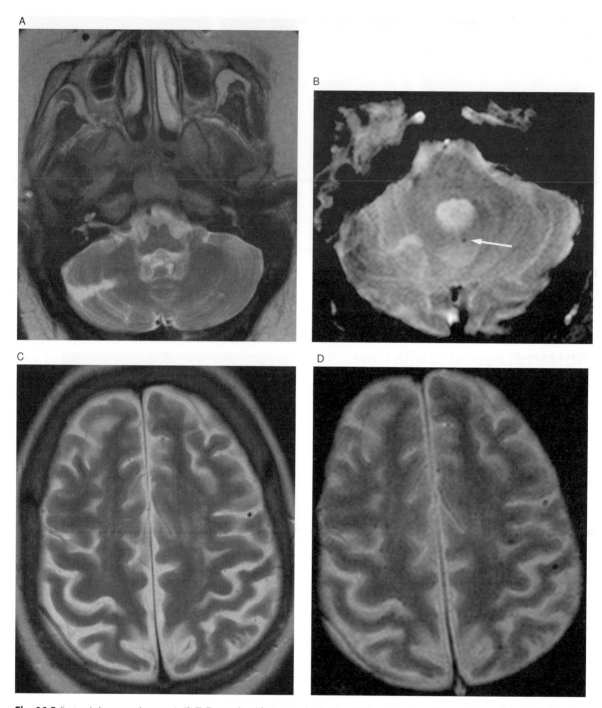

Fig. 16.5 Systemic lupus erythematosis (SLE). T$_2$-weighted fast spin echo (A,C) and T$_2$*-weighted gradient echo sequences (B,D) in a patient with neurological manifestations of SLE. (A) A cerebellar infarct; (B) a cerebellar cerebral microbleed (CMB; arrow); (C) evidence of small vessel disease; (D) multiple CMBs in the subcortical white matter and cortex.

risk. Furthermore, multiple CMBs appeared to confer a higher risk than a single CMB, analogous to the findings in some cohorts of patients after ischemic stroke. The underlying mechanisms of microbleeding in this disease remain unclear. In a single case, a CMB in a patient with moyamoya disease undergoing surgical revascularization was resected [30]; histological analysis showed several associated arterioles, some with disruption of the internal elastic lamina. Overall, the role of CMB imaging in moyamoya disease remains uncertain and requires further larger studies in well-characterized cohorts, directed at addressing clinically relevant questions.

Microbleeds and miscellaneous encephalopathies

A single case of CMBs in limbic encephalitis associated with antibodies to voltage-gated potassium channels has been reported [31]. The patient presented with an acute encephalopathy, and MRI showed typical high-signal abnormality in mesial temporal structures associated with this condition, but also numerous cortical and cortico-subcortical CMBs, which accumulated over the next few months. The development of CMBs was associated with widespread cerebral atrophy. How or if the CMBs were related to the underlying immune-mediated encephalitis remains unclear. Another case report described a man who developed hemiparesis 9 days after receiving a vaccination for influenza. Imaging showed extensive signal hyperintensity in the brainstem, but also widespread CMBs in the brainstem and in both cerebral hemispheres [32]. It was hypothesized that this patient may have had an atypical form of post-vaccination acute disseminated encephalomyelitis, in which foci of demyelination occur, and may have had areas of hemorrhagic necrosis, which could give rise to CMBs. In a patient with African trypanosomiasis, an encephalopathy presumed to be related to melarsoprol treatment was described in which numerous CMBs were detected on GRE T_2*-weighted MRI [33]; autopsy studies of this type of encephalopathy have revealed a leukoencephalopathy with areas of fibrinoid necrosis and hemorrhage related to small vessels.

Cerebral micro- and macrohemorrhages have also been described as a feature of staphylococcal meningitis [34]. It is hypothesized that a vasculitic presentation of this disease can lead to recurrent microhemorrhages, as well as small infarcts (Fig. 16.6).

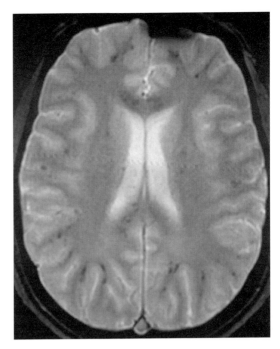

Fig. 16.6 A patient with a history of bacterial meningitis showing multiple hypointense lesions on T_2*-weighted images, some resembling CMBs, predominantly near the gray–white matter junction.

Cerebral microbleeds in renal disease

The brain and kidneys share the same vascular characteristics in that the two organs are subjected to a high flow of blood throughout systole and diastole because they receive a relatively large volume of blood at rest and are exposed to high pulsatile pressure. This has led to interest in how CMBs relate to renal function. Early studies reported frequent CMBs in patients with chronic kidney disease and on hemodialysis [35]. In patients with ischemic stroke, proteinuria of more than 300 mg/l on a spot urine test was strongly associated with the frequency and number of CMBs [36]. In a study of 150 patients with acute ischemic stroke, those with decreased kidney function (defined as an estimated glomerular filtration rate of <60 ml/min per 1.73m^2) were found to have a nearly fourfold increased risk of having CMBs [37]. These studies provide further evidence that cerebral small vessel disease may be part of a systemic microangiopathic disorder. Optimal prevention and treatment of clinically silent chronic kidney disease may help to prevent the consequences of cerebral small vessel damage, including CMBs.

References

1. van den Boom R, Bornebroek M, Behloul F *et al.* Microbleeds in hereditary cerebral hemorrhage with amyloidosis-Dutch type. *Neurology* 2005;**64**: 1288–9.

2. van Rooden S, van der Grond J, van den Boom R *et al.* Descriptive analysis of the Boston criteria applied to a Dutch-type cerebral amyloid angiopathy population. *Stroke* 2009;**40**:3022–7.

3. van Broeckhoven C, Haan J, Bakker E *et al.* Amyloid beta protein precursor gene and hereditary cerebral hemorrhage with amyloidosis. *Science* 1990;**248**: 1120–2.

4. Kiuru S. Gelsolin-related familial amyloidosis, Finnish type (FAF), and its variants found worldwide. *Amyloid* 1998;**5**:55–66.

5. Remes AM, Finnila S, Mononen H *et al.* Hereditary dementia with intracerebral hemorrhages and cerebral amyloid angiopathy. *Neurology* 2004;**63**:234–40.

6. Goren H, Steinberg MC, Farboody GH. Familial oculoleptomeningeal amyloidosis. *Brain* 1980;**103**:473–95.

7. Petersen RB, Goren H, Cohen M *et al.* Transthyretin amyloidosis: a new mutation associated with dementia. *Ann Neurol* 1997;**41**:307–13.

8. Robbins MS, Yasen J. Extensive intracranial microbleeds in transthyretin amyloidosis. *J Am Geriatr Soc* 2008;**56**:1966–7.

9. Gould DB, Phalan FC, van Mil SE *et al.* Role of COL4A1 in small-vessel disease and hemorrhagic stroke. *N Engl J Med* 2006;**354**:1489–96.

10. van der Knaap MS, Smit LM, Barkhof F *et al.* Neonatal porencephaly and adult stroke related to mutations in collagen IV A1. *Ann Neurol* 2006;**59**:504–11.

11. Shah S, Kumar Y, McLean B *et al.* A dominantly inherited mutation in collagen IV A1 (COL4A1) causing childhood onset stroke without porencephaly. *Eur J Paediatr Neurol* 2010;**14**:182–7.

12. Vahedi K, Kubis N, Boukobza M *et al.* COL4A1 mutation in a patient with sporadic, recurrent intracerebral hemorrhage. *Stroke* 2007;**38**:1461–4.

13. Vahedi K, Boukobza M, Massin P *et al.* Clinical and brain MRI follow-up study of a family with COL4A1 mutation. *Neurology* 2007;**69**:1564–8.

14. Vahedi K, Massin P, Guichard JP *et al.* Hereditary infantile hemiparesis, retinal arteriolar tortuosity, and leukoencephalopathy. *Neurology* 2003;**60**:57–63.

15. Lanfranconi S, Markus HS. COL4A1 mutations as a monogenic cause of cerebral small vessel disease. A systematic review. *Stroke* 2010;**41**:e513.

16. Ophoff RA, DeYoung J, Service SK *et al.* Hereditary vascular retinopathy, cerebroretinal vasculopathy, and hereditary endotheliopathy with retinopathy, nephropathy, and stroke map to a single locus on chromosome 3p21.1-p21.3. *Am J Hum Genet* 2001;**69**:447–53.

17. Nandigam RN. Re: "Silent T_2* cerebral microbleeds: a potential new imaging clue in infective endocarditis." *Neurology* 2008 22;**70**:323–4.

18. Klein I, Iung B, Wolff M, *et al.* Silent T_2* cerebral microbleeds: a potential new imaging clue in infective endocarditis. *Neurology* 2007;**68**:2043.

19. Klein I, Iung B, Labreuche J *et al.* Cerebral microbleeds are frequent in infective endocarditis: a case-control study. *Stroke* 2009;**40**:3461–5.

20. Vanacker P, Nelissen N, Van Laere K, Thijs VN. Images in neurology. Scattered cerebral microbleeds due to cardiac myxoma. *Arch Neurol* 2009;**66**:796–7.

21. Herbst M, Wattjes MP, Urbach H *et al.* Cerebral embolism from left atrial myxoma leading to cerebral and retinal aneurysms: a case report. *AJNR Am J Neuroradiol* 2005;**26**:666–9.

22. Jeon SB, Lee JW, Kim SJ *et al.* New cerebral lesions on T_2*-weighted gradient-echo imaging after cardiac valve surgery. *Cerebrovasc Dis* 2010;**30**:194–9.

23. Kim GM, Kim CH, Kim BS. Multiple cerebral infarction and microbleeds associated with adult-onset paroxysmal cold hemoglobinuria. *J Clin Neurosci* 2009;**16**:348–9.

24. Butros LJ, Bussel JB. Intracranial hemorrhage in immune thrombocytopenic purpura: a retrospective analysis. *J Pediatr Hematol Oncol* 2003;**25**:660–4.

25. Lluriu S, Cervera A, Capurro S, Chamorro A. Neurological picture. Familial Sneddon's syndrome with microbleeds in MRI. *J Neurol Neurosurg Psychiatry* 2008;**79**:962.

26. Kikuta K, Takagi Y, Nozaki K *et al.* Asymptomatic microbleeds in moyamoya disease: T_2*-weighted gradient-echo magnetic resonance imaging study. *J Neurosurg* 2005;**102**:470–5.

27. Ishikawa T, Kuroda S, Nakayama N *et al.* Prevalence of asymptomatic microbleeds in patients with moyamoya disease. *Neurol Med Chir (Tokyo)* 2005;**45**:495–500.

28. Mori N, Miki Y, Kikuta K *et al.* Microbleeds in moyamoya disease: susceptibility-weighted imaging versus T_2*-weighted imaging at 3 Tesla. *Invest Radiol* 2008;**43**:574–9.

29. Kikuta K, Takagi Y, Nozaki K *et al.* The presence of multiple microbleeds as a predictor of subsequent cerebral hemorrhage in patients with moyamoya disease. *Neurosurgery* 2008;**62**:104–11, discussion.

30. Kikuta K, Takagi Y, Nozaki K, Okada T, Hashimoto N. Histological analysis of microbleed after surgical resection in a patient with moyamoya disease. *Neurol Med Chir (Tokyo)* 2007;**47**:564–7.

31. Kapina V, Vargas MI, Vulliemoz S *et al.* VGKC antibody-associated encephalitis, microbleeds and progressive brain atrophy. *J Neurol* 2010;**257**:466–8.

32. Turkoglu R, Tuzun E. Brainstem encephalitis following influenza vaccination: favorable response to steroid treatment. *Vaccine* 2009;**27**:7253–6.

33. Checkley AM, Pepin J, Gibson WC *et al.* Human African trypanosomiasis: diagnosis, relapse and survival after severe melarsoprol-induced encephalopathy. *Trans R Soc Trop Med Hyg* 2007;**101**:523–6.

34. Bentley P, Qadri F, Wild EJ, Hirsch NP, Howard RS. Vasculitic presentation of staphylococcal meningitis. *Arch Neurol* 2007;**64**:1788–9.

35. Watanabe A. Cerebral microbleeds and intracerebral hemorrhages in patients on maintenance hemodialysis. *J Stroke Cerebrovasc Dis* 2007;**16**: 30–3.

36. Ovbiagele B, Liebeskind DS, Pineda S, Saver JL. Strong independent correlation of proteinuria with cerebral microbleeds in patients with stroke and transient ischemic attack. *Arch Neurol* 2010;**67**: 45–50.

37. Cho AH, Lee SB, Han SJ *et al.* Impaired kidney function and cerebral microbleeds in patients with acute ischemic stroke. *Neurology* 2009;**73**:1645–8.

Cerebral microbleeds and cognitive impairment

David J. Werring and Mike O'Sullivan

Introduction

Cerebral microbleeds (CMBs) occupy an important position within the spectrum of imaging abnormalities associated with cognitive impairment in that they are linked conceptually both with disorders primarily affecting blood vessels, and with neuropathology of Alzheimer's disease. Consequently, CMBs need to be considered in relation to both of the commonest causes of cognitive impairment – cerebrovascular disease (and consequent *vascular cognitive impairment*) and Alzheimer's disease. This chapter begins with a brief description of how CMBs fit broadly within the spectrum of vascular cognitive impairment, and more specifically with interactions between vascular and degenerative mechanisms, before reviewing the evidence of associations between CMBs and cognitive function across different clinical groups. The extent to which the current evidence supports a direct, causative link is considered and an agenda for future research described.

Cerebral microbleeds and diagnostic groups

Vascular cognitive impairment

Vascular cognitive impairment is a key healthcare challenge facing all aging Western societies. Vascular mechanisms are second only to Alzheimer's neuropathology as a cause of dementia, and vascular cognitive impairment – where vascular mechanisms are considered the predominant cause – is also highly prevalent. Initial concepts of how vascular diseases

affect cognition mainly invoked cortical or subcortical infarction, leading to the terms "multi-infarct dementia" and "post-stroke dementia." However, in recent years, it has become clear that subcortical small vessel disease (often not causing acute or overt clinical symptoms), largely driven by the effects of hypertension on small caliber cerebral vessels, plays a critical role in vascular cognitive impairment. The MRI manifestations of small vessel diseases including white matter hyperintensities (including leukoaraiosis), lacunes and perivascular (Virchow–Robin) spaces have been recognized for many years. The main body of research into small vessel disease and cognition has concentrated on white matter hyperintensities; however, most correlations of these imaging findings with cognition have often been only modest, which may be a reflection of the great pathological heterogeneity of small vessel diseases.

Cerebral microbleeds are commonly found in patients with cerebrovascular diseases, including populations with first-ever or recurrent ischemic or hemorrhagic stroke: CMBs have been found in approximately 35% of patients with first-ever or recurrent ischemic stroke, and approximately 60% of patients with first-ever or recurrent intracerebral hemorrhage (ICH) [1]. In patients meeting current criteria for vascular dementia, the prevalence of CMBs is even greater, 85% in one study [2]. Cerebral autosomal dominant arteriopathy with subcortical infarcts and leukoencephalopathy (CADASIL) is an autosomal dominant disease often considered a genetic model of pure vascular dementia [3]. In these patients, co-existent amyloid angiopathy is unlikely, but the prevalence of CMBs is still high.

Mixed dementia: interaction of vascular mechanisms, amyloid and neurodegeneration

It has also become clear in recent years that the distinction between vascular cognitive impairment and Alzheimer's disease may be an oversimplification since both are diseases of older people and must commonly co-exist. Furthermore, it is recognized that vascular and degenerative processes will have complex interactions and sometimes synergistic or additive effects on brain function. For example, hypertension is a risk factor for developing Alzheimer's disease, and diffuse white matter lesions like those seen in small vessel disease are commonly found on the MRI scans of people with Alzheimer's disease. It has also been hypothesized that pre-existing Alzheimer pathology may make people with stroke more vulnerable to post-stroke cognitive decline. However, exactly how these pathologies are linked remains a critical question in understanding mechanisms of dementia. One intriguing process that could link cerebrovascular disease with Alzheimer's disease is that of cerebral amyloid angiopathy (CAA), a pathological process of vascular amyloid deposition (principally in penetrating leptomeningeal small vessels) that is common with advancing age and a feature of Alzheimer's disease as well as spontaneous ICH in older individuals. One possibility is that vascular amyloid adversely affects cerebrovascular reactivity and small vessel function, causing ischemic damage (white matter ischemia or frank cortico-subcortical small infarcts). Alternatively, ischemic damage to small arteries and veins could lead to impaired clearance of amyloid and its deposition in vessel walls. In either of these scenarios, MRI changes in ischemic small vessel disease (including, for example, white matter changes) may be a useful way to investigate the link between ischemia and amyloid deposition.

Occurrence of CMBs is an attractive target for studying these interactions. In addition to their prevalence in the vascular groups described above, they are found in 20–30% of patients with a clinical diagnosis of Alzheimer's disease and are common in sporadic CAA. There is increasing interest in whether the distribution of CMBs may reliably reflect the underlying type of small vessel disease: it is hypothesized that CMBs in a deep distribution result from hypertensive arteriopathy, while those at the cortico-subcortical boundary of the lobes of the brain result from CAA [4]. Consequently, occurrence and location of CMBs may have considerable promise as an important way to detect and quantify the effects of small vessel disease and amyloid deposition in patients with cognitive impairment. They may be more specific for the underlying pathology than some other imaging manifestations of small vessel diseases (e.g. white matter changes), particularly if their distribution can be mapped.

Cerebral microbleeds and cognitive performance

Studying the impact of microbleeds on cognition: methodological issues

A number of studies in clinical populations have included both quantification of CMBs and some degree of cognitive evaluation. These studies are listed in Table 17.1. A major challenge in any attempt to demonstrate a direct relationship between CMBs and cognitive function is the strong correlation between CMBs and other radiological markers of cerebrovascular diseases, including white matter changes and lacunar lesions [6,14]. The evidence of a direct effect of CMBs on cognitive mechanisms is strengthened if correlations can be found independent of other markers. Some studies have included other markers in modeling the relationship between CMBs and cognition and this is also summarized in Table 17.1.

A direct effect of CMBs on cognitive networks would also be supported if the location of CMBs were found to correspond with the pattern of cognitive deficits seen. This depends not only on accurately surveying CMB location but also on using tests of cognitive function that have a known underlying functional anatomy. The likely functional anatomy is clearer for tests of specific domains or processes (e.g. within the domain of executive function) than for crude, global measures. The correlations found with respect to the tests used are summarized in Table 17.2.

Finally, a much stronger case for a causal link between CMBs and cognitive dysfunction can be made if a temporal relationship can be drawn between incidence and cognitive deficit. However, longitudinal observations of CMB incidence and cognition remain sparse.

Table 17.1 Associations between microbleeds and cognitive function

Study	Design	Clinical Population	Main associations	Associations independent of other MRI markers
Yakushiji et al. 2008 [5]	Cross-sectional	Healthy adults (n = 678); self-funded and self-referring for health screening	Lower scores on MMSE associated with CMBs	WML; logistic regression models were adjusted for this (as well as systolic blood pressure, age, gender, education)
Cordonnier et al. 2006 [6]	Cross-sectional	Memory clinic (n = 772); CMBs found in VaD, AD, MCI and subjective memory complaints	None demonstrated	–
Werring et al. 2004 [7]	Cross-sectional	Neurovascular clinic; group with stroke and transient ischemic attack (n = 25)	Executive dysfunction more common in the group with CMB than in control group	Groups matched for WML (ARWMC rating scale)
Seo et al. 2007 [2]	Cross-sectional	Memory clinic; subgroup with subcortical vascular dementia (n = 86)	CMB associated with MMSE score and tests in a range of cognitive domains with exception of language	WML (Schelten scale), lacunae
Hanyu et al. 2003 [8]	Cross-sectional	Memory clinic; clinical diagnosis of AD (n = 59)	No association with MMSE	–
Petterson et al. 2008 [9]	Cross-sectional	Memory clinic; clinical diagnosis of AD (n = 80)	No association with MMSE or single test of a cognitive test battery	–
Goos et al. 2010 [10]	Cross-sectional	Memory clinic; clinical diagnosis of AD; large cohort population (n = 427) yielded small group (n = 21) with multiple CMB (>8)	Multiple microbleeds associated with lower MMSE score	WMH; no independent association found
Viswanathan et al. 2008 [11]	Cross-sectional	CAH (n = 147)	Association with global measures (MMSE, Mattis Dementia Rating Scale)	WMH, lacunae; no independent association demonstrated except a small strategic effect for caudate/internal capsule CMB
Liem et al. 2009 [12]	Longitudinal, 7-year results	CADASIL (n = 25)	Increase in CMB associated with deterioration on CAMCOG	WMH, lacunae; no independent associations reported
Qui et al. 2010 [13]	Cross-sectional	Healthy older people (AGES-R, n = 3902)	Multiple CMBs associated with slower processing speed and executive function	Adjusted for WMH

AD, Alzheimer's disease; AGES-R, AGES-Reykjavik study; ARWMC, age-related white matter changes; CADASIL, cerebral autosomal dominant arteriopathy with subcortical infarcts and leukoencephalopathy; CAMCOG, cognitive section of the Cambridge Mental Disorders of the Elderly Examination; CMB, cerebral microbleeds; MCI, mild cognitive impairment; MMSE, Mini-Mental State Examination; WMH, white matter hyperintensity; WML, white matter lesions; VaD, vascular dementia.

Normal populations

Cerebral microbleeds have been detected in healthy individuals with no known neurological disorder, with a prevalence ranging from 5% to 40% (see Ch. 9.). The prevalence increases with age, and with the type of imaging method used for CMB detection. Studies of how CMBs could affect cognitive function, however, have been scarce. One recent study included 678 healthy adults who funded their own health screening examination in Japan [5]. Cerebral microbleeds were found in 6.8% of this group, CMBs being mainly

in the cerebral lobes and deep white matter, with a predilection for the frontal lobes. Lower scores on the Mini-Mental State Examination (MMSE) were associated with the presence of CMBs, shorter duration of education and the presence of severe white matter hyperintensities. In particular, "attention and calculation" subscores were lower in those individuals with CMBs than those without. The authors speculated that CMBs may have direct effects of disrupting fronto-subcortical circuits to account for this type of cognitive impairment. One criticism of this study is that, because participants were self-referring

Table 17.2 Neuropsychological tests associated with microbleeds[a]

Study	Tests demonstrating an association	Tests with no significant association	Comments
Stroke/transient ischemic attack Werring *et al.* 2004 [7]	*Executive/working memory:* Stroop, letter fluency, Trail Making B, Modified Card Sorting, Weigl Colour Form Sorting Task	*Memory:* Recognition Memory Test *Language:* Graded Naming Test *Visuospatial/perception:* Visual Object and Space Perception Battery *Speed/attention:* "O" Cancellation Digit Copy, Symbol Digit Modalities Test, Trail Making A	Some inconsistency in which tests for executive/working memory applied to individual patients; no associations with specific single tests or measures reported
Vascular dementia and CADASIL Seo *et al.* 2007 [2]	*Executive/working memory:* Digit Span backwards *Memory:* Seoul Verbal Learning Test, Rey–Osterreith recognition *Visuospatial/perception:* Rey–Osterreith copy	*Language:* Boston Naming Test	
Liem *et al.* 2009 [12]	*Executive/working memory:* Stroop, Trail Making B *Memory:* Wechsler Memory Scale memory quotient	*Speed/attention:* Trail Making A	Note these are longitudinal associations between decline in score and accrual of CMBs
Alzheimer's disease Petterson *et al.* 2008 [9]	None	*Executive/working memory:* letter fluency, Trail Making B, Wisconsin Card Sorting Test *Memory:* California Verbal Learning Test, Wechsler Memory Scale – delayed recall *Language:* Boston Naming Test	Note that letter fluency and Trail Making B have shown associations in other studies
Goos *et al.* 2009 [10]	*Executive/working memory:* Digit Span backwards *Memory:* Visual Association Test object naming *Speed/attention:* Trail Making A, Digit Span forwards	*Executive/working memory:* Trail Making B	Note these are associations found in those with multiple CMBs compared with those with no CMBs

CMB, cerebral microbleeds.

[a] Studies only included if they used neuropsychological testing beyond global screening measures (e.g. Mini-Mental State Examination or Mattis Dementia Rating Scale).

and self-funding, the results may not be generalizable to other populations. In a hospital-based study of 772 patients attending a memory clinic, CMBs were detected in 10% of individuals diagnosed as having "subjective cognitive complaints." However, as in the subgroups thought to have an objective cognitive disorder, no association was found between CMBs and MMSE scores [6].

Cerebrovascular diseases

One study undertaken in a neurovascular clinic population compared detailed cognitive function assessment in consecutive patients with CMBs with that in a control group matched for imaging and clinical factors likely to influence cognition [7]. A difference in the prevalence of executive dysfunction was found, with 60% of patients with CMBs impaired on these tests compared with 30% of patients without CMBs. Executive impairment was also related to CMB location in the frontal lobes or basal ganglia, supporting a possible direct effect of CMBs on fronto-subcortical circuits.

More recently, CMBs have been studied in cohorts of patients with a diagnosis of vascular dementia. Seo *et al.* investigated 86 subjects from a memory clinic with subcortical vascular dementia, using gradient echo T_2*-weighted MRI and neuropsychological testing (MMSE and a clinical dementia rating scale) [2]. The authors reported that CMBs were related to MMSE and to dysfunction in all cognitive domains except language, which showed a trend towards significance. In the large memory clinic population investigated by Cordonnier et al. [6], CMBs were most prevalent in the vascular dementia group (65% of patients compared with 18% of patients with a diagnosis of Alzheimer's disease). In the clinic population as a whole, CMBs were not related to cognition as assessed by the MMSE score.

Alzheimer's disease

Cerebral microbleeds are found in approximately 20–30% of patients with a clinical diagnosis of Alzheimer's disease. However, few studies have examined their relevance to cognitive function. Several studies have reported no evidence of association between CMBs and the MMSE [6,8]. The MMSE is a crude measure of global cognitive performance, but a more recent study with more detailed cognitive testing in a larger sample with Alzheimer's disease (80 individuals) was also negative [9].

One recent study suggested that MMSE scores were lower in patients with Alzheimer's disease and multiple CMBs (in this study, more than eight) than in those with Alzheimer's disease who were free of CMBs [10]. These patients formed a small and highly selective subgroup of individuals with Alzheimer's disease (21 from a total series of 427); consequently, the generalizability of these results to the more common scenario of a single to a few CMBs is questionable. As in the study by Petterson et al. [9], there was an association between CMBs and white matter hyperintensities, and evidence that CMBs have an impact on cognition independent of such other markers is relatively weak.

Cerebral amyloid angiopathy

With respect to CAA, CMBs have attracted most attention as possible diagnostic markers, particularly in demonstrating other silent hemorrhagic lesions in a patient with an incident hemorrhage. Relatively little attention has been paid to a direct role of these lesions in mediating cognitive disturbance, despite evidence that cognitive impairments in patients with CAA result from factors other than symptomatic hemorrhage [15]. In patients with a diagnosis of CAA, visible white matter lesions correlated with cognitive performance, and white matter integrity in the unaffected hemisphere correlated with estimates of premorbid (i.e. prior to symptomatic hemorrhage) cognitive performance [11]. The burden of CMBs cor-

related with the severity of diffuse white matter lesions, but as yet, no independent impact of CMBs on cognition has been delineated. It remains unclear, therefore, whether CMBs have a direct impact through damaging connections important for cognition, or are simply markers of more severe diffuse white matter pathology in this disorder.

CADASIL

Cerebral microbleeds are now an established radiological feature of CADASIL and accumulate as the disease progresses [12]. Interpreting the cognitive impact of CMBs in older cohorts with sporadic cerebrovascular disease is confounded by the possible association with Alzheimer's disease. However, Alzheimer's disease has a prevalence that increases sharply with age, so the impact of microvascular mechanisms can be studied in relative isolation in patients with CADASIL, who often progress to dementia in their 40s or 50s. Furthermore, many patients have florid, multiple CMBs, which increases the power to detect both underlying associations and the potential importance of CMB distribution.

Individuals with CADASIL who meet criteria for dementia have more CMBs than those with milder degrees of cognitive impairment [16]. Further, there is evidence of a graded effect. When global performance is quantified with a measure such as the Mattis Dementia Rating Scale (MDRS), the proportion of patients with four or more CMBs increased from 10% to 41% in the most impaired group. When patients were split into quartiles based on MDRS performance, the most impaired group had a mean of 14 CMBs, compared with a mean of 4 across the whole study sample.

The most comprehensive study to examine the relative impact of CMBs and other MRI markers was performed by the Paris–Munich Study group [16]. This confirmed the univariate associations between CMBs and global cognitive performance but found no evidence for an independent effect of CMBs on cognition, except for evidence of a weak strategic effect in some locations (discussed below). In the 7-year follow-up study, an independent effect was reported only for brain atrophy (increase in ventricular volume).

A temporal link between the incidence of CMBs and cognitive decline has been demonstrated in recent results from 25 patients with CADASIL who underwent imaging and clinical and cognitive assessments over a follow-up interval of 7 years [12]. Over this time, the mean number of CMBs increased from 1.6 to 3.5, an increase that correlated with total score on CAM-COG (cognitive section of the Cambridge Mental Disorders of the Elderly Examination) (and weakly with MMSE, though this trend did not reach the threshold for significance) as well with tests of executive function and episodic memory (Table 17.2).

Cerebral microbleeds have a characteristic distribution in CADASIL that is distinct from that of other lesion types such as lacunae or diffuse white matter lesions [13]. Despite this, there has been little attempt so far to link CMB location with specific aspects of cognitive function. The only study to consider CMB location was unfortunately limited in cognitive evaluation to the MDRS and its subscales [17]; conversely, the 7-year follow-up study of Liem *et al.* included more careful and wide-ranging cognitive evaluation but took no account of lesion location [12]. This study showed that accrual of CMBs was associated with decline on the Weschler Memory Scale Memory Quotient, Trail Making Part B and Stroop Interference, but this pattern of change resembles the characteristic cognitive profile of CADASIL and was also found in association with ventricular volume, so was by no means specific for CMBs.

An interesting feature of the study by Viswanathan *et al.* [11] was an association between global cognitive performance and CMBs in the caudate nucleus or anterior limb of the internal capsule. Approximately half of the effect of caudate lesions was accounted for by reductions in the Mattis Initiation–Perseveration subscale. Caudate CMBs had an independent effect in multivariate analysis. Although the impact of these strategic lesions, considered across the whole cohort, was weak, these findings do suggest that strategic lesions are important in at least a handful of patients.

Conclusions and future directions

A number of studies, in a range of clinical settings, have reported associations between the presence and number of CMBs and cognitive performance. The most consistant pattern that has emerged is an association with executive dysfunction in cohorts with cerebrovascular disease. There is less consistency in studies of clinically defined Alzheimer's disease, and the relevance of CMBs in this group remains unclear.

Several studies have reported associations independent of the two classical manifestations of small vessel disease: white matter hyperintensities and lacunae. However, one important issue is that white matter hyperintensities on conventional (T_2-weighted or fluid attenuated inversion recovery) images do not fully capture the extent of pathological disruption to white matter structure [18], and so these findings are insufficient to attribute a causal role to CMBs. Future research should aim to investigate multiple imaging markers of cerebrovascular disease together, including possible components such as cortical microinfarcts or mesial temporal atrophy. In addition to conventional MRI, quantitative MRI techniques (e.g. diffusion tensor imaging [18], magnetization transfer imaging or relaxation time mapping) should allow the investigation of tissue damage that is not visible on conventional structural MRI.

As yet, lesion location–function relationships have been examined only at a very simple level. Frontal lobe CMBs appear to be more strongly associated with executive deficits in patients with cerebrovascular disease, and there is evidence of a weak strategic effect for caudate CMBs in CADASIL, but otherwise little is known. Careful analysis of lesion distribution has the potential to support a direct, causal role of CMBs in vascular cognitive impairment as the spatial distribution is known to differ from that of lacunes or diffuse white matter lesions. Analysis of lesion topography may also hold the key to distinguishing the effects of microvascular disease and Alzheimer's disease if, as is suspected, CMBs from each of these causes form distinct anatomical distributions. Another factor that would aid this research aim would be a consistent approach to neuropsychological testing and the use of appropriately chosen test batteries rather than adherence to ill-suited screening tests such as the MMSE. Such a strategy has been advocated in vascular cognitive impairment generally [19].

References

1. Cordonnier C, Al-Shahi SR, Wardlaw J. Spontaneous brain microbleeds: systematic review, subgroup analyses and standards for study design and reporting. *Brain* 2007;**130**:1988–2003.

2. Seo SW, Lee BH, Kim EJ *et al.* Clinical significance of microbleeds in subcortical vascular dementia. *Stroke* 2007;**38**:1949–51.

3. Chabriat H, Joutel A, Dichgans M *et al.* Cadasil. *Lancet Neurol* 2009;**8**:643–53.

4. Vernooij MW, van der Lugt A, Ikram MA *et al.* Prevalence and risk factors of cerebral microbleeds:

the Rotterdam Scan Study. *Neurology* 2008;**70**: 1208–14.

5. Yakushiji Y, Nishiyama M, Yakushiji S *et al.* Brain microbleeds and global cognitive function in adults without neurological disorder. *Stroke* 2008;**39**: 3323–8.

6. Cordonnier C, van der Flier WM, Sluimer JD *et al.* Prevalence and severity of microbleeds in a memory clinic setting. *Neurology* 2006;**66**:1356–60.

7. Werring DJ, Frazer DW, Coward LJ *et al.* Cognitive dysfunction in patients with cerebral microbleeds on T_2^*-weighted gradient-echo MRI. *Brain* 2004;**127**: 2265–75.

8. Hanyu H, Tanaka Y, Shimizu S, Takasaki M, Abe K. Cerebral microbleeds in Alzheimer's disease. *J Neurol* 2003;**250**:1496–7.

9. Pettersen JA, Sathiyamoorthy G, Gao FQ *et al.* Microbleed topography, leukoaraiosis, and cognition in probable Alzheimer disease from the Sunnybrook Dementia study. *Arch Neurol* 2008;**65**: 790–5.

10. Goos JD, Kester MI, Barkhof F *et al.* Patients with Alzheimer disease with multiple microbleeds: relation with cerebrospinal fluid biomarkers and cognition. *Stroke* 2009;**40**:3455–60.

11. Viswanathan A, Patel P, Rahman R *et al.* Tissue microstructural changes are independently associated with cognitive impairment in cerebral amyloid angiopathy. *Stroke* 2008;**39**:1988–92.

12. Liem MK, Lesnik Oberstein SA, Haan J *et al.* MRI correlates of cognitive decline in CADASIL: a 7-year follow-up study. *Neurology* 2009 13;**72**: 143–8.

13. Qui C, Cotch MF, Sigurdsson S *et al.* Cerebral microbleeds and dementia: the AGES-Reykjavik study. *Neurology* 2010;**14**:2221–8.

14. Viswanathan A, Chabriat H. Cerebral microhemorrhage. *Stroke* 2006;**37**:550–5.

15. Greenberg SM, Gurol ME, Rosand J, Smith EE. Amyloid angiopathy-related vascular cognitive impairment. *Stroke* 2004;**35**:2616–19.

16. Viswanathan A, Gschwendtner A, Guichard JP *et al.* Lacunar lesions are independently associated with disability and cognitive impairment in CADASIL. *Neurology* 2007;**69**:172–9.

17. Viswanathan A, Godin O, Jouvent E *et al.* Impact of MRI markers in subcortical vascular dementia: a multi-modal analysis in CADASIL. *Neurobiol Aging* 2010;**31**:1629–36.

18. O'Sullivan M, Morris RG, Huckstep B *et al.* Diffusion tensor MRI correlates with executive dysfunction in patients with ischaemic leukoaraiosis. *J Neurol Neurosurg Psychiatry* 2004;**75**:441–7.

19. Hachinski V, Iadecola C, Petersen RC *et al.* National Institute of Neurological Disorders and Stroke-Canadian Stroke Network vascular cognitive impairment harmonization standards. *Stroke* 2006; **37**:2220–41.

Other clinical manifestations of cerebral microbleeds

Simone M. Gregoire and David J. Werring

Introduction

Cerebral microbleeds (CMB) detected on gradient-recalled echo (GRE) T_2^*-weighted MRI have generally been considered as not causing overt clinical symptoms; indeed many reports have referred to them as "silent" or "asymptomatic" [1,2]. Very few studies have investigated whether they have any independent effect on brain function. This chapter considers first the potential mechanisms by which CMBs could cause or be associated with neurological dysfunction. It then considers CMBs in relation to transient neurological symptoms (mainly in the context of cerebral amyloid angiopathy [CAA]) and briefly discusses their association with disability and mortality. Whether CMBs independently influence cognitive function is discussed separately in Ch. 17.

How could microbleeds cause clinical symptoms?

Histopathological studies show that CMBs are associated with surrounding tissue damage [3–6], so they might be expected to disrupt brain function. However, their absolute size is very small, of the order of less than a millimeter, and at most a few millimeters, in diameter. As discussed in Chs. 2 and 3, the absolute size of a CMB is magnified by the blooming effect on T_2^*-weighted or other iron-sensitive images, meaning that the radiological lesions are generally larger than the true extent of the pathology [4]. Nevertheless, lacunes are a clearly accepted cause of acute focal deficits (lacunar syndromes) and are generally considered to be small: <15 mm, with the majority being 2–4 mm in diameter [7]. Absolute measurements of

CMB size are scarce, but they seem to be rather smaller than lacunes: one study in CAA showed that a cut-off of 5.7 mm best separated microbleeds from "macrobleeds" [8], while another in CAA associated with Alzheimer's disease showed that CMBs were mostly around 1 mm in diameter [4]. It might, therefore, be expected that development of a single CMB would be less likely than development of a lacune to produce clinically evident symptoms. However, it is not unreasonable that CMBs could do so if they form rapidly (as has been shown in a recent study in acute stroke [9]), and in a functionally strategic location, for example a small eloquent deep nucleus or white matter tract. The very limited evidence that this can indeed happen is discussed below. Another possibility is that, rather than disrupting function by direct destruction of tissue, microbleeding could disrupt the activity of surrounding neurons, thus affecting local brain function or connectivity. This idea is supported by recent experimental studies showing that small cortical CMBs can indeed adversely affect the function of nearby neurons, as shown by a reduced or absent neural response adjacent to a small experimental hemorrhage (50–200 μm [0.05–0.2 mm]) [10]. Moreover, most CMBs contain hemosiderin, a compound that may affect the electrical activity of cortex [11]. A further possibility is that CMBs are a marker of small vessels with impaired vasoreactivity, which could impair brain function locally or even cause small areas of ischemia.

More likely, perhaps, than such local effects, is that the accumulation of multiple CMBs over time could have a more insidious effect on the brain functions that depend on the integrity of widespread anatomical networks, for example cognition or gait. This hypothesis

---

is analogous to the proposed mechanism for deficits produced by ischemic white matter lesions, including lacunes, of which the majority do not cause acute stroke syndromes but can cumulatively disrupt cognition or gait [12]. This idea is considered in relation to CMBs and cognition in Ch. 17.

A fundamental challenge in studying how CMBs could affect brain function is that they are closely linked to many clinical and imaging manifestations of cerebrovascular disease, including all types of ischemic stroke and intracerebral hemorrhage (ICH), and white matter changes and lacunes on MRI. It is, therefore, difficult to determine whether CMBs have any independent functional effects, and well-designed large studies addressing this remain extremely scarce.

Cerebral microbleeds and transient neurological symptoms

To date, only limited case reports or case series addressing a possible link between CMBs and transient neurological symptoms have been published. In these cases, a causal link between the CMB and a transient event was usually suspected because of the strategic location of the CMB in an anatomical area compatible with the focal symptoms. Most of the cases described have been in patients with clinical features of CAA. As discussed above, there are several ways in which CMBs could theoretically be associated with or cause focal symptoms. First, they could form suddenly, and by a direct tissue-destructive effect cause neurological symptoms, analogous to the acute focal symptoms caused by lacunar infarction. There is only a single published case report suggesting this as a mechanism [13]. In this report, Watanabe and Kobashi described a 72-year-old patient who presented with a lateral gaze disturbance. A CMB was found in the contralateral pontine medial lemniscus when MRI was undertaken 6 months after the onset of symptoms, with no other lesion seen to account for the clinical presentation (Fig. 18.1). An MRI 6 months prior to the symptoms had shown ischemic small vessel changes (multiple lacunar infarcts and leukoaraiosis), but no CMBs. Although the development of the CMB *after* the onset of symptoms cannot be ruled out, the anatomical correlation between the CMB and the symptoms suggests that a single CMB lesion can cause focal neurological symptoms, but this is probably rare in comparison with symptomatic lacunar infarcts.

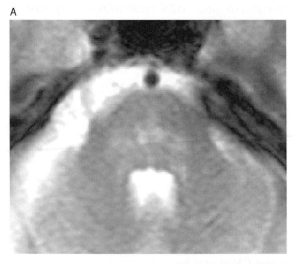

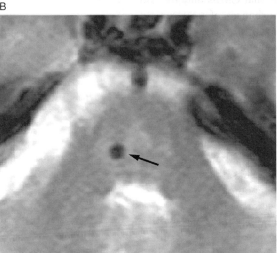

Fig. 18.1 Axial gradient echo T_2*-weighted MR images. (A) The first image showed no cerebral microbleeds in the mid-pontine region. (B) A second image a year later showed a new cerebral microbleed in the mid-pontine region (arrow). (Reproduced with permission from Watanabe and Kobashi, 2005 [13].)

A second way in which CMBs might be associated with focal symptoms is by their association with small areas of ischemia. This possibility has been considered mainly in relation to CAA. Patients with CAA have a propensity to develop ICH, either macroscopic in the form of lobar hemorrhages or microscopic (CMBs). However, recurrent transient neurological symptoms without lobar hemorrhage have also been consistently reported. These symptoms were attributed to recurrent transient ischemic attacks (TIAs), a label implying ischemia as a mechanism, in various case reports [14–17]. In support of this possibility, there is histopathological evidence of areas of infarction in severe CAA [15,18–20]. Increasing neuroimaging evidence with advanced MRI techniques also suggests that small areas of acute infarction occur in a substantial proportion of patients. Kimberly *et al.* recently described subliclinical ischemia on diffusion-weighted MRI in 12 of 78 patients with CAA [21], and a case report has also described the dynamic evolution of ischemic areas in CAA [22]. We have also noted ischemic lesions in approximately 20% of patients with CAA, but in the published reports and our experience these lesions seem mostly to be asymptomatic, so may not be a likely cause of acute focal symptoms. The clinical significance of small areas of ischemia in CAA clearly requires further study.

A third, and perhaps the most likely, possibility is that CMBs may be associated with "electrical" disturbances of nearby tissue: that is, they may cause focal seizures. This possibility is supported by the clinical nature of the transient attacks described in CAA. In a series reported by Greenberg *et al.* [23], four patients subsequently diagnosed with CAA presented initially with transient neurological symptoms. These episodes were multiple, and mostly stereotyped, with focal weakness, paresthesias or numbness and a spreading onset; one patient had visual misperceptions. Although in some respects these events resemble TIAs, the gradual onset and positive neurological phenomena are atypical. Interestingly, three of these patients developed subsequent large ICHs in the cerebral territory corresponding to the location of the preceding transient deficits. The similar location involved in the original spells and in the subsequent macrohemorrhages suggests that in some cases a small lesion (e.g. a CMB) may be a marker for an area of fragile abnormal vessels (perhaps with focal amyloid deposition or microaneurysms) that heralds a larger lobar ICH. Although this hypothesis could not be tested at that time because CMBs as defined currently were not detectable on the imaging available, T_2-weighted and GRE imaging did reveal multiple cortical and subcortical foci of signal loss that correlated anatomically with the symptoms described. More recently, Roch *et al.* [24] described six patients with cognitive complaints and recurrent stereotyped episodes of transient motor or sensory symptoms. Imaging with GRE T_2*-weighted sequences showed multiple CMBs in three of these patients (of which two were subsequently proven to have CAA on histopathological analysis), while the other patients had reduced signal

in cortical sulci compatible with hemosiderin deposition. One patient had a thalamic infarct. Four of these patients responded to anticonvulsant drugs, and two improved with the cessation of antiplatelet therapy. The hypothesis that CMBs could cause seizures or seizure-like attacks is also compatible with the observations that hemosiderin, a key component of CMBs on histopathological studies, can be irritant and epileptogenic when close to cortex [11], and that experimental cortical microhemorrhages cause functional disturbance of adjacent neurons [10]. The response of the transient neurological attacks in some patients to anticonvulsant medication is further evidence of a seizure-like mechanism [24]. It should also be mentioned here that focal convexity atraumatic subarachnoid bleeding is also increasingly recognized as a cause of recurrent stereotyped neurological attacks, described in some cases as rather like migraine auras [25,26]. This pattern of subarachnoid bleeding has also been recognized as a feature of CAA in association with CMBs [26].

In summary, in patients with transient neurological symptoms related to CAA, a seizure-like mechanism may be particularly likely when the symptoms are stereotypical, spread to contiguous cortical regions or resolve with anticonvulsant drugs [24]. By contrast, stroke-like events with more typically "vascular" symptoms (i.e. "negative" phenomena including weakness or sensory loss) and longer-lasting deficits may be more likely attributable to acute "microinfarcts" or the direct effects of new symptomatic CMBs. These presentations may lead to considerable therapeutic dilemmas, because if microbleeding is causing the problems, then antithrombotic treatment should presumably be avoided (Fig. 18.2); if ischemia is the dominant mechanism, then antithrombotic drugs may be warranted; and if the attacks are caused by seizure activity then anticonvulsants are the most logical treatment. With the use of modern MRI techniques, including GRE T_2*-weighted, susceptibility-weighted and diffusion-weighted sequences, it should be possible to differentiate symptomatic ischemic lesions from CMBs with more accuracy, which should increase our understanding of transient focal attacks in CAA and allow the most rational and safe management.

It is important to keep in mind that the limited evidence available suggests that new CMBs do not usually seem to cause acute symptoms. This has been shown in a few longitudinal MRI-correlated observational studies in different patient cohorts. New

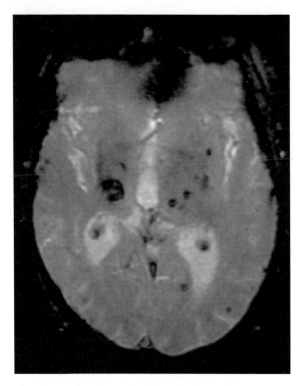

Fig. 18.2 Axial gradient echo T_2*-weighted image from a patient who presented with recurrent transient ischemic attack-like events despite increasingly aggressive antithrombotic treatment. When the antithrombotic therapy was reduced in intensity the frequency of events also reduced, suggesting that the antithrombotic treatment may have exacerbated symptoms related to microbleeding. There are multiple lobar and deep cerebral microbleeds. (Courtesy of Dr Rolf Jager, National Hospital for Neurology and Neurosurgery, London, UK.)

foci of hemosiderin deposition were detected in 38% of patients with lobar hemorrhage (presumed from CAA) followed up over 1.5 years, but all appeared to be clinically silent [27]. In a cohort of patients after stroke and TIA who were followed up at 5.5 years, 50% of those with baseline CMBs had developed new CMBs, compared with only 8% of the CMB-free matched controls, despite most surviving patients remaining clinically stable [28]. In a recent prospective observational study of 19 patients who underwent cardiac valve surgery, 12 developed new lesions, seen by GRE T_2*-weighted sequences, that corresponded to CMBs [29]; only two of these developed transient neurological deficits. In one patient with generalized seizure, facial weakness, irritability and confusion, diffusion-weighted image lesions were found and the relevance of the new microbleeding was unclear. In two other longitudinal studies, no follow-up clinical informa-

tion about neurological events was reported; one of these studies was in a patient cohort with consecutive ischemic stroke [9], the other in a longitudinal study of patients seen in a memory clinic [30].

Cerebral microbleeds, disability and death

The accumulation of CMBs (as well as other cerebrovascular disease markers, including leukoaraiosis or lacunes) might reflect progressive small vessel pathology and so could result in the development of progressive disability (including cognitive dysfunction or reduced mobility) or even be associated with an increased risk of death. Data on this are limited, but a prospective study of 94 patients with spontaneous lobar ICHs showed that the higher the number of baseline CMBs, the higher the 3-year cumulative risk of disability or death [31]. In individuals with more than six CMBs (detected by GRE T_2*-weighted imaging) the cumulative risk of the combined endpoint of cognitive impairment, functional dependence or death was 52% [31]. Occurrence of CMBs has also been associated with clinical disability in the hereditary small vessel disease CADASIL (cerebral autosomal dominant arteriopathy with subcortical infarcts and leukoencephalopathy) [32,33]. The odds ratio for functional dependence (defined as a modified Rankin score of $\geq$3) per additional CMB was 1.16 (95% confidence interval, 1.01–1.34; $p = 0.034$) after adjustment for confounding variables [33]. In a memory clinic population, CMBs had a strong positive predictive value with respect to mortality in adjusted analyses, particularly when numerous CMBs were present [34].

Conclusions

To summarize, although there are plausible mechanisms by which CMBs could cause clinical symptoms, the evidence that CMBs independently affect brain function remains limited. Case reports suggest that CMBs may be a cause of transient neurological attacks, particularly in patients with CAA. These can mimic TIA or ischemic strokes but often seem to be atypical, with gradual onset similar to that seen in partial seizures; they may, therefore, result from "electrical" activity related to CMBs. The evidence that CMBs directly cause focal neurological symptoms through associated tissue damage is even scarcer, but the increasing ability to detect CMBs, together with other advanced neuroimaging methods, should help to determine how important this is as a cause of cerebrovascular events. Some prospective data indicate that new CMBs do not cause obvious symptoms, yet CMBs have been shown to have independent prognostic significance for disability and mortality in different cohorts of patients, including CADASIL, spontaneous lobar hemorrhages and memory clinic populations. The independent contribution of CMBs to disability and death in other groups, including stroke patients, require further investigation.

References

1. Kato H, Izumiyama M, Izumiyama K, Takahashi A, Itoyama Y. Silent cerebral microbleeds on T_2^*-weighted MRI: correlation with stroke subtype, stroke recurrence, and leukoaraiosis. *Stroke* 2002;**33**: 1536–40.

2. Wong KS, Chan YL, Liu JY, Gao S, Lam WW. Asymptomatic microbleeds as a risk factor for aspirin-associated intracerebral hemorrhages. *Neurology* 2003;**60**:511–13.

3. Fazekas F, Kleinert R, Roob G et al. Histopathologic analysis of foci of signal loss on gradient-echo T_2^*-weighted MR images in patients with spontaneous intracerebral hemorrhage: evidence of microangiopathy-related microbleeds. *AJNR Am J Neuroradiol* 1999;**20**:637–42.

4. Schrag M, McAuley G, Pomakian J et al. Correlation of hypointensities in susceptibility-weighted images to tissue histology in dementia patients with cerebral amyloid angiopathy: a postmortem MRI study. *Acta Neuropathol* 2010;**119**:291–302.

5. Tatsumi S, Shinohara M, Yamamoto T. Direct comparison of histology of microbleeds with postmortem MR images: a case report. *Cerebrovasc Dis* 2008;**26**:142–6.

6. Tanaka A, Ueno A, Takayama Y, Takabayashi K. Small haemorrhages and ischemic lesions in association with spontaneous intracerebral hematomas. *Stroke* 1999;**30**:1637–42.

7. Fisher CM. Lacunes: small, deep cerebral infarcts. *Neurology* 1965;**15**:774–84.

8. Greenberg SM, Nandigam RN, Delgado P et al. Microbleeds versus macrobleeds: evidence for distinct entities. *Stroke* 2009;**40**:2382–6.

9. Jeon SB, Kwon SU, Cho AH et al. Rapid appearance of new cerebral microbleeds after acute ischemic stroke. *Neurology* 2009;**73**:1638–44.

10. Cianchetti FA, Nishimura N, Schaffer CB. Cortical microhaemorrhages reduce stimulus-evoked calcium responses in nearby neurons. *J Cerebr Blood Flow Metab* 2009;**29**:S217.

11. Baumann CR, Schuknecht B, Lo RG et al. Seizure outcome after resection of cavernous malformations is better when surrounding hemosiderin-stained brain also is removed. *Epilepsia* 2006;**47**:563–6.

12. Baezner H, Blahak C, Poggesi A et al. Association of gait and balance disorders with age-related white matter changes: the LADIS study. *Neurology* 2008;**70**: 935–42.

13. Watanabe A, Kobashi T. Lateral gaze disturbance due to cerebral microbleed in the medial lemniscus in the mid-pontine region: a case report. *Neuroradiology* 2005;**47**:908–11.

14. Smith DB, Hitchcock M, Philpott PJ. Cerebral amyloid angiopathy presenting as transient ischemic attacks. Case report. *J Neurosurg* 1985;**63**:963–4.

15. Okazaki H, Reagan TJ, Campbell RJ. Clinicopathologic studies of primary cerebral amyloid angiopathy. *Mayo Clin Proc* 1979;**54**:22–31.

16. Chamouard JM, Duyckaerts C, Rancurel G, Poisson M, Buge A. [Transient ischemic attack in amyloid angiopathy.] *Rev Neurol* (*Paris*) 1988;**144**:598–602.

17. Yong WH, Robert ME, Secor DL, Kleikamp TJ, Vinters HV. Cerebral hemorrhage with biopsy-proved amyloid angiopathy. *Arch Neurol* 1992;**49**: 51–8.

18. Cadavid D, Mena H, Koeller K, Frommelt RA. Cerebral beta amyloid angiopathy is a risk factor for cerebral ischemic infarction. A case control study in human brain biopsies. *J Neuropathol Exp Neurol* 2000; **59**:768–73.

19. Olichney JM, Hansen LA, Hofstetter CR et al. Cerebral infarction in Alzheimer's disease is associated with severe amyloid angiopathy and hypertension. *Arch Neurol* 1995;**52**:702–8.

20. Wattendorff AR, Frangione B, Luyendijk W, Bots GT. Hereditary cerebral haemorrhage with amyloidosis, Dutch type (HCHWA-D): clinicopathological studies. *J Neurol Neurosurg Psychiatry* 1995;**58**: 699–705.

21. Kimberly WT, Gilson A, Rost NS et al. Silent ischemic infarcts are associated with hemorrhage burden in cerebral amyloid angiopathy. *Neurology* 2009;**72**: 1230–5.

22. Menon RS, Kidwell CS. Neuroimaging demonstration of evolving small vessel ischemic injury in cerebral amyloid angiopathy. *Stroke* 2009;**40**:e675–7.

23. Greenberg SM, Vonsattel JP, Stakes JW, Gruber M, Finklestein SP. The clinical spectrum of cerebral amyloid angiopathy: presentations without lobar hemorrhage. *Neurology* 1993;**43**:2073–9.

24. Roch JA, Nighoghossian N, Hermier M *et al.* Transient neurologic symptoms related to cerebral amyloid angiopathy: usefulness of T_2^*-weighted imaging. *Cerebrovasc Dis* 2005;**20**:412–14.

25. Izenberg A, Aviv RI, Demaerschalk BM *et al.* Crescendo transient aura attacks: a transient ischemic attack mimic caused by focal subarachnoid hemorrhage. *Stroke* 2009;**40**:3725–9.

26. Kumar S, Goddeau RP, Jr., Selim MH *et al.* Atraumatic convexal subarachnoid hemorrhage: clinical presentation, imaging patterns, and etiologies. *Neurology* 2010;**74**:893–9.

27. Greenberg SM, O'Donnell HC, Schaefer PW, Kraft E. MRI detection of new hemorrhages: potential marker of progression in cerebral amyloid angiopathy. *Neurology* 1999;**53**:1135–8.

28. Gregoire SM, Brown MM, Kallis C *et al.* MRI detection of new microbleeds in patients with ischemic stroke: five-year cohort follow-up study. *Stroke* 2010;**41**:184–6.

29. Jeon SB, Lee JW, Kim SJ *et al.* New cerebral lesions on T_2^*-weighted gradient-echo imaging after cardiac valve surgery. *Cerebrovasc Dis* 2010;**30**: 194–9.

30. Goos JD, Henneman WJ, Sluimer JD *et al.* Incidence of cerebral microbleeds: a longitudinal study in a memory clinic population. *Neurology* 2010;**74**: 1954–60.

31. Greenberg SM, Eng JA, Ning M, Smith EE, Rosand J. Hemorrhage burden predicts recurrent intracerebral hemorrhage after lobar hemorrhage. *Stroke* 2004;**35**: 1415–20.

32. Lesnik Oberstein SA, van den Boom R, van Buchem MA *et al.* Cerebral microbleeds in CADASIL. *Neurology* 2001;**57**:1066–70.

33. Viswanathan A, Guichard JP, Gschwendtner A *et al.* Blood pressure and haemoglobin A1c are associated with microhaemorrhage in CADASIL: a two-centre cohort study. *Brain* 2006;**129**:2375–83.

34. Henneman WJ, Sluimer JD, Cordonnier C *et al.* MRI biomarkers of vascular damage and atrophy predicting mortality in a memory clinic population. *Stroke* 2009; **40**:492–8.

Chapter

19

Cerebral microbleeds and antithrombotic treatment

Yannie O. Y. Soo and Lawrence K. S. Wong

Introduction

Cerebral microbleeds (CMBs), detected by MRI gradient-recalled echo (GRE) sequences, are increasingly recognized as a potential radiological predictor for massive symptomatic intracerebral hemorrhage (ICH). Emerging evidence has increased our understanding on the pathophysiology of this radiological marker [1–3]. Histological analysis of these lesions has shown that they are hemosiderin deposits in macrophages after small vascular leaks, and are related to a small vessel, bleeding-prone microangiopathy [1].

Several cross-sectional studies have shown the connection of CMBs with a number of clinical and imaging vascular risk factors including age, hypertensive vasculopathy, leukoaraiosis, lacunar infarction, cerebral amyloid angiopathy (CAA) and ICH [1,2,4–10]. Accumulating evidence suggests that the location of CMB in the brain is reflective of their underlying origin. Those located in deep subcortical or infratentorial regions are thought to be a result of hypertensive or arteriosclerotic microangiopathy, whereas those occurring strictly in the lobar areas are indicative of CAA [3,11]. While these vascular risk factors are associated with an increased risk of ICH [4,7,8,12–14], they also increase the risk of occlusive cerebral and cardiovascular diseases, which require antithrombotic therapy (Fig. 19.1) [6,15–17]. This creates a clinical dilemma concerning the use of antithrombotic agents in patients with CMBs.

Antiplatelet agents and anticoagulants have proven efficacy in secondary prevention of stroke and other ischemic cardiovascular diseases. However, antithrombotic therapy may disproportionately increase the risk of ICH in patients with CMBs.

With the widespread use of MRI, a crucial question is whether CMBs, a radiological marker of cumulative prior small asymptomatic cerebral vascular leaks, can help to identify individuals at risk of antithrombotic-associated ICH, thus influencing our choice of treatment. The currently available evidence relevant to this question is further considered in this chapter.

Antithrombotic drug exposure and prevalence of cerebral microbleeds

The possible association between antithrombotic drug exposure and presence of CMBs is potentially confounded by the indications for which the drugs are prescribed: as CMBs may be related to the presence of cardiovascular and cerebrovascular diseases in general, antithrombotic drugs may be more often prescribed to persons with an increased risk of developing CMBs unrelated to the use of antithrombotic agents. In the Rotterdam Scan Study, which is a population-based, cross-sectional MRI study in the general elderly community in the Netherlands, CMBs were found in 250 (23.5%) of the 1062 individuals studied. The occurrence of CMBs was significantly more prevalent among users of antiplatelet agents than non-users (odds ratio [OR], 1.71; 95% confidence interval [CI], 1.21–2.41) [11]. After additional adjustment for cardiovascular risk and excluding of persons with a known history of cerebrovascular disease, there was no change in the association between antiplatelet agent usage and presence of CMBs, which further supports the contention that CMBs are more prevalent among antiplatelet users irrespective of potential confounders. Similar findings

Cerebral Microbleeds, ed. David J. Werring. Published by Cambridge University Press. © Cambridge University Press 2011.

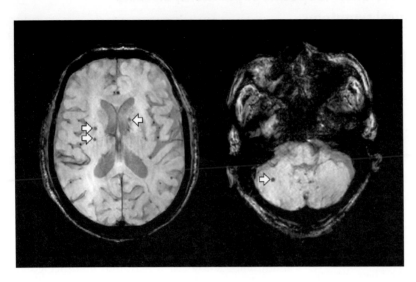

Fig. 19.1 Gradient echo images of a patient with background of hypertension who was admitted for acute ischemic stroke. Multiple cerebral microbleeds (CMBs) (arrows) were found in the subcortical and infratentorial regions, suggesting hypertension as the underlying etiology for these lesions. This patient was treated with aspirin and antihypertensive drugs for secondary stroke prevention.

were also observed in a recent systematic review of CMBs in 1461 patients with ICH and 3817 with ischemic stroke or transient ischemic attacks: CMBs were more frequently noted in antiplatelet users with ICH than non-users with ICH (OR, 1.7; 95% CI, 1.3 0–2.3; $p < 0.001$) as well as in those with ischemic stroke or transient ischemic attack (OR, 1.4; 95% CI, 1.2–1.7; $p < 0.001$) [18].

Another observation in the Rotterdam Study was that strictly lobar CMBs were more prevalent among aspirin users (OR, 2.7; 95% CI, 1.45–5.04) than among those using carbasalate calcium, an alternative antiplatelet agent. As CMBs in different locations may reflect a different underlying vascular condition [3,11], whether aspirin may differentially affect CMB development in CAA (a condition associated with lobar CMBs) needs to be further investigated.

Compared with antiplatelet agents, warfarin has an even stronger association with prevalence of CMBs, but this association was observed only in patients with ICH; CMBs are more frequently found in warfarin users with ICH (OR, 2.7; 95% CI, 1.6–4.4; $p < 0.001$) than in non-users with ICH [18]. However, there was no significant difference in prevalence of CMBs in warfarin users versus non-users in patients with ischemic stroke or transient ischemic attack [18,19].

The underlying pathophysiology for the different associations between antiplatelet agents and anticoagulants with CMBs remains unknown. Although there were more data from antiplatelet users and patients with ischemic stroke or transient ischemic attacks, there was significant heterogeneity in these cohorts, including in imaging techniques, which vary considerably in their sensitivity to detect CMBs (see Chs. 2 and 3) [18]. It also remains unclear if antithrombotic treatment per se causes CMBs, and there is a lack of data evaluating whether dosage and duration of antithrombotic therapy are related to prevalence and lesion load of CMBs. Furthermore, as mentioned above, antithrombotic users are more likely to have a history of hypertension or past stroke than non-users [20], and both risk factors are associated with an increased frequency of CMBs [2,5]. Although currently available data do suggest a positive association between antithrombotic exposure and prevalence of CMBs, further studies with matched risk factor profiles in homogeneous populations are needed to further clarify the causal relationship between antithrombotic therapy and CMBs.

Cerebral microbleeds and antiplatelet-associated intracerebral hemorrhage

In non-cardioembolic ischemic stroke, antiplatelet agents remain the mainstay of treatment for secondary stroke prevention. In general, aspirin is considered as a safe antiplatelet agent for ischemic stroke, carrying only a 1% risk of symptomatic ICH [21]. However, this risk does vary between individuals. Ethnicity, for example, is one of the factors that alters risk, and there is a higher risk of ICH in Asians than in non-Asians

[22]. The higher prevalence of CMBs in antiplatelet users with ICH raises the concern that patients with CMBs could be at higher risk of antiplatelet-associated ICH.

Although the association of CMBs and spontaneous ICH have been shown in a considerable number of cross-sectional studies [4,7,9,16], there are limited data on ICH related specifically to antiplatelet therapy. Among all the antiplatelet agents available for ischemic stroke, aspirin is the most studied agent in patients with CMBs. In an Asian cohort of 21 aspirin users who developed ICH and 21 aspirin users with no history of ICH, CMB in the ICH group was found to be more frequent (19 vs 7; $p < 0.001$) and extensive (13.3 versus 0.4; $p < 0.001$) than in the control group [14]. Similar findings were also observed in a recently published case–control study in a European cohort, which adjusted for confounding factors including age, sex and hypertension. This study comprised 16 antiplatelet users with ICH and 32 antiplatelet users without ICH who were matched for age, sex and hypertension; CMBs were more frequently observed in the ICH group than in the control group (81% versus 45%; $p = 0.03$) [23]. The frequency of lobar microbleeds was also higher in the ICH group than in the control group (69% versus 33%; $p = 0.032$). After adjusting for leukoaraiosis, the number of CMBs (OR, 1.33) and presence of lobar microbleeds (OR, 1.42) were found to be significant independent predictors for antiplatelet-related ICH. In both of these studies, most of the CMBs were found in the cerebral lobes (Fig. 19.2). Previous autopsy studies have suggested that lobar CMBs are the results of previous minor bleeds originating from CAA, where beta-amyloid is deposited in the walls of superficial cortical and leptomeningeal vessels, causing them to become brittle and prone to bleeding. Data from these studies, therefore, support the hypothesis that CAA may play a role in the pathogenesis of antiplatelet-associated ICH [11,24,25]. However, because of the small sample sizes and cross-sectional designs, further studies are needed to confirm the hypothesis.

The largest available prospective study of microbleeds and antithrombotic use included 908 patients with ischemic stroke who were treated with a single antithrombotic agent [17]. Cerebral microbleeds were identified in 27.8% and were most commonly observed in basal ganglia and thalamus, suggesting that hypertension is likely the predominant underlying patho-

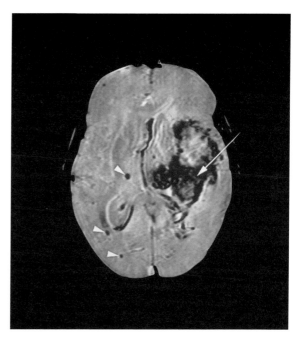

Fig. 19.2 A gradient echo MRI shows an asymptomatic left putaminal hemorrhage (arrow) and multiple asymptomatic microbleeds in the contralateral hemisphere (arrowheads). (Reproduced with permission from Wong *et al.* 2003 [14].)

physiology for CMBs in this cohort [3]. In this study, 93% of the patients were treated with aspirin. Both age and CMB were found to be independent predictors of subsequent ICH. During a mean follow-up of 26 months, it was found that risk of subsequent ICH increased significantly with lesion load of CMBs: 0.6% in patients with no CMB, 1.9% in patients with one CMB, 4.6% in patients with two to four CMBs and 7.6% in patients with five or more CMBs ($p < 0.001$) (Figs. 19.3 and 19.4) [17].

These data support the hypothesis that the risk of ICH varies across different subgroups of patients treated with antiplatelet agents; the presence and quantity of CMB appear to be factors that contribute to the future risk of antiplatelet-associated ICH. However, there are no data that assess if higher dose or longer duration of antiplatelet therapy poses a higher risk of ICH in patients with CMBs.

These data suggest that microbleeds may have promise in helping to assess the risk–benefit ratio of antiplatelet treatment after ischemic stroke, but further prospective studies in other large cohorts are required.

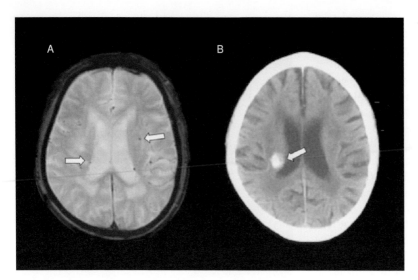

Fig. 19.3 A patient admitted with acute ischemic stroke and treated with aspirin. (A) Gradient echo image showed cerebral microbleeds (CMBs; arrows). (B) He developed symptomatic intracerebral hemorrhage 19 months later, with CT brain showing hematoma at the site of the pre-existing CMB (arrow). (Reproduced with kind permission from Springer Science and Business Media. Reference Soo *et al.* 2008 [17].)

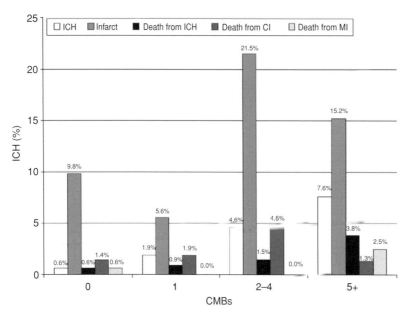

Fig. 19.4 Risk of subsequent intracerebral hemorrhage (ICH), recurrent cerebral infarct (CI) and related mortality in a prospective cohort of 908 patients with ischemic stroke treated with single antithrombotic agent (93% with aspirin) with mean follow-up period of 26 months. CMB, cerebral microbleed; MI, myocardial infarction. (Reproduced with kind permission from Springer Science and Business Media. Reference Soo *et al.* 2008 [17].)

Cerebral microbleeds and warfarin-associated intracerebral hemorrhage

Among patients with ICH, approximately 14% occur in patients who have been treated with warfarin [26]. Given the rising prevalence of atrial fibrillation and the greater use of warfarin, the incidence of oral anticoagulant-associated ICH is expected to rise. Therefore, any means of improving the identification of patients at particular risk is vital, plus it is possible that CMB may be a risk factor for anticoagulant-associated ICH. Unfortunately, there are few CMB studies on warfarin-associated ICH. In a case–control study comparing 24 warfarin users with ICH with 48 warfarin users without ICH, the number of CMBs was much higher for the ICH group (9.0 ± 26.8 versus 0.5 ± 1.03; $p < 0.001$). The lesion load of CMB was significantly correlated with the presence of ICH ($r = 0.299$; $p < 0.001$). Furthermore, increased prothrombin time and the presence of CMBs were both independent predictors of ICH [13]. Data from a recent systematic review of prospective studies also showed a trend towards increased risk of subsequent ICH in patients with CMB among warfarin users (OR, 3.0; 95% CI, 0.5–17.5; $p = 0.23$). However, the analysis was limited by a very small number of outcome events [18]. Occurrence of CMBs in a lobar distribution may be a marker for CAA, which is an increasingly recognized cause of anticoagulant-associated ICH [27]. Unfortunately, there is a lack of data concerning the distribution of CMBs from these studies.

How could treatment with antithrombotic agents amplify the risk of ICH in individuals with CMBs? Theoretically, when vessels rupture, leakage of blood is normally staunched by hemostasis. In patients treated with antithrombotic agents, hemostatic mechanisms are impaired, and a leakage may "snowball" to become a large symptomatic hematoma. Prospective studies are needed to provide more direct evidence about whether or not CMB increases the risk of antithrombotic-associated ICH. So far, existing studies have been limited by containing few warfarin users, having relatively short follow-up periods and having insufficient numbers of outcome events to provide a reliable estimate of the risks of antithrombotic drug use in the presence of CMB [7,17,19,28]. However, the limited prospective data that are available are consistent with the hypothesis that CMBs do increase the risk of ICH as a complication of antithrombotic use.

The potential role of cerebral microbleeds in therapeutic decision making for ischemic stroke

Antithrombotic treatment for ischemic stroke

Antiplatelet and anticoagulant medications have proven efficacy for patients at high risk of ischemic cardiovascular or cerebrovascular disease, but can predispose individuals to ICH. Risk stratifying of patients to individually optimize the balance of anti-ischemic to pro-hemorrhagic effects of antithrombotic drugs remains a major goal of cerebrovascular medicine. With the increasing evidence about the close association of CMBs with ICH, there is growing interest in whether this radiological marker can help to identify patients at high risk of treatment-associated hemor-

rhagic complications and, hence, directly influence the choice of treatment.

Should antithrombotic therapy be avoided in the presence of cerebral microbleeds?

In the BRASIL study, a pooled analysis of 570 patients with ischemic stroke who were given intravenous thrombolysis within 6 hours of onset, there was no significant increase in symptomatic ICH among the 15.1% of patients with CMBs (5.8%) compared with those without CMBs (2.7%) [29]. Although this study is underpowered to detect a statistically significant increase in bleeding, this risk (if present) would still not outweigh the benefit of intravenous thrombolysis. However, there were only 1.1% of patients with more than five CMBs in this study, and the overall prevalence of microbleeds at some centers was much lower than expected, raising questions about whether imaging methods were optimal. Whether patients with multiple CMBs are at increased risk of ICH with thrombolysis remains unanswered. At this stage, there are no data supporting CMB as a contraindication for thrombolysis in acute ischemic stroke. A fuller discussion of this important question can be found in Ch. 20.

Should aspirin be avoided in the presence of cerebral microbleeds?

From the largest prospective cohort in Chinese patients with ischemic stroke and treated with long-term single antiplatelet agent, the risk of subsequent ICH was found to increase substantially to 7.6% among patients with more than five CMBs and resulted in 3.8% mortality (Fig. 19.4) [17]. Comparing with the modest benefit of antithrombotic agents in secondary stroke prevention (absolute risk reduction 0.69 to 2.49% for aspirin in non-cardioembolic stroke) [30], the extra bleeding risk seems to outweigh the benefit of treatment in this subgroup of patients. Although this study is limited by the small number of outcome events, it suggests that in selected patients (e.g. those with high CMB counts) the bleeding risk may differ, thus influencing the benefit–risk balance for antiplatelet therapy. However, given the clear benefit of antiplatelet therapy in secondary stroke prevention, as demonstrated in large randomized controlled trials and meta-analyses [30–33], there are insufficient data at this stage to suggest that antiplatelet therapy should be withheld in patients with CMBs. Of note, most of the CMB studies assessing risk of antiplatelet-associated ICH were performed in patients receiving aspirin as the single antiplatelet agent. The bleeding risk in patients receiving other more potent antiplatelet agents (e.g. clopidogrel) and dual antiplatelet therapy is not known and needs to be investigated.

Should warfarin be avoided in the presence of cerebral microbleeds?

Stroke and systemic thromboembolic events are the most common complications of atrial fibrillation. In patients with atrial fibrillation, the risk of stroke increases with age; other risk factors include hypertension, diabetes mellitus and left ventricular failure. When multiple risk factors are present, the risk of cardioembolic stroke can be up to 18.2% per year [34,35]. Anticoagulation with warfarin remains the most effective prevention for cardioembolic stroke related to atrial fibrillation; in randomized clinical trials, warfarin reduced the relative risk of stroke by 60–70% [36].

Despite the established clinical efficacy of warfarin, intracranial bleeding is the most feared complication and is one of the main reasons limiting its use in clinical practice. In general, anticoagulation with warfarin increases the risk of ICH by two- to fivefold (absolute risk 0.4 to 2.6% per year) depending upon the intensity of anticoagulation [20,37–39]. At present, with the limited available data, there is no reason to suggest that the risk of warfarin-related hemorrhage is high enough to outweigh its benefit and that warfarin should be withheld in patients with CMBs.

Nevertheless, patients with CAA seem to be particularly prone to warfarin-related ICH [20]. The most common clinical presentation of CAA is lobar hemorrhage, with recurrence rates of up to 21% reported [40]. Because of the high recurrence rate, the general current working rule for patients diagnosed with CAA is to avoid anticoagulants, which increase both the frequency (approximately 7- to 10-fold) and severity (approximately 60% mortality) of ICH [41,42]. It should be appreciated that these data are from specialist centers of hospital-based cohort studies and may not necessarily be generalizable to all populations of patients with CAA.

Although strictly lobar CMBs are commonly observed in patients with clinical evidence of CAA, CMBs have not been extensively validated in pathological studies as part of the diagnostic criteria for probable CAA. The presence of CAA should be suspected clinically in patients over the age of 60 who have multiple lobar hemorrhages in the absence of an obvious cause [24]. However, according to proposed Boston criteria for CAA, the disease can be definitely diagnosed only by full autopsy examination of the brain [24,43]. Whether a strictly lobar distribution of CMBs can be used to make the diagnosis in the absence of lobar macrohemorrhage remains to be determined. Until further data are available, warfarin should probably not be withdrawn in patients with CMBs who have a clear indication for anticoagulation. However, for those with predominantly lobar CMBs, measures should be taken to minimize the risk of ICH. General measures such as stringent blood pressure control and close monitoring of clotting (international normalized ratio) would seem to be clinically appropriate in this subgroup of patients. There is an urgent need for more prospective data to address the role of CMBs in decision making about anticoagulation treatment.

Conclusions

Although emerging data support the positive association of CMBs with antithrombotic-associated ICH, many of the findings are based on cross-sectional studies with small sample sizes. Furthermore, most of the CMB studies on patients with stroke were performed among Asian cohorts [17,18,25], which are known to have a higher risk of ICH than Caucasians. Larger longitudinal studies and data from other ethnic groups are needed before these data can be generalized to all populations. Because of the many limitations in study design, sample size and confounding factors, there is still uncertainty about the clinical significance of CMBs for antithrombotic treatment. At this stage, antithrombotic treatment and thrombolysis should not be withheld in ischemic stroke for patients with CMBs and no other reasons for clinical uncertainty, because a clear overall benefit has been established from large randomized trials and meta-analyses. However, with the emergence of novel antithrombotic agents with a potentially lower risk of ICH (e.g. cilostazol and dabigatran) [44,45], further studies are needed to assess if high-risk patients (possibly those with multiple CMBs) may benefit from treatment with antithrombotic agents with lower bleeding risk. Our understanding of CMBs has greatly increased over the past few years; current efforts are dedicated to exploring the benefit–risk balance of various antithrombotic agents in patients with CMBs to guide physicians in choosing a safe and effective treatment for those requiring antithrombotic therapy.

References

1. Fazekas F, Kleinert R, Roob G *et al.* Histopathologic analysis of foci of signal loss on gradient-echo T_2*-weighted MR images in patients with spontaneous intracerebral hemorrhage: evidence of microangiopathy-related microbleeds. *AJNR Am J Neuroradiol* 1999;**20**:637–42.

2. Koennecke HC. Cerebral microbleeds on MRI: prevalence, associations, and potential clinical implications. *Neurology* 2006;**66**:165–71.

3. Sun J, Soo YO, Lam WW *et al.* Different distribution patterns of cerebral microbleeds in acute ischemic stroke patients with and without hypertension. *Eur Neurol* 2009;**62**:298–303.

4. Chen YF, Chang YY, Liu JS *et al.* Association between cerebral microbleeds and prior primary intracerebral hemorrhage in ischemic stroke patients. *Clin Neurol Neurosurg* 2008;**110**:988–91.

5. Cordonnier C, Al-Shahi Salman R, Wardlaw J. Spontaneous brain microbleeds: systematic review, subgroup analyses and standards for study design and reporting. *Brain* 2007;**130**:1988–2003.

6. Fan YH, Mok VC, Lam WW, Hui AC, Wong KS. Cerebral microbleeds and white matter changes in patients hospitalized with lacunar infarcts. *J Neurol* 2004;**251**:537–41.

7. Fan YH, Zhang L, Lam WW, Mok VC, Wong KS. Cerebral microbleeds as a risk factor for subsequent intracerebral hemorrhages among patients with acute ischemic stroke. *Stroke* 2003;**34**:2459–62.

8. Greenberg SM, O'Donnell HC, Schaefer PW, Kraft E. MRI detection of new hemorrhages: potential marker of progression in cerebral amyloid angiopathy. *Neurology* 1999;**53**:1135–8.

9. van den Boom R, Bornebroek M, Behloul F *et al.* Microbleeds in hereditary cerebral hemorrhage with amyloidosis-Dutch type. *Neurology* 2005;**64**:1288–9.

10. Walker DA, Broderick DF, Kotsenas AL, Rubino FA. Routine use of gradient-echo MRI to screen for cerebral amyloid angiopathy in elderly patients. *AJR Am J Roentgenol* 2004;**182**:1547–50.

11. Vernooij MW, van der Lugt A, Ikram MA *et al.* Prevalence and risk factors of cerebral microbleeds: the Rotterdam Scan Study. *Neurology* 2008;**70**:1208–14.

12. Kidwell CS, Greenberg SM. Red meets white: do microbleeds link hemorrhagic and ischemic cerebrovascular disease? *Neurology* 2009;**73**:1614–15.

13. Lee GH, Kwon SU, Kang DW. Warfarin-induced intracerebral hemorrhage associated with microbleeds. *J Clin Neurol* 2008;**4**:131–3.

14. Wong KS, Chan YL, Liu JY, Gao S, Lam WW. Asymptomatic microbleeds as a risk factor for aspirin-associated intracerebral hemorrhages. *Neurology* 2003;**60**:511–13.

15. Jeon SB, Kwon SU, Cho AH *et al.* Appearance of new cerebral microbleeds after acute ischemic stroke. *Neurology* 2009;**73**:1638–44.

16. Nishikawa T, Ueba T, Kajiwara M *et al.* Cerebral microbleeds predict first-ever symptomatic cerebrovascular events. *Clin Neurol Neurosurg* 2009;**111**:825–8.

17. Soo YO, Yang SR, Lam WW *et al.* Risk vs benefit of anti-thrombotic therapy in ischaemic stroke patients with cerebral microbleeds. *J Neurol* 2008;**255**:1679–86.

18. Lovelock CE, Cordonnier C, Naka H *et al.* Antithrombotic drug use, cerebral microbleeds, and intracerebral hemorrhage. A systematic review of published and unpublished studies. *Stroke* 2010;**41**:1222.

19. Orken DN, Kenangil G, Uysal E, Forta H. Cerebral microbleeds in ischemic stroke patients on warfarin treatment. *Stroke* 2009;**40**:3638–40.

20. Rosand J, Eckman MH, Knudsen KA, Singer DE, Greenberg SM. The effect of warfarin and intensity of anticoagulation on outcome of intracerebral hemorrhage. *Arch Intern Med* 2004;**164**:880–4.

21. Sandercock P, Gubitz G, Foley P, Counsell C. Antiplatelet therapy for acute ischaemic stroke. *Cochrane Database Syst Rev* 2003:CD000029.

22. Tokuda Y, Kato J. Aspirin and risk of hemorrhagic stroke. *JAMA* 1999;**282**:732; author reply, 3.

23. Gregoire SM, Jager HR, Yousry TA *et al.* Brain microbleeds as a potential risk factor for antiplatelet-related intracerebral haemorrhage: hospital-based, case-control study. *J Neurol Neurosurg Psychiatry* 2010;**81**:679–84.

24. Greenberg SM. Cerebral amyloid angiopathy: prospects for clinical diagnosis and treatment. *Neurology* 1998;**51**:690–4.

25. Wong KS, Mok V, Lam WW *et al.* Aspirin-associated intracerebral hemorrhage: clinical and radiologic features. *Neurology* 2000;**54**:2298–301.

26. Cordonnier C, Rutgers MP, Dumont F *et al.* Intra-cerebral haemorrhages: are there any differences in baseline characteristics and intra-hospital mortality between hospital and population-based registries? *J Neurol* 2009;**256**:198–202.

27. Greenberg SM, Vernooij MW, Cordonnier C et al. Cerebral microbleeds: a guide to detection and interpretation. *Lancet Neurol* 2009;**8**:165–74.

28. Naka H, Nomura E, Takahashi T et al. Combinations of the presence or absence of cerebral microbleeds and advanced white matter hyperintensity as predictors of subsequent stroke types. *AJNR Am J Neuroradiol* 2006;**27**:830–5.

29. Fiehler J, Albers GW, Boulanger JM et al. Bleeding risk analysis in stroke imaging before thrombolysis (BRASIL): pooled analysis of T_2^*-weighted magnetic resonance imaging data from 570 patients. *Stroke* 2007;**38**:2738–44.

30. **Antithrombotic Trialists' Collaboration**. Collaborative meta-analysis of randomised trials of antiplatelet therapy for prevention of death, myocardial infarction, and stroke in high risk patients. *BMJ* 2002;**324**:71–86.

31. Albers GW, Amarenco P, Easton JD, Sacco RL, Teal P. Antithrombotic and thrombolytic therapy for ischemic stroke: American College of Chest Physicians Evidence-Based Clinical Practice Guidelines (8th Edition). *Chest*. 2008;**133**(6 Suppl):630S-69S.

32. Halkes PH, van Gijn J, Kappelle LJ, Koudstaal PJ, Algra A. Aspirin plus dipyridamole versus aspirin alone after cerebral ischaemia of arterial origin (ESPRIT): randomised controlled trial. *Lancet* 2006;**367**:1665–73.

33. Sacco RL, Diener HC, Yusuf S et al. Aspirin and extended-release dipyridamole versus clopidogrel for recurrent stroke. *N Engl J Med* 2008;**359**:1238–51.

34. van Walraven C, Hart RG, Wells GA et al. A clinical prediction rule to identify patients with atrial fibrillation and a low risk for stroke while taking aspirin. *Arch Intern Med* 2003;163:936–43.

35. Gage BF, Waterman AD, Shannon W et al. Validation of clinical classification schemes for predicting stroke:

results from the National Registry of Atrial Fibrillation. *JAMA* 2001;**285**:2864–70.

36. Albers GW. Atrial fibrillation and stroke. Three new studies, three remaining questions. *Arch Intern Med* 1994;**154**:1443–8.

37. Connolly SJ, Laupacis A, Gent M et al. Canadian Atrial Fibrillation Anticoagulation (CAFA) study. *J Am Coll Cardiol* 1991;**18**:349–55.

38. Stroke Prevention in Atrial Fibrillation Investigators. Bleeding during antithrombotic therapy in patients with atrial fibrillation. *Arch Intern Med* 1996;**156**:409–16.

39. Levine MN, Raskob G, Landefeld S, Kearon C. Hemorrhagic complications of anticoagulant treatment. *Chest* 2001;**119**(1 Suppl):108S-21S.

40. O'Donnell HC, Rosand J, Knudsen KA et al. Apolipoprotein E genotype and the risk of recurrent lobar intracerebral hemorrhage. *N Engl J Med* 2000 27;**342**:240–5.

41. Rosand J, Hylek EM, O'Donnell HC, Greenberg SM. Warfarin-associated hemorrhage and cerebral amyloid angiopathy: a genetic and pathologic study. *Neurology* 2000;**55**:947–51.

42. Hart RG, Boop BS, Anderson DC. Oral anticoagulants and intracranial hemorrhage. Facts and hypotheses. *Stroke* 1995;**26**:1471–7.

43. Greenberg SM, Briggs ME, Hyman BT et al. Apolipoprotein E epsilon 4 is associated with the presence and earlier onset of hemorrhage in cerebral amyloid angiopathy. *Stroke* 1996;**27**:1333–7.

44. Huang Y, Cheng Y, Wu J et al. Cilostazol as an alternative to aspirin after ischaemic stroke: a randomised, double-blind, pilot study. *Lancet Neurol* 2008;**7**:494–9.

45. Connolly SJ, Ezekowitz MD, Yusuf S et al. Dabigatran versus warfarin in patients with atrial fibrillation. *N Engl J Med* 2009;**361**:1139–51.

Cerebral microbleeds and thrombolysis

Chelsea S. Kidwell

Introduction

Thrombolytic therapy remains the only treatment for acute ischemic stroke proven to improve clinical outcome. However, the development of intracerebral hemorrhage (ICH) following treatment remains an important limitation of this therapy and is symptomatic in 2.4–10% of patients depending on the definition used [1–3]. Of note, hemorrhage occurs in 20–30% of patients in a location remote from the acute ischemic field, suggesting an underlying hemorrhage-prone vasculopathy in this subgroup of patients [1,4]. Identifying patients at higher risk for hemorrhagic transformation following thrombolysis is an important goal, and this information, in turn, could increase the overall safety profile of thrombolytic therapy.

Since the 1990s, when MRI increasingly came into use as an imaging modality for acute stroke, a growing body of data has shown that cerebral microbleeds (CMBs) are, in fact, an important marker for a bleeding-prone vasculopathy. Yet, only a few studies have systematically evaluated the risk of ICH following thrombolysis in patients with CMBs. While the results of studies available to date have begun to elucidate the risk, a number of important questions remain. Does the presence of cerebral CMBs increase the risk of hemorrhage with thrombolytic therapies? If there is an increased risk, does this outweigh the benefits? Can patients at the highest risk be identified: is there a threshold number, a pattern of location (e.g. lobar) or other patient characteristics that change the risk–benefit ratio?

In the first report addressing the role of CMBs in thrombolysis-induced symptomatic ICH, Kidwell *et al.* described a series of 41 patients screened with

a baseline MRI followed by intra-arterial thrombolysis for large vessel acute stroke [5]. Five patients had CMBs at baseline; of these, one developed a hemorrhage at the site of a CMB (and remote from the acute infarct). Of note, no further study has evaluated systematically the risk in patients undergoing combined intravenous/intra-arterial or pure intra-arterial thrombolytic therapy. Theoretically, the risk of ICH may be increased with direct intra-arterial injection of the thrombolytic agent (such that the concentration of the drug may be quite high in the cerebral vasculature distal to the injection) as opposed to intravenous treatment (where the agent is diffused throughout the circulation).

Several small case series or individual case reports followed, addressing the potential of an increased risk of hemorrhage related to thrombolytic therapy in the presence of CMBs. Comforto and colleagues reported a patient with multiple cerebral CMBs in the brainstem, cerebellum and basal ganglia found on follow-up MRI [6]. This patient was treated with intravenous tissue plasminogen activator (tPA) without complications. However, Chalela and colleagues reported a symptomatic ICH following intravenous thrombolysis in a patient with multiple CMBs [7]. This group of investigators subsequently altered their criteria for treatment with intravenous thrombolysis for acute stroke such that the presence of multiple CMBs was a relative exclusion criterion [8].

Nighoghossian and colleagues initially reported a case series in which an association between CMBs and subsequent hemorrhage was found following various acute stroke therapies (including antithrombotics and intravenous thrombolysis) [9]. In this first study, 100 patients were included, of whom 20 were found to have

---

Cerebral Microbleeds, ed. David J. Werring. Published by Cambridge University Press. © Cambridge University Press 2011.

one or more CMBs on initial MRI. Only 27 of the 100 patients received thrombolytic therapy, the remainder receiving antithrombotic drugs. A multivariate logistic regression analysis for the whole cohort showed that CMBs, diabetes mellitus and National Institutes of Health Stroke Scale (NIHSS) score were independent predictors of subsequent cerebral hemorrhage.

This same group later performed a retrospective analysis of the impact of CMBs specifically on 44 patients treated with intravenous tPA within 7 hours of symptom onset and screened with MRI [10]. Eight of the patients analyzed had one or more CMBs on baseline MRI. At 24 hours, none of the patients with CMBs had a symptomatic ICH. Three of the eight (37%) developed any hemorrhage, compared with 10 of the 36 (28%) patients without CMBs (p value not significant). At 7 days, symptomatic ICH occurred in one of the eight (12.5%) patients with CMBs versus 2 of the 36 (5.6%) without CMBs, and five of the eight (62.5%) developed any hemorrhage compared with 12 of the 36 (33.3%) without initial CMBs (p values not significant). The authors concluded that patients with a small number of CMBs could be treated safely with thrombolysis but that larger prospective studies were needed.

Fiehler and colleagues also analyzed imaging data from 100 patients treated with thrombolysis within 6 hours of stroke onset [11]. Cerebral CMBs were found in 20–22% of the cohort overall (depending on the reader) and in only one of seven patients with symptomatic ICH. These authors concluded that the presence of cerebral CMBs had low sensitivity (14%) for prediction of ICH following thrombolysis, and also reported that a combination of the presence of CMBs with leukoaraiosis scores did not improve the prediction.

In the Diffusion-weighted Imaging Evaluation for Understanding Stroke Evolution (DEFUSE) study, investigators assessed the impact of CMBs on the frequency of hemorrhagic complications in subjects with acute ischemic stroke who were screened with MRI and treated with intravenous tPA between 3 and 6 hours of symptom onset [12]. Only 11 of 70 patients (16%) with a baseline gradient-recalled echo (GRE) scan had one or more CMB on baseline imaging. None of these 11 patients developed symptomatic ICH (versus 11.9% of patients without CMBs), and none of these patients developed hemorrhagic transformation at the site of a prior CMB. Further, 3 of the 11 (27%) patients with CMBs developed asymptomatic

ICH compared with 22 of the 59 (37%) patients without CMBs (p = 0.52). Of note, of the 11 patients with CMBs, eight had only a single CMB, one had two, one had three, and one had six. The authors concluded that a small number of CMBs on baseline GRE does not increase the risk of hemorrhage following intravenous thrombolysis and should not exclude patients from receiving therapy.

The most comprehensive and informative data on the risk of thrombolysis-induced hemorrhage in the setting of CMBs and acute stroke comes from the Bleeding Risk Analysis in Stroke Imaging before thrombolysis (BRASIL) study [13]. Data were analyzed from a total of 570 patients with ischemic stroke who underwent treatment with intravenous tPA within 6 hours of symptom onset and were screened with MRI (in 29 patients, MRI was obtained after the start of tPA). Scans were analyzed at baseline for CMBs on T_2*-weighted images. The primary endpoint was symptomatic ICH defined as a worsening score of ≥ 4 points on the NIHSS and temporally related to a hematoma on follow-up imaging.

Out of 520 patients, 86 (15%) had one or more CMBs on baseline imaging, with a total of 242 CMBs across the cohort. Median number of CMBs was one (range, 1–77). Only six patients had ≥ 5 CMBs. The rate of symptomatic ICH was 5.8% in the group of patients with CMBs versus 2.7% in those without (p = 0.170 by Fisher's exact test). The odds ratio for symptomatic ICH in patients with CMBs versus without was 2.23 (95% confidence interval, 0.67–6.97). The authors concluded that any increased risk of thrombolytic therapy in the setting of CMBs is likely to be small and unlikely to exceed the benefits of thrombolytic therapy. Because of the very small number of patients with multiple CMBs, no reliable conclusions could be drawn regarding risk in this subgroup. Finally, the authors calculated, based on their data, that a study of 7664 patients would be required to be adequately powered to exclude an increased risk of symptomatic ICH with an odds ratio of 1.5.

It is interesting to note that hemorrhages do occur in regions remote from the acute ischemic stroke field following intravenous thrombolysis for acute stroke (20% of symptomatic ICH in the National Institute of Neurological Disorders and Stroke [NINDS] trial and 33% of parenchymal hematomas in the Safe Implementation of Treatment in Stroke-International Stroke Thrombolysis Register [SITS-ISTR] study) (Fig. 20.1) [1,4]. In patients undergoing thrombolysis for

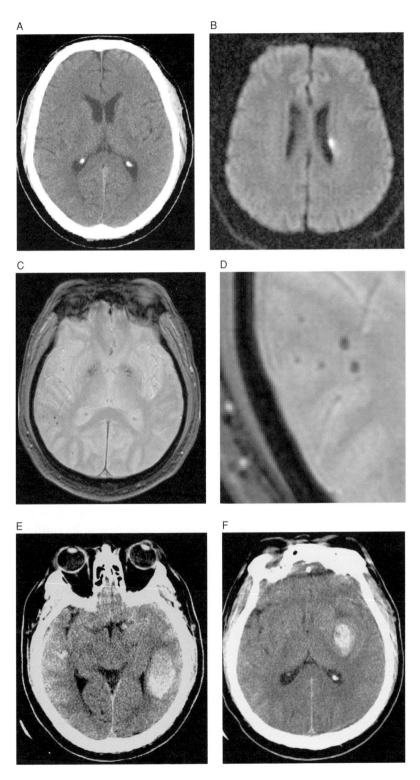

Fig. 20.1 Images from a 52-year-old male who presented 2 hours after onset with clumsy-hand dysarthria syndrome with a National Institutes of Health Stroke Scale score of 3. The patient requested treatment with tissue plasminogen activator (tPA). (A) Baseline CT. (B) Diffusion-weighted image shows an acute left periventricular lacune. (C,D) Baseline gradient-recalled echo sequences, with higher resolution image (D), show multiple temporal lobe cerebral microbleeds (CMBs). Over 30 were visualized throughout the brain. (E,F) CT scan following intravenous tPA shows multiple bilateral intracranial hemorrhages, in some places related to sites of the CMBs, but not in the territory of the acute stroke. This patient was ultimately found to have amyloid angiopathy by biopsy. (Images provided with permission of UCLA Stroke Center.)

cardiac ischemia, the rate of symptomatic hemorrhage is approximately 0.9% [14]; in these cases, the hemorrhage is unlikely to occur at the site of an acute ischemic lesion, although this cannot be ruled out in some cases. In both these scenarios, an alternative underlying vascular pathology besides acute ischemic tissue injury may be the source of the hemorrhage. In these cases, it is certainly possible that CMBs may either be the direct result of vessel injury, and thus the subsequent direct source of the hemorrhage, or occur as a more general marker of vessel fragility.

There are some data to support a differential risk of thrombolysis-related hemorrhage in the setting of CMBs based on the underlying etiology of the CMB (cerebral amyloid angiopathy [CAA]-related versus hypertensive), with CAA harboring the greater increased risk [15]. Winkler and colleagues reported that intravenous thrombolysis led to an increase of microhemorrhages as well as parenchymal and subarachnoid hemorrhages in *APP23* transgenic mice, which display the typical findings of human CAA (cerebrovascular amyloidosis, microhemorrhages and spontaneous intraparenchymal hemorrhages) [16]. Compared with controls, the transgenic mice demonstrated an almost twofold increase in microhemorrhages as well as frank new intraparenchymal hemorrhages (1 of 9 at a dose of 1 mg/kg, 2 of 11 at a dose of 10 mg/kg), which did not occur in the controls.

In CAA, CMBs are located predominantly in lobar regions and the total number of lesions is often significant (10–75 or more). A lobar location is also a more common site for thrombolysis-related hemorrhages. In contrast, CMBs linked to hypertensive small vessel disease are typically located in predominantly deep regions and may be far fewer in number. Further, there is some limited pathological data supporting the role of CAA in thrombolysis-related hemorrhage. As summarized by McCarron and Nicoll from autopsy data, 7 of 10 (70%) patients with thrombolysis-related hemorrhage had autopsy-proven CAA compared with 22% in age-appropriate unselected populations [15]. However, a secondary analysis of the NINDS study did not show an association between the apolipoprotein E (*APOE*) $\varepsilon 4$ genotype and ICH [17]. Since the *APOE* $\varepsilon 4$ allele has been shown to be significantly associated with CAA, this result does not support CAA as a significant source of thrombolysis-related ICH. Prospective, large studies will be needed to sort out the

role of CAA in thrombolysis-related ICH and to determine its role independent of age and leukoaraiosis.

Conclusions

In summary, the evidence suggests that in patients with a small number of CMBs (e.g. less than five), particularly when located in deep structures, the risk of thrombolysis-related ICH (including symptomatic ICH) may be slightly greater than in patients without CMBs, although this risk did not reach statistical significance in studies to date, and it is unlikely that any small increased risk would outweigh the benefit. Therefore, at present, thrombolytic therapy for acute stroke should not be withheld in patients with a small number of CMBs. However, a number of important questions remain unanswered. What is the risk in patients with a primarily lobar pattern of CMBs, or in patients with a substantial burden of CMBs regardless of the location? Is there additional information that could be used to better stratify the risk? While theoretical grounds exist, as well as some limited data, to suggest a greater risk of ICH in patients with CAA as the underlying etiology of CMBs, no definitive data are available to quantify this potential risk. Until these questions are answered, caution must be used in basing treatment decisions on this limited data.

References

1. NINDS rt-PA Stroke Group. Tissue plasminogen activator for acute ischemic stroke. *New Engl J Med* 1995;**333**:1581–7.

2. Furlan A, Higashida R, Wechsler L *et al.* Intra-arterial prourokinase for acute ischemic stroke. The Proact II study: a randomized controlled trial. Prolyse in acute cerebral thromboembolism. *JAMA* 1999;**282**:2003–11.

3. Hacke W, Kaste M, Bluhmki E *et al.* Thrombolysis with alteplase 3 to 4.5 hours after acute ischemic stroke. *N Engl J Med* 2008;**359**:1317–29.

4. Wahlgren N, Ahmed N, Davalos A *et al.* Thrombolysis with alteplase 3–4.5 h after acute ischaemic stroke (SITS-ISTR): an observational study. *Lancet* 2008; **372**:1303–9.

5. Kidwell CS, Saver JL, Villablanca JP *et al.* Magnetic resonance imaging detection of CMBs before thrombolysis: an emerging application. *Stroke* 2002; **33**:95–8.

6. Conforto AB, Lucato LT, Leite Cda C *et al.* Cerebral CMBs and intravenous thrombolysis: case report. *Arq Neuropsiquiatr* 2006;**64**:855–7.

7. Chalela JA, Kang DW, Warach S. Multiple cerebral CMBs: MRI marker of a diffuse hemorrhage-prone state. *J Neuroimaging* 2004;**14**:54–7.

8. Kang DW, Chalela JA, Dunn W, Warach S. MRI screening before standard tissue plasminogen activator therapy is feasible and safe. *Stroke* 2005;**36**:1939–43.

9. Nighoghossian N, Hermier M, Adeleine P *et al.* Old CMBs are a potential risk factor for cerebral bleeding after ischemic stroke: a gradient-echo T2*-weighted brain MRI study. *Stroke* 2002;**33**:735–42.

10. Derex L, Nighoghossian N, Hermier M *et al.* Thrombolysis for ischemic stroke in patients with old CMBs on pretreatment MRI. *Cerebrovasc Dis* 2004; **17**:238–41.

11. Fiehler J, Siemonsen S, Thomalla G, Illies T, Kucinski T. Combination of T2*w and FLAIR abnormalities for the prediction of parenchymal hematoma following thrombolytic therapy in 100 stroke patients. *J Neuroimaging* 2009;**19**:311–16.

12. Kakuda W, Thijs VN, Lansberg MG *et al.* Clinical importance of CMBs in patients receiving iv thrombolysis. *Neurology* 2005;**65**:1175–8.

13. Fiehler J, Albers GW, Boulanger JM *et al.* Bleeding risk analysis in stroke imaging before thrombolysis (BRASIL): Pooled analysis of T2*-weighted magnetic resonance imaging data from 570 patients. *Stroke* 2007;**38**:2738–44.

14. Barron HV, Rundle AC, Gore JM, Gurwitz JH, Penney J. Intracranial hemorrhage rates and effect of immediate beta-blocker use in patients with acute myocardial infarction treated with tissue plasminogen activator. Participants in the National Registry of Myocardial Infarction-2. *Am J Cardiol* 2000;**85**:294–8.

15. McCarron MO, Nicoll JA. Cerebral amyloid angiopathy and thrombolysis-related intracerebral haemorrhage. *Lancet Neurol* 2004;**3**:484–92.

16. Winkler DT, Bondolfi L, Herzig MC *et al.* Spontaneous hemorrhagic stroke in a mouse model of cerebral amyloid angiopathy. *J Neurosci* 2001;**21**: 1619–27.

17. Broderick J, Lu M, Jackson C *et al.* Apolipoprotein e phenotype and the efficacy of intravenous tissue plasminogen activator in acute ischemic stroke. *Ann Neurol* 2001;**49**:736–44.

Index